BLUEPRINTS
FAMILY MEDICINE

Third Edition

BLUEPRINTS
FAMILY
MEDICINE

Third Edition

Martin S. Lipsky, MD
Professor of Family Medicine and
Regional Dean
University of Illinois
College of Medicine, Rockford
Rockford, Illinois

Mitchell S. King, MD
Associate Professor
University of Illinois
College of Medicine, Rockford
Rockford, Illinois

Wolters Kluwer | Lippincott Williams & Wilkins
Health

Philadelphia · Baltimore · New York · London
Buenos Aires · Hong Kong · Sydney · Tokyo

Acquisitions: Charles W. Mitchell
Product Manager: Stacey Sebring
Vendor Manager: Bridgett Dougherty
Cover and Interior Design: Doug Smock
Compositor: MPS Limited, A Macmillan Company

Third Edition

Copyright © 2011 Lippincott Williams & Wilkins, a Wolters Kluwer business.

Wolters Kluwer Health
Two Commerce Square
2001 Market Street
Philadelphia, PA 19103

Printed in China

9 8 7 6 5 4

Library of Congress Cataloging-in-Publication Data

Lipsky, Martin S.
   Blueprints family medicine/Martin S. Lipsky, Mitchell S. King.—3rd ed.
     p.; cm.—(Blueprints)
   Other title: Family medicine
   Includes bibliographical references and index.
   ISBN 978-1-60831-087-6
   1. Family medicine—Outlines, syllabi, etc. 2. Primary care (Medicine)—Outlines, syllabi, etc.
   I. King, Mitchell S. II. Title. III. Title: Family medicine. IV. Series: Blueprints.
   [DNLM: 1. Family Practice—Examination Questions. 2. Primary Health Care—methods—
   Examination Questions. WB 18.2 L767b 2010]
   RC59.B58 2010
   616—dc22

                                                                    2010002515

DISCLAIMER
Care has been taken to confirm the accuracy of the information present and to describe generally accepted practices. However, the authors, editors, and publisher are not responsible for errors or omissions or for any consequences from application of the information in this book and make no warranty, expressed or implied, with respect to the currency, completeness, or accuracy of the contents of the publication. Application of this information in a particular situation remains the professional responsibility of the practitioner; the clinical treatments described and recommended may not be considered absolute and universal recommendations.

The authors, editors, and publisher have exerted every effort to ensure that drug selection and dosage set forth in this text are in accordance with the current recommendations and practice at the time of publication. However, in view of ongoing research, changes in government regulations, and the constant flow of information relating to drug therapy and drug reactions, the reader is urged to check the package insert for each drug for any change in indications and dosage and for added warnings and precautions. This is particularly important when the recommended agent is a new or infrequently employed drug.

Some drugs and medical devices presented in this publication have Food and Drug Administration (FDA) clearance for limited use in restricted research settings. It is the responsibility of the health care provider to ascertain the FDA status of each drug or device planned for use in their clinical practice.

To purchase additional copies of this book, call our customer service department at (800) 638-3030 or fax orders to (301) 223-2320. International customers should call (301) 223-2300.

Visit Lippincott Williams & Wilkins on the Internet: http://www.lww.com. Lippincott Williams & Wilkins customer service representatives are available from 8:30 am to 6:00 pm, EST.

Contents

Contributors to the third edition

Cassandra Lopez, MD
Chief Resident
University of Illinois
College of Medicine, Rockford
Family Medicine Residency Program
Rockford, Illinois

Daniel Cortez
Class of 2010
University of Illinois
College of Medicine, Rockford
Rockford, Illinois

Contributors to the second edition

Adam W. Bennett, MD
Attending Physician
Northwestern Memorial Hospital
Clinical Instructor, Family Medicine
Feinberg School of Medicine
Northwestern University
Chicago, Illinois

Sheila E. Bloomquist, MD
MCH Fellow/FP Physician
PCC Salud Family Health Center
Chicago, Illinois

Sandra V. Doyle, DO
Resident Physician, Family Medicine
McGaw Medical Center of Northwestern University
Glenview, Illinois

Priyah Gambhir, MD
Resident Physician, Family Medicine
Northwestern Memorial Hospital
Chicago, Illinois

Ati Hakimi, MD
Resident Physician, Family Medicine
McGaw Medical Center of Northwestern University
Glenview, Illinois
University of St. Eustatius
Netherlands-Antilles

Leslie Mendoza Temple, MD
Attending Physician
Evanston Northwestern Healthcare
Glenview, Illinois
Clinical Instructor, Family Medicine
Feinberg School of Medicine
Northwestern University
Chicago, Illinois

Purvi Patel, MD
Resident Physician, Family Medicine
McGaw Medical Center of Northwestern University
Glenview, Illinois
Ross University
Dominca, British West Indies

Joanna Turner Bisgrove, MD
Resident Physician, Family Medicine
Evanston Northwestern Healthcare
Glenview, Illinois

Darice Zabak-Lipsky, MD
Clinical Assistant Professor, Family Medicine
University of Illinois
College of Medicine, Rockford
Rockford, Illinois

Contributors to the first edition

Adam W. Bennett, MD
Attending Physician
Northwestern Memorial Hospital
Clinical Instructor, Family Medicine
Feinberg School of Medicine
Northwestern University
Chicago, Illinois

Jasmine Chao, DO
Resident, Family Medicine
McGaw Medical Center of Northwestern University
Glenview, Illinois

Arden Fusman, MD
Resident, Family Medicine
McGaw Medical Center of Northwestern University
Glenview, Illinois

Daria Majzoubi, MD
Resident, Family Medicine
McGaw Medical Center of Northwestern University
Glenview, Illinois

Leslie Mendoza Temple, MD
Attending Physician
Evanston Northwestern Healthcare
Glenview, Illinois
Clinical Instructor, Family Medicine
Feinberg School of Medicine
Northwestern University
Chicago, Illinois

Sanjaya P. Sooriarachchi, MD
Resident, Family Medicine
McGaw Medical Center of Northwestern University
Glenview, Illinois

Reviewers

Melissa Beagle, MD
Resident, Denver Health Hospital
University of Colorado Family Medicine
    Residency Program
Denver, Colorado

Tara Creighton
Class of 2005
University of South Dakota School of Medicine
Vermillion, South Dakota

Joseph W. Gravel, Jr., MD, FAAFP
Assistant Clinical Professor of Family Medicine
    and Community Health
Program Director, Family Medicine Residency
Tufts University School of Medicine
Boston, Massachusetts

Marissa Harris
Resident
Beth Israel Medical Center Residency Program in
    Urban Family Medicine
New York, New York

Celeste Chu Kuo, MD
Resident, Pediatrics
Saint Louis Children's Hospital
St. Louis, Missouri

Amy Marie Little
Class of 2005
Georgetown University
Washington, DC

Kamran Shamsa, MD
Resident, Internal Medicine and Pediatrics
    Combined Program
UCLA Medical Center
Los Angeles, California

Scott Strom
Class of 2004
Michigan State University College of Osteopathic
    Medicine
East Lansing, Michigan

Christine Tsang, DO
Intern, Family Medicine
Crozer-Keystone
Chester, Pennsylvania

Amber M. Tyler, MD
Captain, United States Air Force
Resident, Family Medicine
University of Nebraska
Omaha, Nebraska

Brian J. West, MD
Resident, Family Practice
Shenandoah Valley Family Practice Residency
    Program
Front Royal, Virginia

Preface

In 1997, the first five books in the **Blueprints** series were published as board review for medical students, interns, and residents who wanted high-yield, accurate clinical content for USMLE Steps 2 & 3. More than a decade later, the **Blueprints** brand has expanded into high-quality trusted resources covering the broad range of clinical topics studied by medical students and residents during their primary, specialty, and subspecialty rotations.

The **Blueprints** were conceived as a study aid created by students, for students. In keeping with this concept, the editors of the current edition of the **Blueprints** books have recruited resident contributors to ensure that the series continues to offer the information and the approach that made the original **Blueprints** a success.

Our readers report that **Blueprints** are useful for every step of their medical career—from their clerkship rotations and subinternships to a board review for USMLE Steps 2 & 3. Residents studying for USMLE Step 3 often use the books for reviewing areas that were not their specialty. Students from a wide variety of health care specialties, including those in physician assistant, nurse practitioner, and osteopathic programs, use **Blueprints** either as a course companion or to review for their licensure examinations.

Now in its third edition, **Blueprints** *Family Medicine* has been completely revised and updated to bring you the most current treatment and management strategies. The feedback we have received from our readers has been tremendously helpful in guiding the editorial direction of the third edition. We are grateful to the hundreds of medical students and residents who have responded with in-depth comments and highly detailed observations.

Martin S. Lipsky
Mitchell S. King

Acknowledgments

We would like to thank all of those who helped us make the third edition of this book possible. If our readers feel this book contributes to their understanding of family medicine it is largely due to the many people who played a role in making this new edition possible.

Given all the hair that Olympia Asimacopoulos, Donna Brown, and Karen Morris tore out in working on this project, we thank them for their assistance in organizing the book and in organizing the authors! Ellen Shellhouse, Jeannette Gawronski, and the library staff at the University of Illinois College of Medicine, Rockford deserve our thanks for tracking down references and assuring that the book accurately reflects the latest guidelines and facts.

Finally and most importantly, both of us gratefully acknowledge the support of our family and friends, especially our wives, Darice Zabak-Lipsky and Jackie King. Without Jackie and Darice, this and other projects would not be possible.

Martin S. Lipsky
Mitchell S. King

Abbreviations

AC	acromioclavicular		CHF	congestive heart failure
ACE	angiotensin converting enzyme		CMV	cytomegalovirus
ACL	anterior cruciate ligament		CNS	central nervous system
ACOG	American College of Obstetricians and Gynecologists		COPD	chronic obstructive pulmonary disease
ACS	American Cancer Society		COX-2	cyclooxygenase-2
AD	atopic dermatitis		CPAP	continuous positive airway pressure
AD/HD	attention deficit/hyperactivity disorder		CPK	creatine phosphokinase
ADA	American Diabetes Association		CPR	cardiopulmonary resuscitation
ADLs	activities of daily living		CSF	cerebrospinal fluid
AFP	alpha fetoprotein		CSOM	chronic suppurative otitis media
AGUS	atypical glandular cells of undetermined significance		CT	computed tomography
AIDS	acquired immunodeficiency syndrome		CVA	cerebrovascular accident
AIS	adenocarcinoma in situ		DBP	diastolic blood pressure
AK	actinic keratosis		DEXA	dual-energy x-ray absorptiometry
ALS	amyotrophic lateral sclerosis		DHE	dihydroergotamine
ALT	alanine aminotransferase		DHEA-S	dehydroepiandrosterone sulfate
ANA	antinuclear antibody		DJD	degenerative joint disease
ANCA	antineutrophil cytoplasmic antibody		dsDNA	double-stranded DNA
AOM	acute otitis media		DSM-IV	*Diagnostic and Statistical Manual of Mental Disorders*, fourth edition
ARB	angiotensin receptor blocker		DTaP	diphtheria, tetanus, acellular pertussis
AROM	active range of motion		DTP	diphtheria, tetanus, pertussis
ASCUS	atypical squamous cells of undetermined significance		DTs	delirium tremens
ASO	antistreptolysin O		DUB	dysfunctional uterine bleeding
AST	aspartate aminotransferase		DUI	driving under the influence
AV	arteriovenous		DVT	deep venous thrombosis
BAER	brainstem auditory evoked response		EBV	Epstein–Barr virus
BCC	basal cell carcinoma		ECG	electrocardiogram
BMD	bone mineral density		EDD	estimated date of delivery
BMI	body mass index		EEG	electroencephalogram
BNP	brain natriuretic peptide		EGD	esophagastroduodenoscopy
BP	blood pressure		ELISA	enzyme-linked immunosorbent assay
BPH	benign prostatic hypertrophy		ENT	ear-nose-throat
BPV	benign positional vertigo		ERCP	endoscopic retrograde cholangiopancreatography
BRAT	bananas, rice, applesauce, and toast		ESR	erythrocyte sedimentation rate
BUN	blood urea nitrogen		ET	essential tremor
BV	bacterial vaginosis		FDA	Food and Drug Administration
BZD	benzodiazepine		FSH	follicle-stimulating hormone
CAD	coronary artery disease		FTA-Abs	fluorescent treponemal antibody absorption
CAP	community-acquired pneumonia		FTT	failure to thrive
CBC	complete blood count		G6PD	glucose-6-phosphate dehydrogenase
CFS	chronic fatigue syndrome		GDM	gestational diabetes mellitus
			GERD	gastroesophageal reflux disease

GFR	glomerular filtration rate		MI	myocardial infarction
GGT	gamma-glutamyl transferase		MMR	measles, mumps, rubella (vaccine)
GI	gastrointestinal		MMSE	Mini Mental Status Examination
GnRH	gonadotropin-releasing hormone		MRA	magnetic resonance angiography
HC	homocysteine		MRCP	magnetic resonance
hCG	human chorionic gonadotropin			cholangiopancreatography
Hct	hematocrit		MRI	magnetic resonance imaging
HCTZ	hydrochlorothiazide		MS	multiple sclerosis
HDL	high-density-lipoprotein cholesterol		MSAFP	maternal serum alpha fetoprotein
HEPA	high-efficiency particulate air		MVA	motor vehicle accident
Hib	*H. influenzae* type b		NCAA	National Collegiate Athletic Association
HIV	human immunodeficiency virus		NGU	nongonococcal urethritis
HNKDC	hyperosmolar nonketotic diabetic coma		NH	nursing home
HPF	high-power field		NMDA	N-methyl-D-aspartate
HPV	human papillomavirus		NNRTI	nonnucleoside reverse transcriptase inhibitor
HRT	hormone replacement therapy		NRTI	nucleoside reverse transcriptase inhibitor
HSV	herpes simplex virus		NSAID	nonsteroidal anti-inflammatory drug
HTN	hypertension		NTD	neural tube defect
IADLs	instrumental activities of daily living		OCD	obsessive compulsive disorder
IBD	inflammatory bowel disease		OCPs	oral contraceptive pills
IBS	irritable bowel syndrome		OME	otitis media with effusion
ICU	intensive care unit		OPV	oral polio vaccine
IF	intrinsic factor		OTC	over the counter
IgA	immunoglobulin A		PAC	premature atrial contraction
IgE	immunoglobulin E		PCOS	polycystic ovarian syndrome
IM	intramuscular		PCR	polymerase chain reaction
INR	international normalized ratio		PCV	pneumococcal conjugate vaccine
IPV	injectable polio vaccine		PD	Parkinson disease
ISA	intrinsic sympathomimetic activity		PE	pulmonary embolus
IUD	intrauterine device		PEF	peak expiratory flow
IV	intravenous		PI	protease inhibitor
IVP	intravenous pyelogram		PID	pelvic inflammatory disease
JVD	jugular venous distention		PMI	point of maximal impulse
KOH	potassium hydroxide (stain)		PO	by mouth
LB	Lewy body		PPD	purified protein derivative
LDL-C	low-density-lipoprotein cholesterol		PPE	preparticipation health examination
LEEP	loop electroexcision procedure		PPI	proton pump inhibitor
LES	lower esophageal sphincter		PPV	pneumococcal polysaccharide vaccine
LFT	liver function test		PR	per rectum
LH	luteinizing hormone		PROM	passive range of motion
LH-RH	luteinizing hormone–releasing hormone		PSA	prostate-specific antigen
LMP	last menstrual period		PT	prothrombin time
LN	lymph node		PTCA	percutaneous transluminal coronary
LRI	lower respiratory tract infection			angioplasty
LTC	long-term-care facility		PTT	partial thromboplastin time
LVH	left ventricular hypertrophy		PTU	propylthiouracil
LVSD	left ventricular systolic dysfunction		PVC	premature ventricular contraction
MAOI	monoamine oxidase inhibitor		PVD	peripheral vascular disease
MASH	medications, allergies, surgeries, and		PVL	plasma viral load
	hospitalizations		PVR	postvoid residual
MCTD	mixed connective tissue disease		RA	rheumatoid arthritis
MCV	mean corpuscular volume		RAIU	radioactive iodine uptake
MDI	metered-dose inhaler		RAST	radioallergosorbent test

REM	rapid-eye-movement (sleep)		TIBC	total iron-binding capacity
ROM	recurrent otitis media		TIg	tetanus immunoglobulin
RPR	rapid plasma reagin (test)		TM	tympanic membrane
RSV	respiratory syncytial virus		TMJ	temporomandibular joint
SAH	subarachnoid hemorrhage		TMP/SMX	trimethoprim/sulfamethoxazole
SBE	subacute bacterial endocarditis		TNF	tumor necrosis factor
SBP	systolic blood pressure		TRH	thyrotropin-releasing hormone
SC	subcutaneous		TSH	thyroid-stimulating hormone
SD	standard deviation		UA	urinalysis
SHEP	Systolic HTN in the Elderly Program		UI	urinary incontinence
SIDS	sudden infant death syndrome		URI	upper respiratory tract infection
SIL	squamous intraepithelial lesion		US	ultrasound
SK	seborrheic keratosis		USDHHS	U.S. Department of Health and Human Services
SLE	systemic lupus erythematosus			
SLR	straight leg raising		USPHS	U.S. Public Health Service
SSRI	selective serotonin reuptake inhibitor		UTI	urinary tract infection
STD	sexually transmitted disease		UV	ultraviolet
T3	triiodothyronine		V/Q	ventilation/perfusion
T4	thyroxine		VCUG	voiding cystourethrogram
TB	tuberculosis		VDRL	Venereal Disease Research Laboratory
TBG	thyroxine-binding globulin		VZIG	varicella zoster immune globulin
TCA	tricyclic antidepressant		WBC	white blood cell
Td	tetanus-diphtheria vaccine		WIC	Special Supplemental Nutrition Program for Women, Infants, and Children
TIA	transient ischemic attack			

Chapter

1

Elements of Family Medicine

DEFINITIONS

Family medicine is a medical specialty that provides continuing and comprehensive health care for individuals and families. It is a broad specialty that integrates the biological, clinical, and behavioral sciences. The scope of family medicine encompasses all ages, sexes, organ systems, and disease entities. The specialty evolved as an enhanced expression of general medical practice and is uniquely defined in the family context.

A family physician is a practitioner in the field of family medicine. At present, family physicians complete a 3-year residency in family practice. This prepares them to manage the broad scope of problems involving patients, from newborns to the elderly. On average, about 15% of a family physician's practice is devoted to the care of infants and children. Some family physicians, about 25%, also deliver babies.

Family medicine is one of the primary care specialties. Currently, the most widely accepted definition of primary care is the one developed by the National Academy of Sciences Institute of Medicine in 1996. It defined primary care as the provision of integrated, successful health care services by clinicians who are accountable for addressing a large majority of personal health care needs, helping to sustain partnerships with patients, and practicing in the context of family and community. In addition to family medicine, general pediatrics and general internal medicine are considered primary care fields.

HISTORY OF FAMILY MEDICINE

After World War II, the United States saw a rapid movement toward specialization among physicians. In 1938, about 20% of U.S. physicians designated themselves as specialists and 80% considered themselves generalists. In contrast, by 1970, about 75% of physicians considered themselves specialists. By the late 1960s, this trend toward specialization was noted and the public perceived a need for generalist physicians who could coordinate care and serve as the entry point or "first contact" into the health care system.

The findings of three commissions—the Folsom Report, the Mills Report, and the Willard Report, referred to by the names of their chairmen—were published in 1966. These reports all affirmed the need for general practitioners who could ensure the integration and continuity of all medical services for patients.

In 1969, family practice was approved as the 20th medical specialty and the American Board of Family Practice was established. From these early beginnings, family medicine has grown to become the second largest specialty in the United States, with over 400 residency programs and more than 90,000 physicians, students, and resident members of the American Academy of Family Physicians. Practitioners in family medicine care for more patients each day than do physicians in any other specialty. In the year 2004, family and general physicians managed about one-quarter of patient visits or more than 200 million of the 910 million patient visits made in the United States. In comparison, general internists accounted for 16% of patient visits and pediatricians 13%. Of patients making visits to family physicians, only 6.3% required referral to another discipline.

COMPONENTS OF FAMILY MEDICINE

A successful family physician incorporates several components of patient care, including accessibility, medical diagnosis and treatment, comprehensiveness, communication, coordination of care, continuity of care, and patient advocacy. The family physician is often the patient's first contact and is available if the patient has an urgent or chronic problem. Accessibility includes being financially affordable and geographically accessible.

As the patient's first contact, the family physician must be knowledgeable about a broad array of diseases and have the skill and judgment to determine the scope, site, and pace of medical evaluation. The family physician typically provides a broad range of services, including acute and chronic disease management in the office, hospital, or nursing home, or by telephone. Family medicine incorporates the biological perspective as well as the social and psychological aspects of care. The large number of visits to family physicians for psychosocial and behavioral issues underscores the relationship between emotion and illness.

Communication and coordination of care are also essential elements. These topics are covered in greater detail in Chapter 2.

Continuity is an important component of family medicine. Family physicians typically develop long-term relationships with patients, maintain longitudinal records of patients' problems, and promote healthy lifestyles. These require that the physician see each patient for acute episodes of illness as well as periodically for health maintenance. Continuity nourishes a trusting long-term relationship between patient and physician. This relationship is a valuable tool for improving patient adherence to treatment recommendations. Assessing disease risk, screening for illness, and promoting health to prevent disease and disability are inherent parts of a successful continuous relationship. Early intervention—through health education, behavioral change, and the promotion of a healthy lifestyle—can serve to prevent morbidity and mortality.

Finally, advocacy is a key responsibility for the family physician. Once a patient has been accepted into his or her practice, the family physician must serve as the patient's advocate. In addition, the physician is responsible for educating the patient about treatment outcomes and prognoses, incorporating the patient's preferences into treatment plans, and assuming responsibility for the patient's total care during times of health and illness. This includes helping the patient to make wise health care decisions and to find the needed health care resources.

MEDICAL HOME

A new model of medical care that embraces the components of family medicine is the concept known as the "Medical Home." Also known as the Patient Centered Medical Home (PCMH), the PCMH is defined as comprehensive primary care that facilitates partnerships between patients and physicians by connecting each individual to a personal physician who is trained to provide continuous and comprehensive care. The personal physician serves as the patient's first contact and assumes responsibility for coordinating and integrating an individual's care across the entire spectrum of health care providers, agencies, and facilities with the goal to enhance access while maintaining a focus on quality and safety.

KEY POINTS

- Family medicine is a medical specialty that provides continuing and comprehensive health care for individuals and families, including all ages, sexes, organ systems, and disease entities.

- Practitioners in family medicine care for more patients each day than do physicians in any other medical specialty.

- A successful family physician incorporates several components into caring for his or her patients, including accessibility, medical diagnosis and treatment, comprehensiveness, communication, coordination of care, continuity of care, and patient advocacy.

- Continuity nourishes a trusting long-term relationship between patient and physician. This relationship is a valuable tool for improving patient adherence to treatment recommendations.

Patient Communication and Coordination of Care

Despite advances in technology, effective communication remains the family physician's most powerful diagnostic tool. An old adage is that up to 90% of the time, the diagnosis is made from a complete and accurate history. The key to obtaining a good history is the ability to communicate effectively and empathetically with patients. Good doctor–patient communication also fosters effective treatment. The rule of thirds applies to patient adherence: that is, approximately one-third of the patients will follow recommendations, another one-third will partially follow recommendations, and the remaining one-third will ignore most recommendations. The ability to explain clearly, in lay terms, the results of a test and the available treatment options increases the likelihood that a patient will accept the diagnosis, adhere to the treatment, and return for follow-up. Finally, good communication reduces the risk of malpractice.

In addition to patient–physician communication, the family physician plays a critical role in coordinating patient care. This requires effective communication, both oral and written, with peers, co-workers, and ancillary personnel.

THE PATIENT INTERVIEW

The goal of the patient interview is to obtain information, establish good rapport, and provide an opportunity to educate patients about their health. An important part of this process is projecting a nonjudgmental attitude and creating an environment that allows the patient to feel comfortable and secure about sharing personal information. Establishing good eye contact and maintaining a relaxed manner are important. Nodding occasionally and periodically summarizing what you have been told allow the patient to correct information that you may have misunderstood. Closing the doors of the examination room, minimizing discussion about patients in open areas, and providing written information in the waiting room that explains office procedures are steps that can help to create an atmosphere of confidentiality.

OPEN-ENDED QUESTIONS

The patient interview should begin with an open-ended question. This has two effects: first, it allows patients to express what they feel is important and,

second, it helps provide a global view of their medical and psychological issues. It also allows patients to feel more in control and comfortable with providing personal information. Despite this time-honored principle, numerous studies show that physicians interrupt patients less than 10 seconds into their opening remarks.

TARGETED QUESTIONS

Once a patient expresses his or her chief complaint or the reason for the visit, it is important to start narrowing down the scope of the problem by asking more specific questions. The mnemonic PQRST in Box 2-1 can serve to guide targeted questions for pain symptoms.

New patients must be asked about their medical, surgical, family, and social history. Medications and allergies should be reviewed and a review of systems conducted. If time is limited, obtaining a MASH history (of *m*edications, *a*llergies, *s*urgeries, and *h*ospitalizations) is a way to acquire key information quickly.

PHYSICAL EXAMINATION

Communication can be further enhanced during the physical examination. Ensuring that the patient's physical needs are met (by having a comfortable room temperature and providing appropriate draping) is important for establishing rapport. Subtle clues can also be gleaned from the patient's reaction during an examination. For example, a woman or child with an unusual bruise or burn who gives an evasive answer may very well be the victim of abuse.

PATIENT COUNSELING

Many patients have aspects of their lives that they want to change. Counseling patients about healthy

■ **BOX 2-1** The PQRST Mnemonic
What *p*rovokes and *p*alliates the pain?
What is the *q*uality of the pain?
Does the pain *r*adiate?
What is the *s*everity of the pain?
What is the *t*emporal course of the discomfort?

■ **TABLE 2-1** Patients' Stages of Readiness and Smoking Cessation	
Stage	**Example of Intervention**
Precontemplation	
Not considering quitting smoking	Ask about smoking
May not believe they can quit	Ascertain knowledge about risks
Do not believe they are susceptible to severe illness	
Contemplation	
Considering quitting	Encourage patients to quit
Recognize dangers of smoking	Provide materials about quitting
May be upset about failed attempt	
Preparation	
Ready to make change by setting goal	Encourage patients to set a quit date
	Offer nicotine replacement or other appropriate therapy
Action	
Are in the cessation process	Provide support and positive reinforcement
	Discuss relapse strategies
Maintenance	
Maintain former-smoker status	Continue support and reinforcement
	Be available for help if relapse occurs

lifestyle behaviors requires a systematic approach that evaluates the patient's readiness for change and offers information appropriate to his or her frame of mind. A commonly used approach to behavioral counseling is the "stages of readiness" model shown in Table 2-1, which uses smoking cessation as an example. This model is also widely used to help patients start exercising and changing their diets.

ELDERLY PATIENTS

Communicating with elderly patients poses special challenges due to problems such as hearing loss and cognitive impairment. If you suspect a hearing loss, it is important to sit directly in front of the patient and to speak loudly (do not shout) and clearly. Many hearing-impaired patients unconsciously read lips. Women who work with elderly patients can help by making a special effort to wear lipstick, and men should be careful to ensure that their facial hair is neatly trimmed and does not obscure the mouth. Patients with hearing aids should be instructed to bring them to their office appointments. For cognitively impaired patients, having a family member or other responsible individual present is critical to obtaining an accurate history and planning treatment.

Another key issue to address with elderly patients is advanced directives. These directives are a set of instructions, usually written, intended to allow a patient's current preferences to shape medical decisions

during a future period of incompetence. All patients admitted to a hospital or long-term-care facility should be asked about their treatment preferences in an open fashion should they become unable to speak for themselves. If patients designate a durable power of attorney for health care, it is important that they be encouraged to discuss their treatment preferences with the person who will have this responsibility. The office setting provides the opportunity to initiate discussions about advanced directives when the patient is not acutely ill or otherwise distressed.

INTERPRETERS

Family physicians may encounter patients who do not speak English. Hospitals are required by federal law to offer patients competent interpreters. Patients may decline using an outside interpreter and prefer a family member or friend. However, it is often preferable to use a competent and unbiased interpreter to assure that information is being shared completely. Family members may add their own biases to the translation, which can negatively affect the ability to obtain an accurate history. For example, a husband interpreting for his wife may not be willing to tell the interviewer about her history of a mental disorder, or a family member who is not familiar with medical terminology may translate information incorrectly. Finally, an underage child should not interpret for a parent or older family member.

All physicians' offices should have contact numbers for interpreter agencies or qualified individual interpreters. In the case of deaf patients, a state-licensed sign language interpreter may have to be called in. A useful way to know whether an interpreter will be needed is if the patient enlists a proxy in calling for an appointment. Instruct the receptionist to be alert for such situations and to ask why the patient is not making the call.

INFORMED CONSENT

Patients undergoing surgery or other invasive medical treatments must grant informed consent. The elements of informed consent include describing the nature of the patient's condition and its consequences, such as whether it is life threatening or potentially disabling. Recommended treatment and alternatives should be reviewed, including benefits, risks, costs, discomfort, and side effects. Finally, possible outcomes of nontreatment—including benefits, risks, discomfort, costs, and side effects—should be discussed. Informed consent is one of the cornerstones of preserving patient autonomy and is an important aspect of patient communication and treatment.

COORDINATION OF CARE

"Coordination of care" refers to the organization of health care services in order to meet the needs of the patient. A key element of this is the referral of the patient to a specialist. Although approximately 95% of patient problems seen in the outpatient family practice setting can be handled by a family physician, 5% will need specialist attention.

RESPONSIBILITIES FOR A REFERRING PHYSICIAN

The family physician is responsible for handling several aspects of the referral process, including selection of the desired specialist. The patient may request a certain specialist or may rely on the advice of the family physician for this choice. The family physician must provide required referral information and specify whether he or she wants the specialist to evaluate and treat or to limit the input to a consultation and recommendations about the patient's condition. Referrals should also specify the number of visits and treatments. In this regard, the physician should work with the patient's insurance guidelines as to preauthorization and address in-network versus out-of-network referrals. In the referral, the family physician should provide the consultant with information regarding the nature of the complaint as well as important elements of the history, physical examination, and previously obtained test results. More importantly, the family physician should pose any specific questions he or she wants to have answered by the specialist.

In addition to written information, it is often helpful to call the specialist directly. This gives the family physician the opportunity to discuss the patient with the specialist and allows the specialist to ask specific questions or to request information (e.g., old records) that may be helpful in preparing for the consultation.

SPECIALIST RESPONSIBILITIES

It is the responsibility of the specialist to see any referred patient in a timely fashion. Emergency consultations should be held that day, urgent consultations usually within 24 to 48 hours, and nonurgent consultations within 1 to 2 weeks.

Specialists should attempt to answer any specific questions and offer treatment options if this is requested by the family physician. Specialists should then send a follow-up letter and, when necessary, discuss on phone their findings and recommendations as well as any treatments that might have been initiated.

CASE MANAGEMENT

The family physician often has the difficult but critically important task of coordinating information from several different health care providers, all of whom are participating in the care of one patient. In this situation, it becomes critical that the family physician provide oversight, so that medications and treatments do not interact adversely with one another. In addition, the family physician should review with the patient the findings of other health care providers and specialists and make sure he or she understands and agrees with the treatment options. Often, patients with complex care issues need the support of a trusted personal physician to help guide them through the complexities of modern-day health care.

KEY POINTS

- The rule of thirds applies to patient adherence, that is approximately one-third of patients will follow recommendations, another one-third will partially follow the recommendations, and remaining one-third will ignore most recommendations.
- The goal of the patient interview is to obtain information and to establish good rapport; it should begin with an open-ended question.
- Communicating with elderly patients provides special challenges that must be addressed.
- About 95% of patient problems seen in an outpatient family practice setting can be handled by a family physician, 5% will need specialist attention.

3 Screening

Preventive health care and screening for various diseases are parts of routine medical care at all ages. Disease prevention can be primary, secondary, or tertiary. Primary prevention seeks to prevent a disease or condition from developing. An example of primary prevention is vaccination, whereby many infectious diseases are prevented through immunization. Secondary prevention involves early detection of the disease and is synonymous with screening to limit the effects of the disease. Examples of screening tests are mammography and testing for occult fecal blood (for early detection of breast and colon cancers, respectively), in the hope that early intervention can lead to a cure. Another example of screening is cholesterol and blood pressure testing in order to lower risk for future cardiovascular disease. Included within the context of primary and secondary prevention are screening and counseling for behaviors such as smoking or substance abuse that affect an individual's health.

"Tertiary prevention" refers to rehabilitation as well as efforts to limit complications of a disease after it has developed, such as an exercise program in a patient who recently underwent coronary artery bypass surgery.

CRITERIA FOR USE OF SCREENING TESTS

In order for a screening test to be of value for routine use in patient care, several criteria should be met. First, the disease or condition screened for must be common and have a sufficient impact on an individual's health to justify the risks and costs associated with the testing. Second, effective prevention or treatment measures must be available for the condition, and earlier detection must improve clinical outcome. The screening and treatment benefits should outweigh any risks associated with testing and therapy. Finally, there must be a screening test that is readily available, safe, and accurate. The overall cost-effectiveness of a screening program will be a factor in terms of insurers' and individuals' willingness to pay for the test or procedure. The availability and acceptability of the test affects whether or not patients will actually undergo screening. For example, an individual

may refuse colonoscopy because he or she finds the procedure distasteful.

TEST CHARACTERISTICS

Screening tests should be accurate at detecting the intended disease or condition. Accuracy is a term that considers several different testing measures—namely, sensitivity, specificity, positive predictive value, and negative predictive value (Table 3-1). Sensitivity is a measure of the percentage of cases that a test is able

TABLE 3-1 Determining Sensitivity and Specificity

	Disease Present	Disease Absent
Positive test	a	b
Negative test	c	d
Sensitivity	a/a + c	
Specificity	d/b + d	

TABLE 3-2 Calculating Predictive Values

	Disease Present	Disease Absent
Positive test	9500	4500
Negative test	500	85,500
Sensitivity 9500/9500 + 500 = 95%		positive predictive value 9500/9500 + 4500 = 68%
Specificity 85,500/4500 + 85,500 = 95%		negative predictive value 85,500/500 + 85,500 = 99.4%

Total number of patients = 100,000.

to detect. Specificity measures the percentage of patients testing negative who do not have the disease. These test characteristics are factors in determining the value of screening tests. Desirable characteristics of screening tests include high levels of both sensitivity and specificity.

By combining disease prevalence with these test characteristics, the clinician can determine the predictive values of a screening test. The positive predictive value is the percentage likelihood that a patient with a positive test actually has the disease; conversely, a negative predictive value indicates that a person with a negative test is disease-free. Disease prevalence critically affects the predictive value, as shown by the following example of screening for a disease with a prevalence of 10% in 100,000 patients, using a test that is 95% sensitive and 95% specific. In this instance, the positive and negative predictive values for the test would be 68% and 99.4%, respectively (Table 3-2).

Thus, for every 9500 cases detected, an additional 4500 patients would have to undergo additional testing to determine that they were disease-free. However, a negative test provides 99.4% assurance that the patient is truly disease-free. For diseases with a potentially fatal outcome and where effective treatments are available, this screening would be acceptable. However, if the prevalence of the disease were 1% instead of 10%, the positive predictive value would fall to 16%

TABLE 3-3 Grade Definitions and Suggestions for Practice

Grade	Definition	Suggestions for Practice
A	The USPSTF recommends the service. There is high certainty that the net benefit is substantial	Offer or provide this service
B	The USPSTF recommends the service. There is high certainty that the net benefit is moderate or there is moderate certainty that the net benefit is moderate to substantial	Offer or provide this service
C	The USPSTF recommends against routinely providing the service. There may be considerations that support providing the service in an individual patient. There is at least moderate certainty that the net benefit is small	Offer or provide this service only if other considerations support the offering or providing the service in an individual patient
D	The USPSTF recommends against the service. There is moderate or high certainty that the service has no net benefit or that the harms outweigh the benefits	Discourage the use of this service
I	The USPSTF concludes that the current evidence is insufficient to assess the balance of benefits and harms of the service. Evidence is lacking, of poor quality, or conflicting, and the balance of benefits and harms cannot be determined	Read the clinical considerations section of the USPSTF Recommendation Statement. If the service is offered, patients should understand the uncertainty about the balance of benefits and harms

The USPSTF updated its definitions of the grades it assigns to recommendations and now includes "suggestions for practice" associated with each grade. The USPSTF has also defined levels of certainty regarding net benefit. These definitions apply to USPSTF recommendations voted on after May 2007.

Quality of Evidence

The USPSTF grades the quality of the overall evidence for a service on a three-point scale (good, fair, poor):

Good: Evidence includes consistent results from well-designed, well-conducted studies in representative populations that directly assess effects on health outcomes.

Fair: Evidence is sufficient to determine effects on health outcomes, but the strength of the evidence is limited by the number, quality, or consistency of the individual studies, generalizability to routine practice, or indirect nature of the evidence on health outcomes.

Poor: Evidence is insufficient to assess the effects on health outcomes because of limited number or power of studies, important flaws in their design or conduct, gaps in the chain of evidence, or lack of information on important health outcomes.

From U.S. Preventive Services Task Force Grade Definitions. Rockville, MD: Agency for Healthcare Research and Quality; 2008. Available at: http://www.ahrq.gov/clinic/uspstf/grades.htm.

and the vast majority of patients with positive results would actually be disease-free. The associated health care costs, risks of additional procedures, and patient anxiety may not justify the use of this screening test in this instance, where the disease prevalence and positive predictive value of the test are low.

CLINICAL IMPLEMENTATION OF SCREENING

For preventive health care measures to be effective, health care providers, patients, and society must all agree that screening and prevention are priorities in providing good health care. Conflicting recommendations by government organizations and professional societies have led to uncertainty on the part of physicians regarding both what the actual guidelines are and the effectiveness of the various screening tools. The reasons for these different recommendations include different methods of assessing evidence, different criteria for defining benefit, and different patient populations. In addition, professional interests may play a role. Some authorities may represent groups that treat high-risk individuals, giving them a different perspective or a financial stake in screening. Time constraints and lack of reimbursement for preventive health care are additional barriers to physicians offering screening tests to patients. It is important that family physicians keep abreast of the current preventive health care recommendations and prioritize incorporating screening into their everyday practice. Subsequent chapters will outline recommendations for health screening at different ages. These recommendations are largely based on those of the U.S. Preventive Services Task Force (USPSTF), representing input from the various medical specialties, and utilize an evidence-based approach with analysis of disease prevalence, screening, and treatment effectiveness, as well as overall cost-effectiveness. After evaluating the available information, the USPSTF assigns one of five letter grades to each of its recommendations (A, B, C, D, or I). The task force also grades the strength of evidence behind the recommendation on a three-point scale, good, fair, or poor. Table 3-3 outlines the recommendation grades and evidence levels in greater detail.

To provide primary care to their patients effectively, family physicians must educate their patients regarding preventive health care and the benefits of different screening tests as well as healthy behaviors. This is often accomplished by scheduling a periodic health examination, which comprises a comprehensive prevention-focused history and physical examination. During this visit, the physician can provide counseling about unhealthy behaviors, give immunizations if required, and provide or order indicated screening tests. These issues can also be incorporated into visits triggered by other health concerns.

KEY POINTS

- Primary, secondary, and tertiary preventive strategies can prevent and limit the effects of many diseases.
- Criteria for the use of screening tests include the following: (a) the disease is common and significantly affects individuals and society, (b) effective treatments for the disease are available, and (c) the screening tests or procedures are accurate and reasonable in terms of cost, comfort, and complications.
- Characteristics that measure the accuracy of screening tests include sensitivity, specificity, and positive and negative predictive values.

4 Immunizations

Childhood vaccinations are among the most successful preventive measures of modern medicine. Once-common infections, such as polio, are now rare because of vaccination. Important considerations in deciding whether a vaccine is recommended for routine use are disease prevalence, disease morbidity and mortality, economic costs to society, vaccine efficacy, and adverse reaction to the vaccine. As new vaccines are developed and disease prevalence changes, vaccination recommendations can change. Several organizations, including the American Academy of Family Physicians, provide updates to clinicians about appropriate vaccine schedules.

The schedule of recommended ages for routine administration of currently licensed childhood vaccines is shown in Figure 4-1.

SPECIFIC IMMUNIZATIONS

HEPATITIS B VACCINE

Hepatitis B is a viral infection associated with an acute illness; it can progress to a carrier state or chronic liver disease in about 5% of infected individuals. Since the introduction of universal hepatitis B vaccination of infants, children, and high-risk adults in the United States, there has been a decline in the annual infection rate: 200,000 to 300,000 people per year were infected before 1982, whereas there were only 79,000 reported cases in 2001. Hepatitis B vaccine is available in monovalent form or in combination with other vaccines.

Hepatitis B vaccination can prevent up to 90% of neonatal infections. Infants born to hepatitis B surface antigen–positive mothers should receive both the vaccine and hepatitis B immunoglobulin at separate sites at birth. In addition to universal vaccination for children, adults at higher risk requiring vaccination include those who use intravenous drugs, patients with multiple sexual partners or a history of a sexually transmitted disease, men who have sex with men, those with sexual partners with chronic hepatitis B infection, household contact with hepatitis B carriers, hemodialysis patients, inmates of correctional facilities, people who receive clotting factor concentrates, and health care workers or other individuals who are at occupational risk for exposure to blood.

DIPHTHERIA AND TETANUS VACCINE

The number of tetanus cases has decreased from over 600 per year prior to vaccination to about 40 per year; diphtheria cases have decreased from more than 200,000 annually in 1921 to fewer than 5 annually since 1980. Although each vaccine can be administered alone, most individuals receive both in combination. The vaccine for diphtheria given to children differs from that given to an adult. Before 2005, the only available combined adult booster formulation of tetanus–diphtheria was Td. Today, there are boosters that contain tetanus, diphtheria, and pertussis (Tdap) and after the primary series has been completed, a booster dose of Tdap is recommended at age 11 to 12 years. Adults who did not get Tdap as a teen should get one dose of Tdap instead of a Td when due for their next regularly scheduled tetanus booster. Getting vaccinated with Tdap is especially important for families with new infants. After this one-time dose of Tdap, adults resume getting Td boosters every 10 years.

Fully immunized individuals who have received a booster in the previous 10 years and who sustain a clean, minor wound do not require repeat vaccination. If an individual has a potentially contaminated wound and more than 5 years have lapsed since the last dose, a booster shot should be given. In unimmunized individuals with high-risk wounds, passive immunization with tetanus immunoglobulin (TIg) in addition to starting the primary series is indicated at initial presentation for wound care.

PERTUSSIS VACCINE

Before the introduction of pertussis vaccine, more than 75,000 cases of pertussis per year were reported in the United States. This disease most commonly affected infants and caused pneumonia (22%), seizures (3%), encephalopathy (1%), or death (0.3%).

The older whole-cell vaccine was associated with a higher frequency of adverse reactions, which triggered detailed analysis of risk versus benefit of the vaccine. The newer acellular pertussis vaccine, provided in combination with diphtheria and tetanus (DTaP), has largely eliminated these concerns and provides comparable levels of protection with fewer

Recommended Immunization Schedule for Persons Aged 0 Through 6 Years—United States • 2009

For those who fall behind or start late, see the catch-up schedule

Vaccine ▼ Age ▶	Birth	1 month	2 months	4 months	6 months	12 months	15 months	18 months	19–23 months	2–3 years	4–6 years
Hepatitis B[1]	HepB	HepB		see footnote 1		HepB					
Rotavirus[2]			RV	RV	RV[2]						
Diphtheria, Tetanus, Pertussis[3]			DTaP	DTaP	DTaP	see footnote 3	DTaP				DTaP
Haemophilus influenzae type b[4]			Hib	Hib	Hib[4]	Hib					
Pneumococcal[5]			PCV	PCV	PCV	PCV				PPSV	
Inactivated Poliovirus			IPV	IPV		IPV					IPV
Influenza[6]						Influenza (Yearly)					
Measles, Mumps, Rubella[7]						MMR		see footnote 7			MMR
Varicella[8]						Varicella		see footnote 8			Varicella
Hepatitis A[9]						HepA (2 doses)				HepA Series	
Meningococcal[10]										MCV	

Range of recommended ages

Certain high-risk groups

This schedule indicates the recommended ages for routine administration of currently licensed vaccines, as of December 1, 2008, for children aged 0 through 6 years. Any dose not administered at the recommended age should be administered at a subsequent visit, when indicated and feasible. Licensed combination vaccines may be used whenever any component of the combination is indicated and other components are not contraindicated and if approved by the Food and Drug Administration for that dose of the series. Providers should consult the relevant Advisory Committee on Immunization Practices statement for detailed recommendations, including high-risk conditions: http://www.cdc.gov/vaccines/pubs/acip-list.htm. Clinically significant adverse events that follow immunization should be reported to the Vaccine Adverse Event Reporting System (VAERS). Guidance about how to obtain and complete a VAERS form is available at http://www.vaers.hhs.gov or by telephone, 800-822-7967.

1. Hepatitis B vaccine (HepB). *(Minimum age: birth)*
At birth:
- Administer monovalent HepB to all newborns before hospital discharge.
- If mother is hepatitis B surface antigen (HBsAg)-positive, administer HepB and 0.5 mL of hepatitis B immune globulin (HBIG) within 12 hours of birth.
- If mother's HBsAg status is unknown, administer HepB within 12 hours of birth. Determine mother's HBsAg status as soon as possible and, if HBsAg-positive, administer HBIG (no later than age 1 week).
After the birth dose:
- The HepB series should be completed with either monovalent HepB or a combination vaccine containing HepB. The second dose should be administered at age 1 or 2 months. The final dose should be administered no earlier than age 24 weeks.
- Infants born to HBsAg-positive mothers should be tested for HBsAg and antibody to HBsAg (anti-HBs) after completion of at least 3 doses of the HepB series, at age 9 through 18 months (generally at the next well-child visit).
4-month dose:
- Administration of 4 doses of HepB to infants is permissible when combination vaccines containing HepB are administered after the birth dose.

2. Rotavirus vaccine (RV). *(Minimum age: 6 weeks)*
- Administer the first dose at age 6 through 14 weeks (maximum age: 14 weeks 6 days). Vaccination should not be initiated for infants aged 15 weeks or older (i.e., 15 weeks, 0 days or older).
- Administer the final dose in the series by age 8 months 0 days.
- If Rotarix® is administered at ages 2 and 4 months, a dose at 6 months is not indicated.

3. Diphtheria and tetanus toxoids and acellular pertussis vaccine (DTaP). *(Minimum age: 6 weeks)*
- The fourth dose may be administered as early as age 12 months, provided at least 6 months have elapsed since the third dose.
- Administer the final dose in the series at age 4 through 6 years.

4. Haemophilus influenzae type b conjugate vaccine (Hib). *(Minimum age: 6 weeks)*
- If PRP-OMP (PedvaxHIB® or Comvax® [HepB-Hib]) is administered at ages 2 and 4 months, a dose at age 6 months is not indicated.
- TriHiBit® (DTaP/Hib) should not be used for doses at ages 2, 4, or 6 months but can be used as the final dose in children aged 12 months or older.

5. Pneumococcal vaccine. *(Minimum age: 6 weeks for pneumococcal conjugate vaccine [PCV]; 2 years for pneumococcal polysaccharide vaccine [PPSV])*
- PCV is recommended for all children aged younger than 5 years. Administer 1 dose of PCV to all healthy children aged 24 through 59 months who are not completely vaccinated for their age.

- Administer PPSV to children aged 2 years or older with certain underlying medical conditions (see *MMWR* 2000;49[No. RR-9]), including a cochlear implant.

6. Influenza vaccine. *(Minimum age: 6 months for trivalent inactivated influenza vaccine [TIV]; 2 years for live, attenuated influenza vaccine [LAIV])*
- Administer annually to children aged 6 months through 18 years.
- For healthy nonpregnant persons (i.e., those who do not have underlying medical conditions that predispose them to influenza complications) aged 2 through 49 years, either LAIV or TIV may be used.
- Children receiving TIV should receive 0.25 mL if aged 6 through 35 months or 0.5 mL if aged 3 years or older.
- Administer 2 doses (separated by at least 4 weeks) to children aged younger than 9 years who are receiving influenza vaccine for the first time or who were vaccinated for the first time during the previous influenza season but only received 1 dose.

7. Measles, mumps, and rubella vaccine (MMR). *(Minimum age: 12 months)*
- Administer the second dose at age 4 through 6 years. However, the second dose may be administered before age 4, provided at least 28 days have elapsed since the first dose.

8. Varicella vaccine. *(Minimum age: 12 months)*
- Administer the second dose at age 4 through 6 years. However, the second dose may be administered before age 4, provided at least 3 months have elapsed since the first dose.
- For children aged 12 months through 12 years the minimum interval between doses is 3 months. However, if the second dose was administered at least 28 days after the first dose, it can be accepted as valid.

9. Hepatitis A vaccine (HepA). *(Minimum age: 12 months)*
- Administer to all children aged 1 year (i.e., aged 12 through 23 months). Administer 2 doses at least 6 months apart.
- Children not fully vaccinated by age 2 years can be vaccinated at subsequent visits.
- HepA also is recommended for children older than 1 year who live in areas where vaccination programs target older children or who are at increased risk of infection. See *MMWR* 2006;55(No. RR-7).

10. Meningococcal vaccine. *(Minimum age: 2 years for meningococcal conjugate vaccine [MCV] and for meningococcal polysaccharide vaccine [MPSV])*
- Administer MCV to children aged 2 through 10 years with terminal complement component deficiency, anatomic or functional asplenia, and certain other high-risk groups. See *MMWR* 2005;54(No. RR-7).
- Persons who received MPSV 3 or more years previously and who remain at increased risk for meningococcal disease should be revaccinated with MCV.

The Recommended Immunization Schedules for Persons Aged 0 Through 18 Years are approved by the Advisory Committee on Immunization Practices (www.cdc.gov/vaccines/recs/acip), the American Academy of Pediatrics (http://www.aap.org), and the American Academy of Family Physicians (http://www.aafp.org).

DEPARTMENT OF HEALTH AND HUMAN SERVICES • CENTERS FOR DISEASE CONTROL AND PREVENTION

Figure 4-1 • Pediatric immunizations

adverse local and systemic reactions. The acellular vaccine is recommended for U.S. children younger than 7 years of age who do not have a contraindication to vaccination. Since there are several vaccines available, it is recommended that the same brand of pertussis vaccine be used whenever possible, because there are few data on safety or efficacy when different formulations are interchanged. Formerly pertussis vaccine was given in combination with diphtheria and tetanus toxoids as DTP (diphtheria, tetanus, pertussis); however, new vaccines are now available, including combinations with *Haemophilus influenzae*. One such is DTaP–conjugate Hib (*H. influenzae* type b) (TriHIBIT); another is a combination with hepatitis B and polio (DTaP–hepatitis B–IPV) (injectable polio vaccine) (Pediatrix).

While the pertussis vaccine is highly effective and saves many lives, the protection it offers begins to decline after a few years. Although childhood is the time of greatest risk, waning immunity has resulted in the emergence of a large pool of susceptible adults and adolescents. In addition to creating a primary reservoir for pertussis, there has also been an increasing number of pertussis infections among adults. Coupled with the development of a safer vaccine, health authorities now recommend giving a pertussis booster in combination with tetanus and diphtheria to preteens and adults, except to those individuals with contraindications to pertussis.

Contraindications to pertussis vaccination include an immediate anaphylactic reaction to the vaccine or any of its components or the occurrence of encephalopathy within 7 days of vaccination. Relative contraindications include seizure with or without fever that occurs within 3 days of vaccination, persistent inconsolable screaming, or any of the following within 48 hours of vaccination: crying for 3 or more days, a shocklike state, and unexplained temperature of greater than or equal to 40.5°C (104.8°F). These relative contraindications and benefits should be discussed with the parent prior to administration of the vaccine.

POLIOVIRUS VACCINE

The last reported case of wild poliovirus infection was in 1979, although there were approximately eight cases per year of vaccine-related infection due to the live attenuated oral vaccine. As a result, in January 2000, authorities recommended switching to the inactivated IPV from the oral polio vaccine (OPV) to eliminate the risk of vaccine-associated paralytic poliomyelitis in the United States. IPV is available either in monovalent form or in combination as DTaP–hepatitis B–IPV. Mild local reactions such as redness and swelling are the primary adverse effects, although in rare instances more serious reactions may occur in those allergic to the trace amounts of antibiotics (streptomycin, neomycin, polymyxin B)

present in the vaccine. Since IPV is a killed vaccine, it can be given to immunodeficient persons and their household contacts.

MEASLES, MUMPS, AND RUBELLA (MMR) VACCINE

Mumps is a childhood viral illness associated with orchitis, pancreatitis, myocarditis, and encephalitis. These complications are unusual and death and long-term sequelae from mumps are rare. Measles is associated with significant morbidity and mortality. Some 1 to 3 patients per 1000 of those with measles infections die as a result of respiratory and neurologic complications. Rubella is associated with congenital anomalies in the children of infected women. These children are born with ophthalmologic, cardiac, and neurologic defects, including mental retardation. The vaccines for these three illnesses have led to a 99% reduction in the incidence of infection. They were once administered as a single vaccine dose; however, outbreaks of measles in the late 1990s led to a recommendation for a second booster shot administered prior to school entry at the age of 4 to 6 years. Individuals born after 1956 or those previously receiving killed measles vaccine must be given two doses of live attenuated measles vaccine at least 1 month apart before being considered immune.

MMR is a live attenuated virus vaccine and should not be given to pregnant women or immunocompromised persons. Because measles can cause severe and even fatal disease in patients infected with human immunodeficiency virus (HIV), MMR is recommended for children with HIV who are not severely immunocompromised and for their household contacts who lack immunity to measles. Other contraindications include allergic reactions to any vaccine component. Children who are severely allergic to eggs are considered at risk for anaphylactic reactions in measles-containing vaccines. MMR should be delayed for 3 months or longer following the administration of blood products or immunoglobulin. If indicated, a tuberculin skin test should be given either before or together with MMR because the vaccine may temporarily suppress tuberculin sensitivity.

VARICELLA VACCINE

Varicella, or chickenpox, is generally a self-limited childhood infection. However, despite its reputation as a benign childhood disease, it once, prior to implementation of varicella vaccination, caused approximately 4 million cases of disease, 11,000 hospitalizations, and a number of deaths each year in the United States. Physicians should give the live attenuated varicella vaccine (Varivax) to children age 12 months and older or adults who do not have a confirmed history of chickenpox and have no contraindication to vaccination. Varicella vaccine is 95% or more effective against severe disease. The absolute duration of immunity is unknown, although exposure to wild-type varicella zoster virus boosts antibody levels. The varicella vaccine should not be given to patients with a history of hypersensitivity. Pregnant and immunocompromised or immunosuppressed individuals should not generally receive the vaccine. The immune response is less in those over age 12 years; in this group, two doses 1 month apart are recommended, in contrast to the single dose administered to children aged 1 to 12 years. Adverse reactions to the vaccine include fever, occurring in up to 15% of recipients; local reactions, seen in 20% of recipients; and a varicella-like rash containing virus that develops in 3% to 5% of recipients and can be spread to others by direct contact with lesions.

An additional vaccine for all adults over age 60 years without contraindications for receiving live attenuated viral vaccines is the Herpes zoster vaccine. This is a one-time administration regardless of prior history of Herpes zoster infection. The intent with the vaccine is to decrease the incidence of subsequent zoster infections. Adverse reactions are uncommon and largely include local reactions at the site of administration.

PNEUMOCOCCAL VACCINE

Streptococcus pneumoniae is a bacterium that can cause respiratory infection, bacteremia, and meningitis in both adults and children. It is one of the most common bacterial causes of community-acquired pneumonia and meningitis in addition to being the predominant bacterium causing sinusitis and otitis media. Prevnar, the pneumococcal conjugate vaccine (PCV7), has been found safe and reduces the risk of invasive disease by about 90% from the seven pneumococcal serotypes contained in the vaccine. The heptavalent vaccine is recommended for all children up to 2 years of age. These vaccines are well tolerated, with local reactions as the primary adverse effect. The PCV7 vaccine should not be given to adults. Instead, Pneumovax, the pneumococcal polysaccharide vaccine (PPV), is given to older children and adults. PPV is not indicated in children below 2 years of age because it is poorly immunogenic in this age group. Children 2 to 5 years of age who are at moderate-to-high risk for invasive pneumococcal disease may receive PPV, usually 8 weeks following the final dose of PCV.

PPV is recommended for all persons 65 years of age and over and those 2 years of age and over with chronic illnesses such as cardiovascular disease, pulmonary disease, diabetes mellitus, alcoholism, liver disease, cerebrospinal fluid leaks, or cochlear implants. It is also indicated for patients with functional or anatomic asplenia and for those living in special environments or social settings, such as Alaskan natives, American Indians, and residents of long-term-care facilities. It should be given at least 2 weeks prior to elective splenectomy or the initiation of immunosuppressive therapy.

INFLUENZA VACCINE

The influenza virus generally causes mild respiratory illness in young healthy adults; however, in high-risk groups of older patients (over age 65), children under 2 years of age, and those with cardiac disease, chronic respiratory illness, renal disease, diabetes mellitus, or cancer, it may lead to severe respiratory illness, pneumonia, and death. Each year in the United States there is an estimated 36,000 deaths and 226,000 hospitalizations from seasonal influenza. The vaccine must be administered annually due to the antigenic variation in the influenza viruses from year to year. The vaccine's efficacy will vary based on the accuracy of the antigen match for the particular year, with an efficacy of approximately 70% to 80%. In February of 2008, Centers for Disease Control and Prevention (CDC) and the Advisory Committee on Immunization Practice voted to recommend the annual vaccination of all children aged 6 months to 18 years along with the current recommendation of immunization for all adults. While the flu vaccine is recommended for all adults without a contraindication, it is especially important for persons who are at high risk for influenza complications, including those 65 years of age or older; residents of chronic-care facilities; adults and children with chronic cardiovascular or pulmonary problems (including asthma); adults and children with chronic metabolic diseases such as diabetes mellitus, renal disease, hemoglobinopathies or immunosuppression (e.g., HIV); women who will be in the second or third trimester of pregnancy during flu season; and those requiring chronic aspirin therapy. Health care workers and persons providing care to individuals in high-risk groups and household contacts with persons at risk should also be given the influenza vaccine.

Local reactions occur in up to 20% of patients; however, serious reactions are rare. Those with severe egg allergies should forego vaccination and use chemoprophylaxis or undergo formal allergy evaluation. The recently introduced nasal influenza vaccine contains live attenuated virus and is indicated for healthy individuals (i.e., those who do not have underlying medical conditions that predispose them to influenza complications) between the ages of 2 and 49 years. While the live attenuated virus may be more effective than the trivalent inactivated vaccine, it is also more expensive and should not be administered to children under age 5 years who have recurrent wheezing. This vaccine should be avoided in health care workers and immunocompromised individuals as well as those with close contact with immunocompromised patients, since the virus can be shed for up to 7 days after administration.

HEPATITIS A VACCINE

Hepatitis A is a viral infection that usually causes a mild, self-limited illness. There is no chronic form of this illness. Vaccination is recommended for unvaccinated adults traveling to or living in areas with high endemic rates of disease, users of illicit drugs, and men who have sex with men. Universal recommendation is recommended for all children aged 1 year and is given as 2 doses at least 6 months apart. Catch-up vaccination is also recommended for older children who are at increased risk of infection. The vaccine has an efficacy of 94% to 100% and causes local reactions as the primary adverse effect. Recently, a combination product of hepatitis A and hepatitis B vaccine has been introduced into the market.

MENINGOCOCCAL VACCINE

Neisseria meningitidis causes invasive bacterial disease and meningitis in 1 per 100,000 in the population. Although not a common disease, meningococcal disease is associated with very high morbidity and mortality and tends to occur in outbreaks. Recently, a new polysaccharide-conjugate vaccine (Menactra) was introduced and universal vaccination at 11 to 12 years of age, at high school entry, or for college freshman living in dormitories is now recommended. The vaccine is now licensed for use in children from 2 to 10 years of age and also recommended for high-risk groups such as patients with anatomic or functional asplenia, military recruits, those with complement component deficiencies, and travelers to endemic regions. Vaccine administration does not substitute for antimicrobial chemoprophylaxis for close contacts of an infected individual.

ROTAVIRUS VACCINE

Rotavirus can cause severe diarrhea, mostly in infants and young children, often accompanied by vomiting. Each year in the United States, rotavirus results in more than 200,000 emergency room visits, approximately 60,000 hospitalizations, and between 20 and 60 deaths. An earlier vaccine was taken off the market in the late 1900s because of an association with intussusception. However, the newer vaccines have not been associated with intussusception.

HUMAN PAPILLOMAVIRUS

Human papillomavirus (HPV) is the most common sexually transmitted disease in the United States. It can cause anogenital warts and low-grade cervical cytological changes. HPV infections are often subclinical and while most resolve without significant sequelae, some HPV infection can cause cervical cancer, anogenital malignances, and associated precancerous lesions. Since 2006, a quadravalent vaccine that protects against HPV types 16 and 18, which account for 70% of the cases of cervical cancer, and types 6 and 11, which are responsible for 90% of cases genital warts, has been available. The vaccine is composed of surface proteins, contains no viral DNA, and is not infectious. The vaccine is recommended for girls age 11 to 12 years and is given as a series of three shots that can be given with other recommended vaccines. The rationale for immunization at 11 to 12 years of age is that to be maximally effective it should be given before a woman becomes sexually active. Women aged 13 to 26 years who have not previously been immunized or have not completed the full vaccine series should still be offered the HPV vaccine even if they have been sexually active. Sexually active women can benefit even if they have been exposed to HPV already since they probably have not been exposed to all four vaccine strains. The vaccine is not a substitute for recommended cervical cancer screening and individuals should be educated that it does not prevent other sexually transmitted diseases.

KEY POINTS

- The implementation of routine childhood vaccinations is one of the most successful preventive measures in modern-day medicine.
- Considerations in deciding whether a vaccine is recommended for routine use are disease prevalence, disease morbidity and mortality, economic cost to society, vaccine efficacy, and adverse reactions to the vaccine.

5

Preventive Care: 19 to 64 Years

The focus of preventive care is age-dependent, reflecting the changes in disease prevalence across the adult life span. While many available guidelines can assist practitioners in making decisions about appropriate preventive care, they should not replace medical judgment. In addition to primary prevention, secondary prevention to prevent or limit future disease is important. A common dilemma for secondary prevention of an asymptomatic illness such as hypertension is that the consequences may not be seen for years after a person develops high blood pressure. For example, blood pressure evaluation and treatment is a preventive measure for future disease that may not manifest itself until the patient is 70 years of age or beyond.

19 TO 39 YEARS

The most common causes for death in young adults are accidents, homicides, and suicides. In addition, diseases that increase in prevalence and contribute to morbidity and mortality in this age range include HIV infection, heart disease, and some forms of cancer. Lifestyle assessment is important since young adults often acquire habits that may jeopardize their current health or place them at risk for future disease. For example, promiscuity may result in sexually transmitted diseases, including HIV. Smoking may lead to a lifelong habit and increased risk for stroke, heart disease, and lung disease. Alcohol and drug abuse may place the individual at risk for hepatitis, liver disease, and accidents or injuries.

Many patients will begin regular preventive care visits after age 30. There is a debate as to the value of routine visits in this age group. If patients are not coming to the office for preventive care, preventive care issues must be addressed when they are in the office for other reasons. For example, when a woman comes for a Pap smear, she may be instructed to come in after fasting in order to check her lipid profile. At each visit, height, weight, and blood pressure should be checked and any issues regarding blood pressure or weight elevation addressed. Those presenting with an acute injury may be reminded about injury prevention measures, such as the use of helmets and seat belts. Inquiring about domestic violence is important for women seen for acute injuries.

Past medical history may indicate a need for vaccination (e.g., hepatitis B, MMR; see Figure 5-1). Patients with medical problems such as diabetes or asthma should receive pneumococcal and influenza vaccines. Those who have never had chickenpox may wish to consider the varicella vaccine. In addition to reviewing the past medical history, family history, and social history will provide information that may lead to counseling or screening measures. For example, individuals with a family history of premature coronary artery disease or hyperlipidemia should be screened for hyperlipidemia. Patients with a family history of skin cancer and those with fair skin should be counseled about limiting sun exposure. Individuals with a history of substance abuse or smoking should be counseled about the potential consequences associated with these behaviors. Sexually active individuals require counseling about contraception and the prevention of sexually transmitted diseases. Those who own firearms should be counseled about their safe storage. Women should be counseled about adequate calcium intake and supplemented if needed, and those who desire pregnancy can be counseled about supplementation with folate to prevent birth defects. Screening for cervical cancer should start within 3 years of sexual activity or at age 21, which ever comes first. While recommendations vary, a common practice is to screen for cervical cancer every two to three years in women age 30 and older who are sexually active, have a cervix, and who have had three consecutive normal Pap tests. Higher risk women merit more frequent screening. Patients should be reminded about good dental care and the importance of regular dental visits. Other routine screening measures may be recommended in this age group including cholesterol screening in men over age 35 and periodic screening of blood pressure for men and women over age 21.

40 TO 64 YEARS

Many physicians recommend that their patients begin annual preventive care visits at age 40 years. Screening for cardiovascular risk factors and malignancy becomes of greater concern as individuals age. Heart disease is the leading cause of death in the

Recommended Adult Immunization Schedule
UNITED STATES · 2009
Note: These recommendations *must* be read with the footnotes that follow
containing number of doses, intervals between doses, and other important information.

Figure 1. Recommended adult immunization schedule, by vaccine and age group

VACCINE ▼ AGE GROUP▶	19–26 years	27–49 years	50–59 years	60–64 years	≥65 years
Tetanus, diphtheria, pertussis (Td/Tdap)[1,*]	Substitute 1-time dose of Tdap for Td booster; then boost with Td every 10 yrs				Td booster every 10 yrs
Human papillomavirus (HPV)[2,*]	3 doses (females)				
Varicella[3,*]	2 doses				
Zoster[4]				1 dose	
Measles, mumps, rubella (MMR)[5,*]	1 or 2 doses		1 dose		
Influenza[6,*]	1 dose annually				
Pneumococcal (polysaccharide)[7,8]	1 or 2 doses				1 dose
Hepatitis A[9,*]	2 doses				
Hepatitis B[10,*]	3 doses				
Meningococcal[11,*]	1 or more doses				

*Covered by the Vaccine Injury Compensation Program.

For all persons in this category who meet the age requirements and who lack evidence of immunity (e.g., lack documentation of vaccination or have no evidence of prior infection)	Recommended if some other risk factor is present (e.g., on the basis of medical, occupational, lifestyle, or other indications)	No recommendation

Report all clinically significant postvaccination reactions to the Vaccine Adverse Event Reporting System (VAERS). Reporting forms and instructions on filing a VAERS report are available at www.vaers.hhs.gov or by telephone, 800-822-7967.

Information on how to file a Vaccine Injury Compensation Program claim is available at www.hrsa.gov/vaccinecompensation or by telephone, 800-338-2382. To file a claim for vaccine injury, contact the U.S. Court of Federal Claims, 717 Madison Place, N.W., Washington, D.C. 20005; telephone, 202-357-6400.

Additional information about the vaccines in this schedule, extent of available data, and contraindications for vaccination is also available at www.cdc.gov/vaccines or from the CDC-INFO Contact Center at 800-CDC-INFO (800-232-4636) in English and Spanish, 24 hours a day, 7 days a week.

Use of trade names and commercial sources is for identification only and does not imply endorsement by the U.S. Department of Health and Human Services.

Figure 2. Vaccines that might be indicated for adults based on medical and other indications

INDICATION ▶ VACCINE ▼	Pregnancy	Immuno-compromising conditions (excluding human immunodeficiency virus [HIV])[13]	HIV infection[3,12,13] CD4+ T lymphocyte count		Diabetes, heart disease, chronic lung disease, chronic alcoholism	Asplenia[12] (including elective splenectomy and terminal complement component deficiencies)	Chronic liver disease	Kidney failure, end-stage renal disease, receipt of hemodialysis	Health-care personnel
			<200 cells/µL	≥200 cells/µL					
Tetanus, diphtheria, pertussis (Td/Tdap)[1,*]	Td	Substitute 1-time dose of Tdap for Td booster; then boost with Td every 10 yrs							
Human papillomavirus (HPV)[2,*]		3 doses for females through age 26 yrs							
Varicella[3,*]	Contraindicated			2 doses					
Zoster[4]	Contraindicated			1 dose					
Measles, mumps, rubella (MMR)[5,*]	Contraindicated			1 or 2 doses					
Influenza[6,*]	1 dose TIV annually								1 dose TIV or LAIV annually
Pneumococcal (polysaccharide)[7,8]	1 or 2 doses								
Hepatitis A[9,*]	2 doses								
Hepatitis B[10,*]	3 doses								
Meningococcal[11,*]	1 or more doses								

*Covered by the Vaccine Injury Compensation Program.

For all persons in this category who meet the age requirements and who lack evidence of immunity (e.g., lack documentation of vaccination or have no evidence of prior infection)	Recommended if some other risk factor is present (e.g., on the basis of medical, occupational, lifestyle, or other indications)	No recommendation

These schedules indicate the recommended age groups and medical indications for which administration of currently licensed vaccines is commonly indicated for adults ages 19 years and older, as of January 1, 2009. Licensed combination vaccines may be used whenever any components of the combination are indicated and when the vaccine's other components are not contraindicated. For detailed recommendations on all vaccines, including those used primarily for travelers or that are issued during the year, consult the manufacturers' package inserts and the complete statements from the Advisory Committee on Immunization Practices (www.cdc.gov/vaccines/pubs/acip-list.htm).

The recommendations in this schedule were approved by the Centers for Disease Control and Prevention's (CDC) Advisory Committee on Immunization Practices (ACIP), the American Academy of Family Physicians (AAFP), the American College of Obstetricians and Gynecologists (ACOG), and the American College of Physicians (ACP).

DEPARTMENT OF HEALTH AND HUMAN SERVICES CDC
CENTERS FOR DISEASE CONTROL AND PREVENTION

Figure 5-1 • Recommended adult immunization schedule by vaccine and age group. (Reprinted from the Centers for Disease Control and Prevention. Recommended Adult Immunization Schedule—United States, 2009. *MMWR* 2008; 57:53, with permission.)

Footnotes

Recommended Adult Immunization Schedule—UNITED STATES · 2009

For complete statements by the Advisory Committee on Immunization Practices (ACIP), visit www.cdc.gov/vaccines/pubs/ACIP-list.htm.

1. Tetanus, diphtheria, and acellular pertussis (Td/Tdap) vaccination

Tdap should replace a single dose of Td for adults aged 19 through 64 years who have not received a dose of Tdap previously.

Adults with uncertain or incomplete history of primary vaccination series with tetanus and diphtheria toxoid-containing vaccines should begin or complete a primary vaccination series. A primary series for adults is 3 doses of tetanus and diphtheria toxoid-containing vaccines; administer the first 2 doses at least 4 weeks apart and the third dose 6–12 months after the second. However, Tdap can substitute for any one of the doses of Td in the 3-dose primary series. The booster dose of tetanus and diphtheria toxoid-containing vaccine should be administered to adults who have completed a primary series and if the last vaccination was received 10 or more years previously. Tdap or Td vaccine may be used, as indicated.

If a woman is pregnant and received the last Td vaccination 10 or more years previously, administer Td during the second or third trimester. If the woman received the last Td vaccination less than 10 years previously, administer Tdap during the immediate postpartum period. A dose of Tdap is recommended for postpartum women, close contacts of infants aged less than 12 months, and all health-care personnel with direct patient contact if they have not previously received Tdap. An interval as short as 2 years from the last Td is suggested; shorter intervals can be used. Td may be deferred during pregnancy and Tdap substituted in the immediate postpartum period, or Tdap may be administered instead of Td to a pregnant woman after an informed discussion with the woman.

Consult the ACIP statement for recommendations for administering Td as prophylaxis in wound management.

2. Human papillomavirus (HPV) vaccination

HPV vaccination is recommended for all females aged 11 through 26 years (and may begin at 9 years) who have not completed the vaccine series. History of genital warts, abnormal Papanicolaou test, or positive HPV DNA test is not evidence of prior infection with all vaccine HPV types; HPV vaccination is recommended for persons with such histories.

Ideally, vaccine should be administered before potential exposure to HPV through sexual activity; however, females who are sexually active should still be vaccinated consistent with age-based recommendations. Sexually active females who have not been infected with any of the four HPV vaccine types receive the full benefit of the vaccination. Vaccination is less beneficial for females who have already been infected with one or more of the HPV vaccine types.

A complete series consists of 3 doses. The second dose should be administered 2 months after the first dose; the third dose should be administered 6 months after the first dose.

HPV vaccination is not specifically recommended for females with the medical indications described in Figure 2, "Vaccines that might be indicated for adults based on medical and other indications." Because HPV vaccine is not a live-virus vaccine, it may be administered to persons with the medical indications described in Figure 2. However, the immune response and vaccine efficacy might be less for persons with the medical indications described in Figure 2 than in persons who do not have the medical indications described or who are immunocompetent. Health-care personnel are not at increased risk because of occupational exposure, and should be vaccinated consistent with age-based recommendations.

3. Varicella vaccination

All adults without evidence of immunity to varicella should receive 2 doses of single-antigen varicella vaccine if not previously vaccinated or the second dose if they have received only one dose unless they have a medical contraindication. Special consideration should be given to those who 1) have close contact with persons at high risk for severe disease (e.g., health-care personnel and family contacts of persons with immunocompromising conditions) or 2) are at high risk for exposure or transmission (e.g., teachers; child care employees; residents and staff members of institutional settings, including correctional institutions; college students; military personnel; adolescents and adults living in households with children; nonpregnant women of childbearing age; and international travelers).

Evidence of immunity to varicella in adults includes any of the following: 1) documentation of 2 doses of varicella vaccine at least 4 weeks apart; 2) U.S.-born before 1980 (although for health-care personnel and pregnant women, birth before 1980 should not be considered evidence of immunity); 3) history of varicella based on diagnosis or verification of varicella by a health-care provider (for a patient reporting a history of or presenting with an atypical case, a mild case, or both, health-care providers should seek either an epidemiologic link with a typical varicella case or to a laboratory-confirmed case or evidence of laboratory confirmation, if it was performed at the time of acute disease); 4) history of herpes zoster based on health-care provider diagnosis or verification of herpes zoster by a health-care provider; or 5) laboratory evidence of immunity or laboratory confirmation of disease.

Pregnant women should be assessed for evidence of varicella immunity. Women who do not have evidence of immunity should receive the first dose of varicella vaccine upon completion or termination of pregnancy and before discharge from the health-care facility. The second dose should be administered 4–8 weeks after the first dose.

4. Herpes zoster vaccination

A single dose of zoster vaccine is recommended for adults aged 60 years and older regardless of whether they report a prior episode of herpes zoster. Persons with chronic medical conditions may be vaccinated unless their condition constitutes a contraindication.

5. Measles, mumps, rubella (MMR) vaccination

Measles component: Adults born before 1957 generally are considered immune to measles. Adults born during or after 1957 should receive 1 or more doses of MMR unless they have a medical contraindication, documentation of 1 or more doses, history of measles based on health-care provider diagnosis, or laboratory evidence of immunity.

A second dose of MMR is recommended for adults who 1) have been recently exposed to measles or are in an outbreak setting; 2) have been vaccinated previously with killed measles vaccine; 3) have been vaccinated with an unknown type of measles vaccine during 1963–1967; 4) are students in postsecondary educational institutions; 5) work in a health-care facility; or 6) plan to travel internationally.

Mumps component: Adults born before 1957 generally are considered immune to mumps. Adults born during or after 1957 should receive 1 dose of MMR unless they have a medical contraindication, history of mumps based on health-care provider diagnosis, or laboratory evidence of immunity.

A second dose of MMR is recommended for adults who 1) live in a community experiencing a mumps outbreak and are in an affected age group; 2) are students in postsecondary educational institutions; 3) work in a health-care facility; or 4) plan to travel internationally. For unvaccinated health-care personnel born before 1957 who do not have other evidence of mumps immunity, administering 1 dose on a routine basis should be considered and administering a second dose during an outbreak should be strongly considered.

Rubella component: 1 dose of MMR vaccine is recommended for women whose rubella vaccination history is unreliable or who lack laboratory evidence of immunity. For women of childbearing age, regardless of birth year, rubella immunity should be determined and women should be counseled regarding congenital rubella syndrome. Women who do not have evidence of immunity should receive MMR upon completion or termination of pregnancy and before discharge from the health-care facility.

6. Influenza vaccination

Medical indications: Chronic disorders of the cardiovascular or pulmonary systems, including asthma; chronic metabolic diseases, including diabetes mellitus, renal or hepatic dysfunction, hemoglobinopathies, or immunocompromising conditions (including immunocompromising conditions caused by medications or human immunodeficiency virus [HIV]); any condition that compromises respiratory function or the handling of respiratory secretions or that can increase the risk of aspiration (e.g., cognitive dysfunction, spinal cord injury, or seizure disorder or other neuromuscular disorder); and pregnancy during the influenza season. No data exist on the risk for severe or complicated influenza disease among persons with asplenia; however, influenza is a risk factor for secondary bacterial infections that can cause severe disease among persons with asplenia.

Occupational indications: All health-care personnel, including those employed by long-term care and assisted-living facilities, and caregivers of children less than 5 years old.

Other indications: Residents of nursing homes and other long-term care and assisted-living facilities; persons likely to transmit influenza to persons at high risk (e.g., in-home household contacts and caregivers of children aged less than 5 years old, persons 65 years old and older and persons of all ages with high-risk condition[s]); and anyone who would like to decrease their risk of getting influenza. Healthy, nonpregnant adults aged less than 50 years without high-risk medical conditions who are not contacts of severely immunocompromised persons in special care units can receive either intranasally administered live, attenuated influenza vaccine (FluMist®) or inactivated vaccine. Other persons should receive the inactivated vaccine.

7. Pneumococcal polysaccharide (PPSV) vaccination

Medical indications: Chronic lung disease (including asthma); chronic cardiovascular diseases; diabetes mellitus; chronic liver diseases, cirrhosis; chronic alcoholism, chronic renal failure or nephrotic syndrome; functional or anatomic asplenia (e.g., sickle cell disease or splenectomy [if elective splenectomy is planned, vaccinate at least 2 weeks before surgery]); immunocompromising conditions; and cochlear implants and cerebrospinal fluid leaks. Vaccinate as close to HIV diagnosis as possible.

Other indications: Residents of nursing homes or long-term care facilities and persons who smoke cigarettes. Routine use of PPSV is not recommended for Alaska Native or American Indian persons younger than 65 years unless they have underlying medical conditions that are PPSV indications. However public health authorities may consider recommending PPSV for Alaska Natives and American Indians aged 50 through 64 years who are living in areas in which the risk of invasive pneumococcal disease is increased.

8. Revaccination with PPSV

One-time revaccination after 5 years for persons with chronic renal failure or nephrotic syndrome; functional or anatomic asplenia (e.g., sickle cell disease or splenectomy); and for persons with immunocompromising conditions. For persons aged 65 years and older, one-time revaccination if they were vaccinated 5 or more years previously and were aged less than 65 years at the time of primary vaccination.

9. Hepatitis A vaccination

Medical indications: Persons with chronic liver disease and persons who receive clotting factor concentrates.

Behavioral indications: Men who have sex with men and persons who use illegal drugs.

Occupational indications: Persons working with hepatitis A virus (HAV)-infected primates or with HAV in a research laboratory setting.

Other indications: Persons traveling to or working in countries that have high or intermediate endemicity of hepatitis A (a list of countries is available at wwwn.cdc.gov/travel/contentdiseases.aspx) and any person seeking protection from HAV infection.

Single-antigen vaccine formulations should be administered in a 2-dose schedule at either 0 and 6–12 months (Havrix®), or 0 and 6–18 months (Vaqta®). If the combined hepatitis A and hepatitis B vaccine (Twinrix®) is used, administer 3 doses at 0, 1, and 6 months; alternatively, a 4-dose schedule, administered on days 0, 7 and 21 to 30 followed by a booster dose at month 12 may be used.

10. Hepatitis B vaccination

Medical indications: Persons with end-stage renal disease, including patients receiving hemodialysis; persons with HIV infection; and persons with chronic liver disease.

Occupational indications: Health-care personnel and public-safety workers who are exposed to blood or other potentially infectious body fluids.

Behavioral indications: Sexually active persons who are not in a long-term, mutually monogamous relationship (e.g., persons with more than 1 sex partner during the previous 6 months); persons seeking evaluation or treatment for a sexually transmitted disease; current or recent injection-drug users; and men who have sex with men.

Other indications: Household contacts and sex partners of persons with chronic hepatitis B virus (HBV) infection; clients and staff members of institutions for persons with developmental disabilities; international travelers to countries with high or intermediate prevalence of chronic HBV infection (a list of countries is available at wwwn.cdc.gov/travel/contentdiseases.aspx); and any adult seeking protection from HBV infection.

Hepatitis B vaccination is recommended for all adults in the following settings: STD treatment facilities; HIV testing and treatment facilities; facilities providing drug-abuse treatment and prevention services; health-care settings targeting services to injection-drug users or men who have sex with men; correctional facilities; end-stage renal disease programs and facilities for chronic hemodialysis patients; and institutions and nonresidential daycare facilities for persons with developmental disabilities.

If the combined hepatitis A and hepatitis B vaccine (Twinrix®) is used, administer 3 doses at 0, 1, and 6 months; alternatively, a 4-dose schedule, administered on days 0, 7 and 21 to 30 followed by a booster dose at month 12 may be used.

Special formulation indications: For adult patients receiving hemodialysis or with other immunocompromising conditions, 1 dose of 40 μg/mL (Recombivax HB®) administered on a 3-dose schedule or 2 doses of 20 μg/mL (Engerix-B®) administered simultaneously on a 4-dose schedule at 0, 1, 2 and 6 months.

11. Meningococcal vaccination

Medical indications: Adults with anatomic or functional asplenia, or terminal complement component deficiencies.

Other indications: First-year college students living in dormitories; microbiologists who are routinely exposed to isolates of *Neisseria meningitidis*; military recruits; and persons who travel to or live in countries in which meningococcal disease is hyperendemic or epidemic (e.g., the "meningitis belt" of sub-Saharan Africa during the dry season [December–June]), particularly if their contact with local populations will be prolonged. Vaccination is required by the government of Saudi Arabia for all travelers to Mecca during the annual Hajj.

Meningococcal conjugate (MCV) vaccine is preferred for adults with any of the preceding indications who are aged 55 years or younger, although meningococcal polysaccharide vaccine (MPSV) is an acceptable alternative. Revaccination with MCV after 5 years might be indicated for adults previously vaccinated with MPSV who remain at increased risk for infection (e.g., persons residing in areas in which disease is epidemic).

12. Selected conditions for which *Haemophilus influenzae* type b (Hib) vaccine may be used

Hib vaccine generally is not recommended for persons aged 5 years and older. No efficacy data are available on which to base a recommendation concerning use of Hib vaccine for older children and adults. However, studies suggest good immunogenicity in persons who have sickle cell disease, leukemia, or HIV infection or who have had a splenectomy; administering 1 dose of vaccine to these persons is not contraindicated.

13. Immunocompromising conditions

Inactivated vaccines generally are acceptable (e.g., pneumococcal, meningococcal, and influenza [trivalent inactivated influenza vaccine]), and live vaccines generally are avoided in persons with immune deficiencies or immunocompromising conditions. Information on specific conditions is available at www.cdc.gov/vaccines/pubs/acip-list.htm.

United States and is more prevalent in patients over 40 years of age. The prevalence of many different forms of cancer also increases in older populations, making cancer one of the common causes of morbidity and mortality in persons over age 40.

Identification and, if possible, treatment of risk factors for various diseases is a focus of routine health care visits. For some diseases there are no recommendations to screen for the actual disease, but there are recommendations to screen for risk factors. For example, routine screening for heart disease is not recommended, but screening for cardiac risk factors is recommended. Risk factors for heart disease include modifiable factors such as smoking, hypertension, diabetes mellitus, obesity, and hyperlipidemia. For other diseases, such as osteoporosis, screening is recommended only for those with risk factors. Some nonmodifiable risk factors for osteoporosis are white race, slight build, and family history of osteoporosis. Modifiable risk factors for osteoporosis include smoking, menopause, sedentary lifestyle, heavy alcohol and coffee consumption, and low calcium intake. In the case of some diseases—such as breast, cervical, and colon cancer—screening is recommended for all patients of a certain age in order to detect such diseases early. For other cancers—such as lung, oral, and skin cancers—no specific recommendations are made regarding disease detection, but counseling regarding risk factor modification may be beneficial. For example, smoking cessation is advised to prevent lung and oral cancers, and limiting sun exposure is suggested to prevent skin cancers.

Blood pressure should be checked every 1 to 2 years to screen for hypertension. Cholesterol screening is recommended in men every 5 years beginning at age 35 and women every 5 years beginning at age 45. Assessment of substance use can be addressed during the history taking, and any concerns should prompt counseling regarding the associated risks. Measurements of height and weight to calculate the body mass index (BMI) can be performed along with the testing of vital signs; a dietary history will help to screen for potential obesity as well as the risk for osteoporosis. After age 40, women should aim for a daily calcium intake of 1200 to 1500 mg. Diabetes screening is recommended, with a fasting glucose obtained every 3 years beginning at age 45. Other preventive measures include screening for depression and recommending aspirin for the primary prevention of cardiovascular events in high risk individuals and for secondary prevention in those with established disease.

Cancer screening assumes a greater role in preventive care after age 40. Cancer screening in women continues to include Pap smears and yearly mammograms beginning at age 50 (or earlier in those at risk). There are no recommendations for ovarian or uterine cancer screening. For men, the risk and benefits of annual prostate cancer screening should be discussed and screening individualized. For both men and women, colon cancer screening with colonoscopy every 10 years or annual fecal occult blood testing plus sigmoidoscopy every 3 to 5 years is recommended beginning at age 50. In patients with a first-degree relative with colon cancer, colonoscopy should be performed every 5 to 10 years beginning at age 40. There are no formal recommendations for routine screening for lung, skin, or oral cancers. Counseling to perform self-examination for testicular and breast cancer may be beneficial.

Immunizations should be updated. During this age period, annual seasonal flu vaccine is recommended and is especially important for those with chronic illnesses such as diabetes or chronic lung disease that place an individual at higher risk for complications from an influenza infection. Tetanus and diphtheria should be provided every 10 years with a one-time administration of TdaP to boost immunity to pertussis. A single dose of herpes zoster is recommended for individuals age 60 or above. In patients with underlying medical diseases—such as lung disease, heart disease, or diabetes—pneumococcal vaccine should be considered. Patients at risk because of occupational or travel exposures can be given hepatitis A or B vaccines. Figure 5-1 provides detailed information regarding adult vaccination schedules.

Reinforcement of other healthy behavioral measures should also be incorporated into the visit. Healthful eating and exercise should be encouraged. Prevention of unintended pregnancies and sexually transmitted diseases is an issue that should still be discussed with many patients in this age group.

KEY POINTS

- The most common causes of death in adults aged 19 to 40 years are accidents, homicides, and suicides.
- Screening for cardiovascular risk factors and malignancy becomes a focus of health care visits for individuals over age 40.

Each year more than 25 million Americans undergo surgery. Family physicians are often asked to evaluate these patients preoperatively. This evaluation is not just to "clear" patients but also to identify and to intervene, as appropriate, in higher-risk patients requiring surgical procedures. The physician must understand the risk factors associated with the surgical procedure and incorporate this information into the evaluation and treatment recommendations for the individual patient.

At least one surgical complication occurs in 17% of patients undergoing surgery. Surgical morbidity and mortality generally fall into one of three categories: cardiac, respiratory, or infectious complications. These complications are increased for certain populations of patients. Identification of at-risk patients and preparation may help to reduce the risks of surgery.

RISK FACTORS

Patients with angina, recent myocardial infarction (MI), arrhythmias, congestive heart failure (CHF), and diabetes are at significantly increased risk for perioperative MI, heart failure, or arrhythmias. An increased risk for cardiac complications is also present in elderly patients and those with abnormal electrocardiograms (ECGs), low functional capacity, history of stroke, and uncontrolled hypertension.

Surgeries may be classified as high-, intermediate-, or low-risk procedures. Those posing a high risk for cardiac complications (greater than 5% cardiac risk) include vascular surgeries, emergency surgeries, and surgeries associated with increased blood loss or large fluid shifts. Intermediate-risk surgeries (1% to 5% cardiac risk) include most intrathoracic, intraperitoneal, and orthopaedic procedures. Low-risk procedures (less than 1% cardiac risk) include cosmetic procedures, cataract operations, and endoscopies.

Patients at risk for pulmonary complications include those with lung disease—for example, asthma or chronic obstructive pulmonary disease (COPD)—obesity, a history of smoking, and undiagnosed cough or dyspnea. Procedures that increase the risk for pulmonary complications are primarily abdominal or thoracic surgeries, with the rule being that the closer the surgery is to the diaphragm, the higher the risk of complications.

Wound infections are the most common infectious complications following surgery, followed by pneumonia, urinary tract infections, and systemic sepsis. Diabetes and vascular disease are patient factors associated with an increased risk for wound infections. Surgeries with potential spillage of infectious material, such as abscess drainage or gastrointestinal surgery, pose a higher risk of postoperative infections. Instrumentation of the urinary tract, as occurs during bladder catheterization or genitourinary surgery, can lead to the development of urinary tract infections.

CLINICAL EVALUATION

Preoperative evaluation consists of a thorough history and physical examination as well as a risk assessment, which then directs preoperative testing and perioperative medical management. If possible, the preoperative evaluation for elective surgery should take place a few weeks before the scheduled procedure to allow time to correct any conditions that might preclude surgery. For example, if the preoperative examination revealed a previously undiagnosed atrial fibrillation, the condition could be stabilized before surgery and thus avoid rescheduling.

The history should include information about the patient's current condition requiring surgery, past surgical procedures, and experience with anesthesia. It is important to assess the patient's exercise tolerance or functional level. In children, past medical history—including birth history, perinatal complications, congenital chromosomal or anatomic malformations, and recent infections, particularly upper respiratory infections or pneumonia—are important elements of the preoperative evaluation. The physician must inquire about any chronic medical conditions, particularly those involving the heart and lungs. Medications, including over-the-counter medications, must be noted. Medication dosing may have to be adjusted in the perioperative period. Aspirin and other nonsteroidal anti-inflammatory drugs (NSAIDs) should generally be discontinued 1 week prior to surgery to avoid excessive bleeding.

During the evaluation, immunization status can be assessed and updated, if necessary. A history of tobacco, alcohol, and drug use should be elicited;

ideally, the patient should quit smoking 8 or more weeks preoperatively to minimize the risk of pulmonary complications. A functional assessment should be made, and the physician should review the patient's social supports and potential need for assistance after hospital discharge. For example, a patient undergoing hip replacement who has only limited assistance available at home may require home services or temporary placement in a rehabilitation facility. Planning for these needs can occur prior to hospitalization.

The physician must pay particular attention during the physical examination to the bedside cardiopulmonary assessment. More than 20% of patients undergoing elective surgery have some form of cardiovascular disease. Key features that may warrant further evaluation include elevated blood pressure, heart murmurs, chest pain, signs of CHF, shortness of breath, and lung disease (most commonly obstructive lung disease). After assessment or therapy, patients with identified cardiopulmonary disease may warrant a second examination just prior to hospitalization and surgery. In children with recent upper respiratory infections, a second visit to assess the current state of the infection can allow the clinician to identify persistent fever, wheezing, or significant nasal discharge; this may, after consultation with the surgeon, result in postponement of the surgery.

DIAGNOSTIC EVALUATION

Clinical studies during the last 15 years have led to changes in preoperative screening. Although preoperative laboratory tests once routinely included the ordering of a complete blood count (CBC), chemistry profiles, a urinalysis (UA), prothrombin time (PT), partial thromboplastin time (PTT), an ECG, and chest x-rays, recent studies demonstrate that extensive testing does not reduce morbidity and mortality. Among the small percentage of patients with unexpected abnormal results, patient management was rarely affected. Current recommendations call for selective ordering of laboratory tests based on patient-specific indications.

Generally, preoperative testing will include hemoglobin, UA, and—in patients over age 40—a serum glucose and ECG. Urine pregnancy tests should be considered in women of childbearing age and a chest x-ray, blood urea nitrogen (BUN), creatinine, and CBC in patients above 75 years of age. Other testing should be directed by specific indications prompted by the history and physical examination.

Patients with risk factors for cardiac complications undergoing elective or semielective surgeries may require preoperative cardiac evaluation (Figure 6-1). Those requiring emergency surgery will need to have postoperative cardiac assessment and management. In addition to an ECG, an echocardiogram may be used to evaluate murmurs, left ventricular (LV) function, hypertrophy, and wall motion abnormalities. While evaluation of LV function is not warranted in all patients, it is reasonable to assess LV function in patients with dyspnea of unknown function, those with current or prior heart failure (if not assessed within 12 months), and those with a questionable history of a cardiomyopathy. Patients with major clinical predictors—such as decompensated CHF, unstable angina, recent MI, severe valvular disease, or arrhythmias—warrant cardiology consultation and possibly angiography. For the remainder of patients, assessment of functional capacity can assist with decision making. Patients with good functional capacity can climb two flights of stairs, walk up a hill effortlessly, or walk four or more blocks easily. Patients with poor functional capacity are limited to activities such as personal care, walking indoors around the house, or walking slowly on level ground. Patients with intermediate predictors (history of MI, angina, compensated CHF, diabetes, renal disease) and poor functional capacity should have stress testing performed, as should patients with intermediate predictors undergoing high-risk procedures, such as vascular surgery. For patients with minor clinical predictors, only those with poor functional capacity who are undergoing high-risk procedures require stress testing. Those with positive stress test results warrant cardiologic consultation prior to proceeding with surgery.

A baseline chest x-ray may be helpful in patients at risk for pulmonary complications. Guidelines for ordering pulmonary function tests have been published but have not been shown to be predictive of complications. Pulmonary function testing may be helpful in diagnosing and assessing disease severity. Other than for lung resection surgery, there are currently no preoperative guidelines that absolutely define prohibitive lung function.

PROPHYLACTIC THERAPIES

Prophylaxis against postoperative infections, namely wound or surgical site infections, includes using antibiotics 30 minutes before the start of surgery and, for prolonged procedures, may include additional doses of antibiotics during the procedure. The administration of postoperative antibiotics is controversial, although many surgeons give one additional postoperative dose of antibiotic. Additional doses should generally be used only for those with suspected or documented infection. Antibiotic selection depends on the type of surgery. For most surgeries, cefazolin or vancomycin is used to cover skin flora, specifically *Staphylococcus aureus*, which is commonly responsible for wound infections. Gram-negative coverage is recommended for gastrointestinal, oral, head and neck, and genitourinary surgeries, and anaerobic coverage should be provided for gastrointestinal and oral surgeries. Cefoxitin is commonly used for gastrointestinal

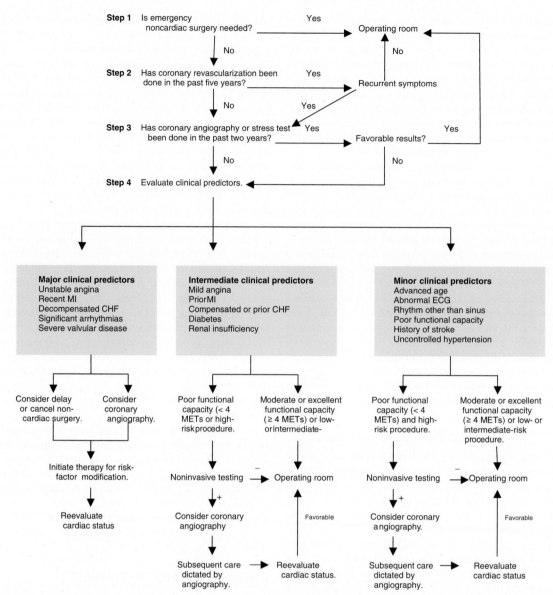

Figure 6-1 • Preoperative cardiac evaluation. (Modified from Eagle KA, Berger PB, Calkins H, et al. ACC/AHA guideline update for perioperative cardiovascular evaluation for noncardiac surgery: executive summary. *J Am Coll Cardiol.* 2002;39:542–553, with permission. Copyright 2002, American College of Cardiology Foundation.)

surgeries and ciprofloxacin for genitourinary procedures; the combination of gentamicin and clindamycin is commonly recommended for head and neck surgeries.

Endocarditis prophylaxis may be indicated for selected individuals. Newer guidelines reflect a consensus that only people at greatest risk of bad outcomes from infective endocarditis should receive short-term preventive antibiotics before common, routine dental and medical procedures. Table 6-1 lists conditions associated with highest risk. Since prophylaxis was preventing only an extremely small number of cases of

infective endocarditis, the emerging consensus is that preventive antibiotics in lower-risk situations do more harm than good due to the associated risks of antibiotic side effects, allergic reactions, and the increasing antibiotic resistance. Not all dental procedures require antibiotic prophylaxis. For example, prophylaxis should be considered for procedures involving the manipulation of gingival tissue, the periapical region of teeth, or perforation of the mucosa and is not indicated for routine injection or placement of orthodontic appliances. Routine prophylaxis of genitourinary (GU) or gastrointestinal (GI) endoscopic procedures in those

■ **TABLE 6-1** Cardiac Conditions Associated with the Highest Risk of Adverse Outcome from Endocarditis for Which Prophylaxis with Dental Procedures is Reasonable

Prosthetic cardiac valve or prosthetic material used for cardiac valve repair
Previous infective endocarditis (IE)
Congenital heart disease (CHD)a
Unrepaired cyanotic CHD, including palliative shunts and conduits
Completely repaired congenital heart defect with prosthetic material or device, whether placed by surgery or by catheter intervention, during the first 6 months after the procedureb
Repaired CHD with residual defects at the site or adjacent to the site of a prosthetic patch or prosthetic device (which inhibit endothelialization)
Cardiac transplantation recipients who develop cardiac valvulopathy

aExcept for the conditions listed above, antibiotic prophylaxis is no longer recommended for any other form of CHD.
bProphylaxis is reasonable because endothelialization of prosthetic material occurs within 6 months after the procedure.
Used with permission from *Circulation*. 2007;116:1736–1754. Copyright 2007, American Heart Association, Inc.

without active infection is not indicated. Table 6-2 lists dental regimens.

Planning for surgery should also include deep venous thrombosis (DVT) prophylaxis and efforts to maximize the patient's pulmonary function. Prophylaxis to prevent venous thromboembolism and pulmonary embolism should be provided to most surgical patients. Risk for developing DVT is approximately 15% to 30% in the general surgical patient and increases to 50% to 60% for patients undergoing hip surgery. Risk factors for developing DVT include age over 40, obesity, orthopaedic surgery, CHF, prior or family history of DVT, stroke, malignancy, immobiliza-

tion, trauma, and estrogen use. Accepted prophylactic therapies for lower-risk patients include early ambulation, gradient compression stockings, pneumatic compression stockings, and low-dose subcutaneous unfractionated or low-molecular-weight heparin. For high-risk patients, either low-molecular-weight heparin or warfarin should be considered. In cases where the risk of bleeding may be too high to permit the use of anticoagulants (e.g., certain neurosurgical procedures), pneumatic compression stockings are generally used. Maximizing preoperative pulmonary function in at-risk patients (e.g., those with COPD) may include treatment of any apparent infections and

■ **TABLE 6-2** Regimens for a Dental Procedure

Situation	Agent	Regimen: Single Dose 30 to 60 Minutes Before Procedure	
		Adults	**Children**
Oral	Amoxicillin	2 g	50 mg/kg
Unable to take oral medication	Ampicillin **OR** Cefazolin **OR** Ceftriaxone	2 g IM or IV 1 g IM or IV	50 mg/kg IM or IV 50 mg/kg IM or IV
Allergic to penicillin or ampicillin–oral	Cephalexina,b **OR** Clindamycin **OR** Azithromycin **OR** Clarithromycin	2 g 600 mg 500 mg	50 mg/kg 20 mg/kg 15 mg/kg
Allergic to penicillin or ampicillin and unable to take oral medication	Cefazolin **OR** Ceftriaxoneb **OR** Clindamycin	1 g IM or IV 600 mg IM or IV	50 mg/kg IM or IV 20 mg/kg IM or IV

aOr other first- or second-generation oral cephalosporin in equivalent adult or pediatric dosage.
bCephalosporins should not be used in an individual with a history of anaphylaxis, angioedema, or urticaria with penicillins or ampicillin.
IM indicates intramuscular; IV indicates intravenous.

the use of bronchodilators, with or without corticosteroids, in those with reversible airway disease. High-risk patients should be trained in the use of incentive spirometry before surgery.

Beta-blocker therapy may reduce myocardial ischemia and mortality in appropriate patients. Current recommendations are that beta blockers should be continued in patients currently receiving beta blockers for coronary artery disease, symptomatic arrhythmias, and hypertension. Beta blockers are also indicated for patients undergoing vascular surgery who are at high cardiac risk (e.g., those with evidence of ischemia on preoperative testing or the presence of coronary heart disease), who are undergoing high-risk or intermediate-risk surgery. The usefulness of therapy for patients undergoing vascular surgery with no clinical risk factors or for those undergoing intermediate-risk procedures or vascular surgery with a single risk factor is uncertain. Contraindications to beta blockers include asthma, heart block greater than first degree, and bradycardia and caution should be exercised in patients with heart failure. Ideally, beta blockers should be started a couple of days or weeks before surgery and the dosage adjusted to a resting heart rate of 60.

KEY POINTS

- Routine preoperative evaluation includes a thorough history and physical examination, with additional testing based on patient characteristics.
- Risk factors for cardiac disease, the type of surgery, and the patient's functional status determine the need for cardiac evaluation.
- Incentive spirometry and smoking cessation can help to limit pulmonary complications.
- Laboratory testing for the otherwise healthy patient includes a hemoglobin and urine analysis and, in those over age 40, a serum glucose and ECG.
- Antibiotic prophylaxis is warranted for procedures with high infection rates, those involving implantation of prosthetic devices, and those in which the consequences of infection are particularly serious.
- DVT prophylaxis is warranted for most surgical patients.

Family Violence: Awareness and Prevention

Family violence poses serious public health risks and manifests itself in various forms, including child abuse, domestic violence between intimate partners, and elder abuse or neglect. Abuse may be physical, sexual, or emotional, with the abuser exerting control over the victim.

EPIDEMIOLOGY

Domestic violence causes a spectrum of health risks, particularly for women, ranging from minor injuries to death. Recent studies estimate that 2 to 4 million women each year suffer injuries from domestic violence, and more than 1 million seek medical attention for such injuries. Approximately 30% of all female homicides in the United States are the result of domestic violence.

Approximately 900,000 abused and neglected children are identified in the United States each year; in 2002, an estimated 1400 children died of abuse and neglect. Many cases of child abuse are unreported. Intentional injury is the number one cause of injury-related death in children under 1 year of age. Children who have been abused physically or sexually are significantly more likely to be sexually active as teens, to abuse tobacco and alcohol, to attempt suicide, and to exhibit violent or criminal behavior.

Owing to factors such as patient denial and underreporting by patients, caregivers, and physicians, the full extent of elder mistreatment in the United States is unknown. However, it is estimated that over 2.5 million older adults are mistreated each year. Abusers are most likely to be caregivers, such as adult children or a spouse. Neglect is the most common form of elder mistreatment, followed by physical abuse, financial exploitation, and emotional and sexual abuse.

Victims of domestic violence are more likely to be young women between the ages of 12 and 35 years; from a lower income group; single, separated, or divorced; not to have attended college; to have experienced abuse as children; and have a partner who abuses alcohol or drugs. The single most-common risk factor in domestic violence is whether the victim

■ **BOX 7-1** Risk Factors for Domestic Violence
Medical
Alcoholism/substance abuse
Mental or physical disability
Relationships
Past history of abusive relationships
Witness to parental violence as a child or adolescent
Rigid family rules or conflicted roles
Social isolation
External Stressors
Poverty, financial struggle
Losses
Work stress
Life cycle changes

witnessed parental violence as a child or an adolescent. This risk factor is consistently associated with being a victim of domestic violence from a spouse.

Domestic violence is associated with poorer pregnancy outcomes. Up to one-third of pregnant women are abused during pregnancy, making battery far more common than the combined incidence of rubella, Rh and ABO (blood type) incompatibility, hepatitis, and gestational diabetes. Pregnant women who are battered are more likely to register late for prenatal care, suffer preterm labor or miscarriage, and have low-birth-weight infants. Box 7-1 summarizes the factors that increase the risk of domestic violence.

PATHOGENESIS

Domestic violence often results from one partner's need to achieve dominance and control. The abuser learns that violence is an effective way to maintain control. Abusers tend to blame family stress and unfulfilled expectations in their partners. Typically, there is a cycle of violence in which an assault is followed by a time when the batterer is remorseful and often loving. Following this is a tension-building period, which then culminates in another episode. Over time, the episodes become more frequent and severe.

CLINICAL MANIFESTATIONS

HISTORY

Identifying victims of abuse is challenging in all but the most obvious cases. The chief complaint can be related to an injury or extend to any organ system. In many cases, abused patients may present with non-traumatic diagnoses, such as upper respiratory tract symptoms or abdominal pain.

Many studies have identified provider barriers to the identification of battered women, which include lack of knowledge or training, time limitations, inability to offer lasting solutions, and fear of offending the patient. Health care providers may have personal experiences that contribute to their reluctance to broach the issue of abuse. Class elitism, racial prejudice, and sexism may also act as barriers to the proper identification and treatment of victims of domestic violence.

PHYSICAL EXAMINATION

Certain types of injury patterns suggest family violence. These include injuries to the face, abdomen, and genitals. Also, multiple injuries in various stages of healing suggest possible abuse. Since many women seen in the emergency room for trauma are victims of abuse, there should be a high index of suspicion for any acute injury that does not have a clear cause. Burns in children are often a tip-off for abuse, particularly burn patterns that suggest an immersion injury or a cigarette burn. Weight loss in the elderly is the most reliable indicator of malnutrition and may be an indicator of neglect. Other signs of abuse in the elderly may be multiple bruises or fractures, welts, bite marks, burns, decubitus ulcers, poor hygiene, and a generally unkempt appearance. Poor cognition is a strong risk factor for mistreatment and should be assessed.

SCREENING

DOMESTIC VIOLENCE SCREENING

Studies have shown that direct questioning of patients at risk for domestic violence yields better information than a written questionnaire. Three important questions to ask are:

1. Have you been hit, kicked, punched, or otherwise hurt by someone within the past year? If so, by whom?
2. Do you feel safe in your current relationship?
3. Is there a partner from a previous relationship making you feel unsafe now?

The first question regarding physical violence is nearly as sensitive and specific as the combination of all three questions. Thus, the problem of identifying women involved in abusive relationships may be simplified by the use of routine screening tools like the questions above.

CHILD ABUSE SCREENING

Screening for child abuse during the interview is difficult, and standardized questions have not been shown to be sensitive or specific in detecting child abuse. Open-ended questions about parenting and discipline may be useful, however, in eliciting evidence of child abuse. For example, the health care provider may ask, "What do you do when he or she misbehaves? Have you ever been worried that someone was going to hurt your child?" Box 7-2 lists clues for suspecting that an injury is due to abuse. Neglect is another type of abuse and can take the form of medical, physical, or emotional neglect. Poor supervision, such as leaving a young child alone without adequate adult oversight, is another type of abuse.

ELDER ABUSE SCREENING

Screening for elder abuse can be difficult. The elderly patient may be unable to provide information due to cognitive impairment or may fear either retaliation from the abuser or ultimate placement in a nursing home. Asking open-ended questions about the patient's perception of safety at home is a good way to begin an interview. More specific questions should focus on incidents of rough handling, confinement, withholding of food and/or medicine, improper touching, and verbal or emotional abuse. Other red flags are a history of delay in seeking medical care, conflicting or improbable accounts of events, and a history of similar or other suspicious events.

■ **BOX 7-2** Clues to Child Abuse
The story given by the parents does not seem to explain the injury
The explanation given by the parent or caretaker is inconsistent or contradictory
There is a long interval between the injury and seeking care
The parent's reaction to the injury is inappropriate
The parent's interaction with the child seems inappropriate

TREATMENT AND INTERVENTION

The most important and most easily provided intervention is the simple message that no one deserves to be hurt and that the victim is not to be blamed for the behavior of the perpetrator.

DOMESTIC VIOLENCE INTERVENTION

Battered women report that the most desirable behaviors by physicians with whom they interact include listening, providing emotional support, and reassuring them that being beaten was not their fault. Women in the same study reported that the most undesirable behaviors include treatment of physical injuries without inquiry as to how they occurred.

Once a patient has been identified as a victim of abuse, it is important to address safety needs, such as ascertaining whether there are guns or other weapons in the house. Simply asking patients whether they feel safe in going home can yield valuable information. Questions about the safety of children are crucial, because as many as 70% of batterers also abuse children. Patients should be encouraged to begin making plans to be safe whether or not they plan to leave their relationship or home situation.

Referral to community services is an important part of treatment for battered women. Shelters provide much more than refuge for victims of domestic violence. Women there can take advantage of child services, counseling, and legal and employment services. The physician can offer to contact the police unless required by law to do so; in that case, the patient should understand the physician's duty to report. Victims should be informed that battering is a crime throughout the United States and that there is help available from the judicial system. Civil protection orders (stay-away orders) are available in every jurisdiction. In addition to barring contact between the perpetrator and the victim, these orders can include temporary custody of children and mandate rent or mortgage payments by the batterer even if he is not allowed to live in the home. **The worst thing the physician can do is nothing.** Even if the patient refuses any help, it is still critical to acknowledge the patient's disclosure and assign responsibility to the abuser. Supportive statements emphasizing that this is not the patient's fault and that violence is not an acceptable means of conflict resolution can be helpful. It is important to remember that terminating an abusive relationship is often a long process. Continuous support, follow-up, and accessibility are critically important for those individuals who choose to remain in an abusive relationship.

CHILD ABUSE INTERVENTION

Intervention studies in child abuse have concentrated on primary prevention. Home visits to high-risk families early in a child's life have been shown to decrease the rate of child abuse and the need for medical visits. Unfortunately, most clinicians do not have the option of providing this level of intervention, much less extending this type of treatment for long periods of time. In up to 60% of cases, there may be recurrent abuse despite interventions.

ELDER ABUSE INTERVENTION

Effective interventions for elder abuse may also be limited, in large part because the abuser is often an overworked primary caregiver. The patient's cognition should be assessed; if he or she is competent, the patient should be an active participant in treatment. In some cases nursing home placement may be the best or the only option, but often a multidisciplinary team approach can be taken. Members of such teams include geriatricians, social workers, case management nurses, and representatives from legal, financial, and adult protective services. Team members can work together with the patient and caregiver and come up with solutions to eliminate the abuse.

DOCUMENTATION

Medical records must document abuse accurately and legibly, since these records are readily admissible at civil and criminal trials. They can provide objective diagnoses that can substantiate a victim's assertion of harm. These records can be used even when the victim is unable or unwilling to testify. Whenever possible, the patient's own words should be used. The relationship of the perpetrator to the victim should also be clearly stated. If possible, the record should include photographs, because these are particularly valuable as evidence. Areas of tenderness, even in the absence of visible injury, should be documented in writing as well as on a body map. Attention to detail is invaluable when one is attempting to recreate the circumstances of abuse for the criminal justice system. A well-documented medical record improves the likelihood of successful prosecution without testimony from the health care provider.

REPORTING

In all states, suspected cases of child abuse or neglect must be reported to local child protective services agencies. In most states, suspected elder abuse must also be reported. Almost all states mandate reporting injuries that result from the use of a gun, knife, or other deadly weapon. It is unknown whether mandatory reporting improves patient/victim outcomes. Nevertheless, health care providers must be familiar with local laws and comply with them. A few states now require that health care workers report cases of suspected domestic violence. The reporting of abuse is **not** a substitute for proper intervention and management of child abuse, domestic violence, or elder abuse.

BATTERERS

Information on batterers is limited. This is particularly worrisome because the solution to the problem of abuse lies largely in changing perpetrator behavior. Current theories hold that the cycle of battery, particularly in intimate partner violence, revolves around the batterer having total control of the victim. The primary goal of intervention should be to break this cycle. However, more data are needed to establish which specific interventions are most helpful with batterers.

KEY POINTS

- Approximately 30% of all female homicides in the United States are the result of domestic violence.

- Children who have been abused physically or sexually are significantly more likely to be sexually active as teens, to abuse tobacco and alcohol, to attempt suicide, and to exhibit violent or criminal behavior.

- The most common form of elder abuse is neglect, followed by physical abuse, financial exploitation, emotional abuse, and sexual abuse.

- The chief complaint can be related to an injury; however, in many cases abused patients may present with nontraumatic diagnoses, such as upper respiratory tract symptoms or abdominal pain.

- The most important and most easily provided intervention is the simple message that no one deserves to be hurt and that the victim is not to blame for the behavior of the perpetrator.

Chapter

8 Allergies

The term **allergy** can be defined as an immunoglobulin E (IgE)-mediated hypersensitivity to an antigen. Type I hypersensitivity reactions include allergic rhinitis, atopic dermatitis, conjunctivitis, asthma, food allergies, and systemic anaphylaxis.

EPIDEMIOLOGY

Allergic rhinitis affects up to 20% of the population, and 10% to 20% of children suffer from atopic dermatitis. Asthma occurs in 5% to 7% of the population and is associated with significant morbidity and an increasing number of deaths. Allergic rhinitis and asthma often coexist and more than half of the asthma cases in the United States can be attributed to seasonal allergies. In some cases allergic rhinitis and asthma may be thought of as manifestations of the same disease. Food allergies, although less common, occur in a significant number of individuals.

PATHOGENESIS

In allergic rhinitis, allergens bind to IgE on mast cells on the nasal mucosa of a sensitized individual. This causes mast cells to degranulate, releasing chemical mediators such as histamines, leukotrienes, and bradykinins, which cause vasodilatation, fluid transudation, and swelling. Common seasonal allergens include pollens from trees, grasses, and weeds. Perennial rhinitis, which occurs throughout the year, is caused primarily by indoor allergens such as house dust, animal dander, and molds.

IgE-mediated reactions can also trigger asthma. Environmentally important allergens leading to asthma include air pollution, dust mites, and cockroaches, which may explain the increasing prevalence of asthma in the inner city.

Cutaneous, respiratory, or gastrointestinal exposure to allergens may cause symptoms in the exposed organ system or produce more generalized symptoms. Common skin manifestations of allergies include urticaria and eczema. Gastrointestinal symptoms associated with allergen exposure include nausea, vomiting, diarrhea, and abdominal pain. Foods most commonly found to be allergenic in children are milk, eggs, peanuts, soy, wheat, tree nuts, fish, and shellfish. In adults, peanuts, tree nuts, shellfish, and fish are the most common.

A severe, life-threatening systemic allergic reaction called **anaphylaxis** can occur from food allergies (e.g., to peanuts), during blood transfusions, from medications, or from insect stings of the Hymenoptera order (bees, wasps, and ants).

CLINICAL MANIFESTATIONS

HISTORY

The symptoms of allergic rhinitis include runny nose (rhinorrhea), sneezing, nasal congestion, conjunctivitis, and itching of the ears, eyes, nose, and throat. Nonproductive cough, nasal congestion with headaches, plugged or itchy ears, diminished smell and taste, or sleep disturbances may all be symptoms of allergies. Timing of the symptoms is important. Tree pollens tend to affect people more in the early spring, grasses in mid-May to June, and ragweed from August until the first frost. Those who are allergic to pollens typically have worse symptoms during the day and improve at night. The common perennial allergens are house dust, feathers, animal dander, and molds. In these patients the symptoms may be worse at night. Continual waxing and waning throughout the year suggest a combination of perennial and seasonal allergies. Genetic factors appear to play a role, and patients with allergies often have a family history of atopy.

Food allergies often affect the skin and the gastrointestinal system. Food allergies may present with urticaria, usually within an hour of ingesting the offending agent. Patients should be asked whether they have ever experienced symptoms suggestive of more severe or anaphylactic reactions. Manifestations of anaphylaxis include agitation, palpitations, paresthesias, pruritus, difficulty swallowing, cough, and wheezing. Patients with these symptoms need emergency care, since the initial symptoms may progress rapidly and even lead to cardiovascular collapse.

PHYSICAL EXAMINATION

The physical examination should focus on the eyes, nose, throat, lungs, and skin. Patients may have conjunctivitis and increased lacrimation. The nasal mucosa may appear swollen and pale. The turbinates should be inspected to rule out any nasal polyps, which are common in patients with allergies. The term "allergic shiners" describes the darkening of the infraorbital skin in people with chronic allergies. Some patients may have a nasal crease across the bridge of the nose due to the frequent nose rubbing ("allergic salute") to relieve itching. The sinuses should be examined for tenderness and the lungs for wheezing.

Skin reactions such as eczema and urticaria are common in children with food allergies. Atopic dermatitis in infants and young children is usually an exudative eruption with oozing and crusting primarily occurring in the head and neck areas, diaper area, forearms, and wrists. In preschool and school children the rash is typically drier and scalier. Similar to adults, the rash is often found in the large flexures and the skin is dry, thickened, and lichenified with frequent evidence of scratch marks. An abdominal examination should be performed in patients presenting with gastrointestinal symptoms so as to exclude other causes for their symptoms.

DIFFERENTIAL DIAGNOSIS

The differential diagnosis depends on the presenting complaint. In allergic conjunctivitis, it is important to differentiate between viral, bacterial, allergic, and irritant causes of conjunctivitis. Viral and bacterial conjunctivitis are discussed in Chapter 27. Allergic conjunctivitis is often seasonal and occurs during periods of high exposure. Patients may also develop red eyes due to irritants such as dust and smoke.

Rhinorrhea can be due to a common cold, vasomotor rhinitis, atrophic rhinitis, rhinitis medicamentosa, or sinusitis. In common cold, the mucosa is usually red with thickened discharge, whereas with allergies the nasal mucosa appears pale and boggy or bluish. In nonallergic rhinitis, there is no pruritus. Patients with vasomotor rhinitis present with chronic nasal congestion with watery rhinorrhea, which may be intensified by sudden changes in temperature, humidity, or odors. Atrophic rhinitis is a condition seen in elderly patients and is characterized by marked atrophy of the nasal mucosa, chronic nasal congestion, and a bad odor. Rhinitis medicamentosa is caused by chronic use of cocaine or topical nasal decongestants. In sinusitis, the nasal discharge may be purulent and accompanied by headaches, nasal congestion, facial pain, and tenderness over the sinuses. Other causes of rhinitis include foreign bodies, nasal polyps, tumors, and nasal congestion associated with hormonal causes such as pregnancy, the use of birth control pills, and hypothyroidism. Wegener granulomatosis, midline granuloma, and sarcoidosis are rare but serious causes of nasal discharge.

The symptoms of food allergies include skin reactions and gastrointestinal symptoms. Urticarial lesions, or hives, are characterized by pruritic erythematous raised lesions, which may be migratory. Atopic dermatitis is an eczematous rash that is flat, erythematous, pruritic, and scaly and can be confused with contact dermatitis or lichen simplex chronicus. On rare occasions a skin biopsy is needed to exclude other conditions. Evaluation of the gastrointestinal symptoms requires a thorough history and physical examination as well as an association of symptoms with the suspected allergen.

DIAGNOSTIC EVALUATION

The diagnosis of allergic disease is usually made on the basis of the history and physical examination. In most patients, treatment may be started without any diagnostic tests; if the patient responds to therapy, no further testing is needed.

Eosinophils found on microscopic examination of nasal smears are characteristic of allergic rhinitis. However, this test is not commonly performed because of its poor sensitivity and specificity. In patients who do not respond to empiric therapy, allergy testing is helpful. The radioallergosorbent test (RAST) tests the blood for the presence of IgE to different allergens. The test is sensitive but not specific; thus, many individuals may be positive on the RAST but may not be having clinical symptoms from the allergen identified by it. Skin-prick testing involves injecting a small amount of allergen into the skin and observing for local responses. This test is more specific but less sensitive than the RAST and is usually performed by an allergist. Identifying offending allergens is useful for directing avoidance therapy. If no allergens are identified and the patient continues to have symptoms, flexible nasolaryngoscopy may be performed to rule out any anatomic or pathologic abnormalities. In patients with food allergies, the history should help formulate a possible list of allergenic foods. Avoidance and challenge testing can assess for different food allergies.

TREATMENT

The first treatment for any allergic disorder is allergen avoidance. Examples include staying indoors during a high-pollen day or reducing household dust by frequent cleaning, vacuuming using a high-efficiency particulate air (HEPA) filter, and removing dust-collecting items such as books or shag rugs. Pharmacologic therapy includes antihistamines, oral and topical decongestants, intranasal and oral corticosteroids, antileukotriene therapy with a selective leukotriene receptor antagonist (LTRA) and intranasal cromolyn sodium. Antihistamines are the first-line therapy for allergic rhinitis and are also helpful for other forms of allergy. They block the H_1 receptors, preventing the release of histamine, and help reduce sneezing, rhinorrhea, and itching. The main side effect of these drugs is sedation. However, newer nonsedating antihistamines are now available. A topical antihistamine nasal spray (azelastine) is also available but is expensive compared to generic oral antihistamines. Topical

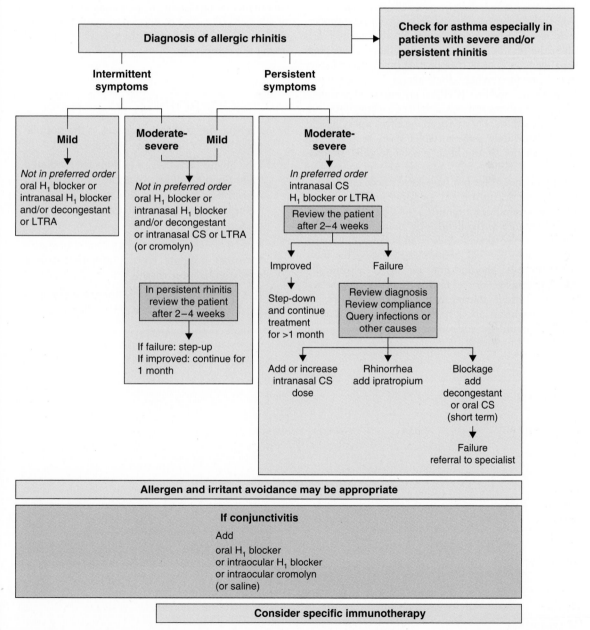

Figure 8-1 • Algorithm for allergic rhinitis diagnosis and management. (Reprinted from Bousquet et al. *Allergy.* 2008;63(suppl 86):8–160, with permission.)

nasal decongestant sprays have a very limited role in allergic rhinitis because of the risks of tachyphylaxis and rebound nasal congestion. Oral decongestants, such as pseudoephedrine, can relieve nasal congestion but should be used with caution in patients with hypertension, thyroid disease, diabetes, and difficulty in urination.

Intranasal steroids are the treatment of choice for most patients with moderate-to-severe persistent allergic rhinitis because of their effectiveness and minimal side effects. Oral corticosteroids are potent medications but have significant long-term side effects; therefore, their use should generally be restricted to 3 to 7 days. Cromolyn, which stabilizes mast cells, is available as an over-the-counter nasal spray. Cromolyn is only moderately effective but is very safe and well tolerated. It is often the first line of treatment in children and pregnant women. Topical therapies or oral antihistamines may provide relief for allergic conjunctivitis. Leukotriene modifiers (LTRAs) are also used to reduce allergic symptoms and may also benefit those with concomitant asthma. They have an excellent safety profile, and because they come in tablet form, are easier for some patients to use than nasally inhaled steroids. Intranasal anticholinergics may be helpful in cases of persistent rhinorrhea but have little effect on obstructive symptoms. Figure 8-1 presents an overview of treatment for allergic rhinitis.

For patients with allergic skin manifestations, oral antihistamines, topical steroids, and cool colloid baths may be helpful. Oral steroids can be used for acute urticaria but should not be used chronically. Moisturizing lotions and creams to avoid dryness and to repair the skin barrier may improve symptoms. As with other forms of allergy, avoidance of any known triggers should be advised as well as avoiding skin irritants such as woolen or abrasive clothing. Patients with food allergies should avoid the foods that bring on the symptoms.

Therapy for patients with asthma is outlined in Chapter 38. In cases of anaphylaxis, the treatment of choice is epinephrine. Patients who have a history of anaphylaxis should carry injectable epinephrine. They should wear an "alert" bracelet and have an emergency action plan that describes the signs and symptoms of anaphylaxis and emergency instructions.

In recalcitrant cases, immunotherapy may be tried. In this process, patients are exposed to the allergen by subcutaneous injections of increasing concentrations of allergens. The goal of immunotherapy is to induce a tolerance in the patient for the specific allergen triggering the symptoms.

KEY POINTS

- Allergies are common diseases in the population and their prevalence is increasing.
- Type I hypersensitivity reactions are mediated by antigen binding to IgE on mast cells and basophils; this causes the mast cell or the basophil to release mediators of the allergic response.
- Intranasal steroids are the treatment of choice for most patients with moderate-to-severe persistent allergic rhinitis.
- The first and definitive treatment for any allergic disorder is avoidance of the allergens.

9 Back Pain

Approximately two-thirds of all adults experience back pain at some time in their lives. It is the second most-common reason for physician visits after respiratory tract infection.

PATHOGENESIS

Ligaments, vertebral bones, facet joints, intervertebral disks, nerve roots, and muscles are all potential sources of back pain. The most common causes of back pain are muscular injuries and age-related degenerative processes in the intervertebral disks and facet joints. Muscle fibers of the paraspinal muscles may tear under strenuous activity, such as twisting or heavy lifting. This results in bleeding and spasm, causing local swelling and tenderness. Obesity and poor conditioning contribute to the problem. Age-related degenerative changes in the intervertebral disks and facet joints are the result of chronic stress on the lumbosacral spine. Weakening of the fibrous capsule can cause the disk to bulge or herniate beyond the interspace. Disk herniation is responsible for 95% of cases of nerve root impingement. The most common site of disk herniation is the L5–S1 level, followed by L4–5. Table 9-1 reviews the symptoms and deficits associated with the different levels of nerve impingement. Back pain may also result from visceral structures near the spine, such as the aorta, kidneys, pancreas, and gallbladder.

CLINICAL MANIFESTATIONS

HISTORY

The history should elicit the onset of pain as well as its severity, location, and character; aggravating and relieving factors; past medical history, previous injuries; and psychosocial stressors. "Red flags" such as fever, night pain, weight loss, and bone pain suggest something other than mechanical low back pain. The presence of sciatica, a sharp pain that radiates down the back or side of the leg past the knee, is often a sign of disk herniation with nerve root irritation. Difficulty urinating, fecal incontinence, progressive weakness, and saddle anesthesia are symptoms of the cauda equina syndrome, a surgical emergency.

Spinal stenosis, a degenerative disease of the spine, is usually seen after age 50. Patients typically complain of back pain and may experience pseudoclaudication, or pain/paresthesias of the lower extremities or back, that worsens with standing or back extension.

The evaluation of a child with back pain requires the presence of a parent or caretaker. Sports participation may cause injuries. For example, back handsprings or walkovers in gymnastics and hyperextension in football are associated with spondylolysis and spondylolisthesis, which can cause pain. As a general rule, pain from spondylolysis, spondylolisthesis, Scheuermann disease, muscle disease, and overuse problems improves with

■ TABLE 9-1 Impingement of Nerve Roots and Symptoms			
Level	**Nerve Root**	**Deficits**	**Sciatica**
L3–4	L4	Patellar jerk (reflex) dorsiflexion of foot (motor) medial aspects of tibia (sensory)	Uncommon
L4–5	L5	Extensor of great toe (motor) dorsum of foot/base of first toe (sensory)	Common
L5–S1	S1	Ankle jerk (reflex) plantar flexion (motor) buttock, post thigh, calf, lateral ankle, and foot (sensory)	Common

■ **TABLE 9-2** Clinical Manifestations of Back Pain

Type	Onset	Trigger	Symptoms
Muscular	Acute	Heavy lifting	Lateralized back pain, pain in buttock and posterior upper thigh
Disk herniation	Recurrent	Trivial stress	Nerve root L5, S1 impingements, frequent sciatica
Spinal stenosis	Old age or congenital	OA[a] or congenital	Pseudoclaudication[a]
Spondylolisthesis[b]	Chronic	OA, spondylolysis	Nerve root L5, S1 impingement hyperextension activities
Compression fracture (fx)	Acute	Osteoporosis	Pain limited in middle-to-lower spine steroid use or myeloma
Neoplasms	Insidious	Neoplasms[c]	Night pain, not relieved with supine position
Cauda equina syndrome	Old age	Massive disk herniation	Overflow incontinence (90%), saddle anesthesia[d] (75%), decreased anal sphincter tone
Osteomyelitis	Acute	Back procedure	Fever, spinal tenderness
Inflammatory diskitis	Young age	*S. aureus*	Refusal to walk, fever, signs of sepsis; disk space narrowing, sclerosis per radiograph
Ankylosing spondylitis	Young age	HLA-B27	Morning spinal stiffness, history of inflammatory bowel disease (dz) sacroiliitis, chest expansion <2.5 cm, "bamboo-spine" in radiograph
Spondylolysis	>10 years	Hyperextension	Back, buttock pain with lordosis with activity, tight hamstrings
Scheuermann disease	Young age	Fatigue	Round back, vertebral wedging, end plate irregularity per radiograph

[a]OA (osteoarthritis); pseudoclaudication is pain in the lower extremity worsened by walking and relieved by sitting down that mimics vascular insufficiency.
[b]Spondylolisthesis is forward subluxation of a vertebral body, usually in L4–5 or L5–S1.
[c]Neoplasm include primary (i.e., multiple myeloma, spinal cord tumor) or metastatic to the spine (i.e., breast, lung, prostate, gastrointestinal, genitourinary neoplasms).
[d]Saddle anesthesia is reduction in sensation over the buttocks, upper posterior thighs, and perineum.

rest. In contrast, tumor, infection, or inflammatory diseases can cause nighttime wakening due to pain and do not improve with bed rest.

The clinical manifestations of back pain are summarized in Table 9-2.

PHYSICAL EXAMINATION

A back examination should include (1) inspecting the back for deformity; (2) checking for leg-length discrepancy; (3) checking spinal motion; (4) palpating for focal tenderness suggestive of tumor, infection, fracture, or disk herniation; (5) performing a neurologic examination to identify motor or sensory deficits; and (6) testing straight leg raising (SLR). SLR is positive if sciatica is reproduced with elevation of the leg less than 60 degrees. Ipsilateral SLR is more sensitive for a herniated disk, whereas contralateral SLR (with the symptoms of sciatica in the leg opposite to the examined leg) is more specific for a herniated disk.

Examination of the abdomen, rectum, groin, pelvis, and the peripheral pulses is also important in patients with back pain. Other signs of systemic diseases are fever, breast mass, pleural effusion, enlarged prostate nodule, lymphadenopathy, and joint inflammation.

■ **BOX 9-1** Differential Diagnosis of Acute Low Back Pain

Mechanical Low Back Pain (97%)
Lumbar strain (70%), degenerative processes in the intervertebral disks and facet joints (10%), herniated disk (4%), compression fx (4%), spinal stenosis (3%), spondylolisthesis (2%), spondylolysis, trauma, congenital diseases
Nonmechanical Spinal Conditions (1%)
Neoplasia (0.7%), infections (0.01%), inflammatory arthritis (0.3%), Scheuermann disease, Paget disease
Visceral Diseases (2%)
Diseases of pelvic organs (prostatitis, endometriosis, chronic PID), renal diseases (nephrolithiasis, pylonephritis, perinephritic abscess), aortic aneurysm, gastrointestinal disease (pancreatitis, cholecystitis, penetrating ulcer)

■ **BOX 9-2** Indications for X-Rays in Patients with Back Pain

Age >50
History of significant trauma
Neurologic deficit
Systemic symptoms
Chronic steroid use
Possible hereditary condition
History of drug or alcohol abuse
History of osteoporosis
Immunodeficient state
Pain persisting >6 weeks

DIFFERENTIAL DIAGNOSIS

Box 9-1 lists the differential diagnosis of back pain. In general, the history and physical examination should help place patients with back pain into one of the following three broad categories: nonspecific low back pain, back pain associated with a radiculopathy or stenosis, and back pain associated with an underlying cause. Unfortunately, a large percentage of patients have nonspecific pain and cannot be given a definitive diagnosis. Often they are classified as having a lumbar strain or mechanical low back pain. Only a small fraction of patients have a serious problem such as a fracture, malignancy, infection, or visceral disease as a cause of low back pain. Systemic diseases that may present as back pain include metastatic cancer, multiple myeloma, and osteoporosis.

DIAGNOSTIC EVALUATION

Box 9-2 lists indications for obtaining spinal x-rays. For most patients x-rays are not recommended unless the pain persists beyond 6 weeks. Negative plain films do not rule out the possibility of significant disease.

Both magnetic resonance imaging (MRI) and computed tomography (CT) are more sensitive than plain films for detecting spinal infections, cancers, herniated disks, and spinal stenosis; they have largely replaced myelography. Because these two tests are highly sensitive and frequently demonstrate "abnormalities" in normal individuals, the American College of Physicians and the American Pain Society discourage routine imaging in patients with nonspecific low back to avoid overdiagnosis and recommend that imaging should be ordered only if there is strong suspicion of disease. Electromyography and measurement of somatosensory-evoked potentials may help to define the extent of neurologic involvement.

Blood tests are not necessary for most patients with back pain. A CBC, UA, calcium, phosphorus, erythrocyte sedimentation rate (ESR), and alkaline phosphatase may be considered in patients with suspected systemic disease, older individuals, and those who fail conservative treatment. A CBC screens for infection, anemia associated with multiple myeloma, or occult malignancy. The ESR may be elevated in patients with malignancy, infection, or a connective tissue disease. Patients who may require long-term NSAIDs may require baseline renal and liver function tests.

TREATMENT

Serious nonmechanical causes of low back pain—such as infection, malignancy, or fracture—require treatment of the underlying problem. Patients with a progressive neurologic finding need hospital admission and prompt consultation.

Most patients with mechanical low back pain will get better with conservative treatment consisting of pain control, education, reassurance, and appropriate activity. About 80% to 90% will recover within 6 weeks. Bed rest is generally not recommended unless the pain is severe enough to preclude normal activities; even then, it should be limited to 2 to 3 days. Longer periods of bed rest result in deconditioning. During the acute phase of an attack, the patient should be encouraged to continue normal activities, including work as tolerated, but told to avoid heavy lifting (>25 lb), twisting, prolonged sitting, driving for long periods, and heavy vibration. Traction and analgesic injection are usually not helpful in the acute stage.

Although there are no well-controlled studies demonstrating the value of heat, ice, or massage, many clinicians and patients feel that these treatments are helpful and pose little risk.

Medications are important for relieving pain. Acetaminophen is safe and inexpensive. It is a good first choice alone or in combination with an NSAID. NSAIDs can relieve pain and have an anti-inflammatory effect. However, they should be used with caution in patients with a history of gastritis, ulcers, hypertension, chronic renal failure, or CHF. For younger patients and those at low risk of cardiovascular disease who cannot tolerate traditional NSAIDs, the cyclooxygenase-2 (COX-2) inhibitors have fewer gastrointestinal (GI) side effects, although they still have the same adverse effects on the kidneys and on fluid balance. COX-2 inhibitors also increase the risk of heart attack and stroke. Although Vioxx is most closely associated with cardiac disease, this may be a class effect of COX-2 inhibitors. Narcotic pain relievers are often prescribed in the acute setting and while they may be useful in the first few days of treatment, the benefit of opioids for the long-term management of chronic low back pain remains questionable. Concerns related to long-term use include tolerance, medication misuse, hypogonadism, constipation, and hyperalgesia that paradoxically can cause an increase in pain over time.

Muscle relaxants are occasionally helpful for individuals in whom spasm plays a major role. However, they frequently cause dizziness, drowsiness, and may inhibit a return to normal activities. Comparison studies have not shown one agent to be superior to another. Patients with radicular low back pain may benefit from antiepileptic drugs such as gabapentin and patients with chronic low back pain may benefit from tricyclic antidepressants. Surgical treatment is indicated for cauda equina syndrome and for patients with intractable pain and worsening of neurologic deficits. For patients with herniated disks not responding after 4 to 6 weeks of conservative therapy, a diskectomy may be considered. For spinal stenosis, surgery may be of benefit to those who do not respond to conservative care and have disabling symptoms.

Patients with persistent or frequent recurrences of back pain merit referral. Physical therapy or epidural steroid injections benefit some patients, although evidence to support the use of spinal injections is limited. If the pain persists for more than 6 months, it is considered chronic and requires a different approach. Consultation with a physiatrist or chronic pain management specialist is often helpful and ensures that no remediable cause of back pain has been overlooked. Individuals who have not returned to work after 6 months due to back pain have only a 50% chance of ever being employed again.

KEY POINTS

- The majority of cases of acute low back pain are due to mechanical factors and resolve within 4 to 8 weeks with conservative treatment.

- SLR is positive if sciatica (not tightened hamstring) is reproduced with elevations of the leg less than 60 degrees.

- Surgical treatments are indicated for cauda equina syndrome and for patients with intractable pain, with worsening of neurologic deficits.

- "Red flags" such as fever, night pain, weight loss, and bone pain suggest something other than mechanical back pain.

10 Chest Pain

The primary concern for patients with chest pain is whether or not the pain is of cardiac origin. In addition to cardiac disease, chest pain may be due to pulmonary, GI, musculoskeletal, or psychological diseases. Emergent causes of chest pain include MI, aortic dissection, pulmonary embolus (PE), and pneumothorax. Patients with these diagnoses usually present to the emergency room but may on occasion present in the outpatient setting. Chest pain in the office setting is most commonly due to musculoskeletal, GI, and cardiac causes. Approximately 15% of patients with chest pain do not fit into any diagnostic category and remain undiagnosed despite evaluation.

PATHOGENESIS

Chest pain may emanate from inflammation or injury to the structures in and around the thoracic cavity. Muscular chest pain is common and may occur when there is inflammation from overuse or injury to the muscles of the chest wall. The costochondral joints may also become inflamed from overuse or injury or in association with viral illnesses. Rib fractures may produce significant pain and are generally due to trauma, but they may also occur as a result of metastatic cancer.

Gastroesophageal reflux disease (GERD) and esophageal motility disorders are common causes of chest pain. The reflux of acidic gastric contents into the lower esophagus may produce esophagitis and chest pain that is indistinguishable from cardiac chest pain. The symptoms of gastritis and peptic ulcer disease may also be perceived by some patients as a substernal pain. Cholelithiasis and cholecystitis, which usually cause right-upper-quadrant pain, may also produce substernal pain.

Cardiac chest pain results from an insufficient oxygen supply to myocardial tissue, usually from coronary artery disease. The initial step in the development of atherosclerotic heart disease is the fatty streak. Over time, the fatty streak can enlarge into a calcified plaque, eventually narrowing the vessel lumen and impairing blood flow. If the plaque ruptures, lipids and tissue factors are released from the plaque, triggering a series of events that ultimately result in intravascular thrombosis and MI. If the plaque does not rupture, a gradual narrowing of the lumen can cause anginal chest pain. This is typically brought on by exertion as the myocardial oxygen demand exceeds the supply.

Since lung tissue does not have pain fibers, inflammation or irritation of the parietal pleura is responsible for the chest pain from pulmonary diseases such as pneumonia or PE.

Other causes of chest pain include psychological and neurologic diseases, such as herpes zoster and cervical or thoracic radiculopathies. Patients with herpes zoster may experience pain before the rash appears. Disk herniation or osteoarthritic narrowing of the cervical or thoracic foramen may result in nerve compression and chest pain following a radicular pattern. Patients with psychological disease, such as anxiety and panic disorder, may present with a variety of chest symptoms—including palpitations, dyspnea, and chest pain—as part of their symptom complex.

CLINICAL MANIFESTATIONS

HISTORY

Patients with chest pain should be asked about its severity, quality, location, and duration; aggravating factors; relieving factors; radiation of pain; and other associated symptoms. Myocardial pain is often described as substernal chest tightness or pressure that radiates to the left arm, shoulders, or jaw. Patients may also complain of diaphoresis, shortness of breath, nausea, and vomiting. Anginal pain is typically brought on by exercise, eating, or emotional excitement. The pain usually lasts from 5 to 15 minutes and disappears with rest or nitroglycerin. Pain that lasts less than 1 minute or longer than 30 minutes should not be considered anginal. Pericardial pain is often persistent, sharp, severe, and relieved by sitting up. Breathing, lying back, or coughing may aggravate the pain. The pain of aortic dissection is anterior and severe; it often has a ripping or tearing quality, with radiation to the back or the abdomen.

Tracheobronchitis may cause a burning pain in the upper sternal area associated with a productive cough. Pain with pneumonia commonly occurs in the overlying chest wall and is aggravated by breathing and coughing. In pneumothorax, the pain is of sudden onset, sharp, unilateral, pleuritic, and associated with shortness of breath. Pleurisy is a sharp pleuritic chest pain, often in association with a preceding viral illness.

GERD causes a burning pain that radiates up the sternum. It is worsened by large meals and lying down. Antacids may relieve the pain. The pain of esophageal spasm, which is usually associated with swallowing, may be indistinguishable from cardiac pain. Since nitroglycerin relaxes smooth muscle, it may relieve the pain.

Musculoskeletal pain from costochondritis can often be reproduced on palpation. Patients are also reluctant to take a deep breath, since this aggravates the pain.

Patients with generalized anxiety will often complain of chest pain. However, this pain is nonspecific. Associated symptoms include overwhelming fear, palpitations, breathlessness, and tachypnea.

PHYSICAL EXAMINATION

Vital signs help to assess the urgency of the patient's complaints. Hypotension can occur with myocardial ischemia, pericardial tamponade, PE, and GI bleeding. Tachycardia may indicate severe illness, and arrhythmias can occur with cardiac or pulmonary causes of chest pain. The presence of fever suggests an infectious cause, such as pneumonia. Inspection and palpation may reveal ecchymosis from an injury, the rash of shingles, crepitus associated with rib fractures, and the sharply localized tenderness of intercostal muscle pain or costochondritis.

A thorough cardiopulmonary examination is warranted for all patients with chest pain. Patients with myocardial ischemia may have an audible S_4 or signs of congestive heart failure, such as an S_3 and pulmonary rales. Pericarditis may cause a friction rub and pulsus paradoxus. Beck's triad—consisting of jugular venous distention, muffled heart sounds, and decreased blood pressure—suggests cardiac tamponade, which may be seen in severe cases of pericarditis. In aortic dissection, patients may have hypotension, absence of peripheral pulses, and a murmur of aortic insufficiency. Patients with pneumonia will have crackles on inspiration, dullness to percussion, and egophony, indicating consolidation. Signs of pneumothorax include hyperresonance to percussion, tracheal deviation, decreased breath sounds, and decreased tactile and vocal fremitus. Patients with pulmonary embolism will likely have normal auscultatory findings but may be tachycardic, tachypneic, and have lower extremity edema.

Patients with acute cholecystitis may have right-upper-quadrant abdominal tenderness. GERD and gastritis will often cause epigastric pain on deep palpation. Esophageal spasm and psychogenic chest pain typically do not produce abnormal physical findings.

DIFFERENTIAL DIAGNOSIS

Common causes of chest pain are presented in Box 10-1. In the outpatient setting, musculoskeletal disease is present in over one-third of patients with chest pain. GI disease occurs in approximately 20% of patients seen in the office with chest pain, followed in frequency by cardiac, psychogenic, and pulmonary causes. Cardiac and pulmonary diseases, although not the most common in the outpatient setting, must be considered in any patient presenting with chest pain because of the potentially life-threatening diseases these represent.

DIAGNOSTIC EVALUATION

The history and physical examination help to classify the chest pain into cardiac, pulmonary, GI, musculoskeletal, or psychogenic causes. An ECG is a critical element for evaluating chest pain.

■ BOX 10-1 Causes of Chest Pain

| Cardiac Chest Pain |
| Myocardial infarction |
| Angina pectoris |
| Pericarditis |
| Aortic dissection |
| Pulmonary Causes of Chest Pain |
| Pulmonary embolus |
| Pneumothorax |
| Pneumonia |
| Tracheobronchitis |
| Musculoskeletal Causes |
| Costochondritis |
| Muscular Strain |
| Gastrointestinal Causes |
| GERD |
| Esophageal spasm |
| Cholelithiasis |
| Psychogenic Causes |
| Somatization disorders |
| Anxiety disorders (including panic disorder) |
| Neurogenic Causes |
| Herpes zoster |
| Cervical or thoracic disease |

Although an ECG can be normal in patients with heart disease, ST-segment elevation or depression is indicative of myocardial ischemia. Diffuse ST-segment elevation is consistent with pericarditis, while Q waves can indicate an old or recent MI. Cardiac markers such as creatine phosphokinase (CPK), troponin, and myoglobin are intracellular macromolecules that diffuse from damaged cardiac myocytes into the circulation. These markers are sensitive tests for determining whether myocardial injury or infarction is present. Troponins are the first enzymes to rise and remain elevated for 5 to 14 days. They are the most sensitive and specific for MI. The MB fraction of CPK-MB serves as another sensitive test; it begins to rise within 4 hours and peaks at 24 hours after an MI. It is important to obtain serial cardiac markers, since the first set of cardiac markers is negative in 25% to 50% of patients with an acute MI. However, by 8 hours after the onset of symptoms, up to 95% of patients will have a positive test for CPK-MB or one of the troponins. A negative troponin between 6 and 72 hours after the onset of chest pain is strong evidence against MI and acute coronary syndrome, particularly if the ECG is normal or near normal.

In stable patients with suspected cardiac disease, outpatient exercise stress testing is indicated. Patients should have a baseline ECG to detect abnormalities such as a conduction defect or strain pattern that make interpreting a stress test difficult. Patients with baseline ECG abnormalities or a positive exercise stress test should undergo radionuclide testing, a stress echocardiogram, and/or coronary angiography. If an individual is unable to exercise, then a chemical stress test using either adenosine or dobutamine to achieve a target heart rate may be necessary.

An echocardiogram can detect wall motion abnormalities in areas damaged by ischemic myocardial disease, pericardial effusions, and valvular heart disease. If the cause of pericarditis is not evident, an antinuclear antibody, blood urea nitrogen, creatinine, thyroid-stimulating hormone (TSH), and tuberculosis skin test are indicated.

A chest x-ray can detect pneumonia, pneumothorax, or other lung pathology. If PE is suspected, a ventilation/perfusion scan or a spiral computed tomography scan (CT scan) is generally indicated. Spiral CT scanning is the preferred test in those with abnormal chest x-ray findings due to underlying diseases such as COPD. Newer algorithms for assessing patients with possible pulmonary embolism utilize testing blood levels of D-dimer. A totally normal D-dimer level in a low-risk patient is strong evidence against a pulmonary embolism. Patients with suspected PE should also have a venous Doppler to rule out DVT.

Patients suspected of having musculoskeletal chest pain might not require any diagnostic testing. Evaluation for GI causes is discussed in Chapter 17.

TREATMENT

Any patient with suspected MI, unstable angina, or PE should be hospitalized for evaluation. Patients who present with MI should be stabilized initially with oxygen, nitroglycerin, and morphine for pain control. Aspirin alone has been shown to reduce the mortality from acute MI by more than 20%, and all patients with suspected MI should receive aspirin as soon as possible. In patients allergic to aspirin, clopidogrel may be used. Other drugs used to treat an acute MI include beta blockers, heparin, nitrates, angiotensin-converting enzyme (ACE) inhibitors, and thrombolytics. Ideally, the systolic blood pressure should be maintained at 100 to 120 mmHg (except in patients with previously severe hypertension) and the heart rate kept at about 60 beats per minute. Thrombolytics should be considered in patients below 75 years of age with ST-segment elevation and a history consistent with an acute MI who present within 6 hours of the onset of chest pain. Recent studies suggest that treatment within 12 hours after the onset of pain may still be beneficial for older patients. Contraindications for thrombolytics include active internal bleeding, history of cerebrovascular disease, recent surgery, intracranial neoplasm, arteriovenous malformation, aneurysm, bleeding diathesis, or severe uncontrolled hypertension. Percutaneous transluminal coronary angioplasty (PTCA) is emerging as an alternative to thrombolytic therapy in institutions that can provide emergent catheterization. Glycoprotein inhibitors are useful when added to heparin in patients with unstable angina and non-Q-wave infarctions.

Patients with stable angina may be treated in the outpatient setting and started on aspirin and sublingual nitroglycerin for anginal episodes. Beta blockers reduce the frequency of symptoms, increase anginal threshold, and reduce the risk of a subsequent MI in patients with a previous MI. Long-acting nitrates reduce anginal pain but do not increase longevity and require a daily nitrate-free period to avoid tolerance. For patients who continue to have angina despite maximal therapy with beta blockers and nitrates, calcium channel blockers may aid in controlling symptoms. Aggressive treatment of risk factors such as hypertension, inactivity, and lipids is also an important component of long-term management. Evidence-based guidelines from the Adult Treatment Panel III (ATP III) of the National Cholesterol Education Program recommend lowering the low-density-lipoprotein cholesterol (LDL-C) to <100 mg/dL in individuals with coronary artery disease. Newer evidence suggests that an LDL-C <75 mg/dL may even be a more appropriate target in patients with coronary artery disease.

Aortic dissection is an emergency and requires hospitalization and surgical consultation. Pericarditis may improve with aspirin or other NSAIDs. Steroids should be considered in severe cases. PE requires anticoagulation. Warfarin is started concomitantly with heparin; once the international normalized ratio (INR) reaches the therapeutic level, heparin may be discontinued. A smaller pneumothorax (<30%) in a stable individual can be managed conservatively; a larger pneumothorax requires chest tube insertion. Treatment for patients with pneumonia or bronchitis is outlined in Chapter 29. Costochondritis is treated with NSAIDs. The management of chest pain due to GERD and GI causes is outlined in Chapter 17. Psychogenic disorders are discussed in Chapter 31.

KEY POINTS

- Chest pain can be due to pulmonary, GI, cardiac, musculoskeletal, or psychological causes.

- The most common emergent causes of chest pain include MI, unstable angina, aortic dissection, PE, and pneumothorax.

- Cardiac chest pain that lasts more than 30 minutes is most probably secondary to infarction.

- Beck's triad—jugular venous distention, muffled heart sounds, and decreased blood pressure—indicates cardiac tamponade.

- Signs of pneumothorax include hyperresonance to percussion, tracheal deviation, decreased breath sounds, and decreased tactile and vocal fremitus.

- A patient who presents with MI should be stabilized initially with oxygen, nitroglycerin, and morphine for pain control.

- Contraindications to thrombolytics include active internal bleeding, history of cerebrovascular disease, recent surgery, intracranial neoplasm, arteriovenous malformation, aneurysm, bleeding diathesis, and severe uncontrolled hypertension.

11 Constipation

Constipation most often occurs in patients at the extreme ages of life. Most individuals eating an average diet will pass at least three stools per week, making it useful to define constipation clinically as the passage of less than three stools per week. Other criteria that can be used to define constipation include lumpy or hard stools, straining, a sensation of incomplete evacuation, and the need to use manual maneuvers such as digital extraction to facilitate defecation.

PATHOGENESIS

The passage of stool depends on stool volume, colonic motility, and patency of the colon's lumen. Defecation requires a complex interaction between the central nervous system and the muscles that increase intra-abdominal pressure, relax the sphincter, and open the canal. Alteration of any one of these components can cause constipation. Anorectal disorders such as anal fissures or thrombosed hemorrhoids that cause pain can also lead to constipation by causing avoidance of defecation. Mechanical obstruction—as seen in cancer, strictures, or external compression—is another cause of constipation.

Patients with diminished fluid and fiber intake have decreased stool volume and can experience constipation. Colonic motility can be inhibited by a variety of medical conditions including hypothyroidism, hypercalcemia, hypokalemia, scleroderma, diabetes, and neurologic disorders such as multiple sclerosis, Parkinson disease, and paraplegia. Medications such as calcium channel blockers (e.g., verapamil), narcotics, and anticholinergics commonly cause a delay in colonic motility. Irritable bowel syndrome (IBS) is characterized by abnormal colonic motility, with delayed colonic transit followed by periods of more frequent and looser stools. A sedentary lifestyle or bed rest (e.g., postoperative patients) results in significant slowing of fecal matter through the colon. Congenital disorders such as Hirschsprung disease may also lead to delayed emptying.

CLINICAL MANIFESTATIONS

HISTORY

Since many patients have misconceptions regarding normal stool patterns, the frequency of bowel movements and consistency of stool must be accurately determined. It is important to inquire about symptoms such as pain with defecation, abdominal distention, gas, nausea, emesis, abdominal discomfort, and the presence of blood in the stool. A dietary history should include questions about the type and quantities of liquid, fruits, vegetables, and fiber as well as any recent change in diet.

Past medical history, previous surgeries, exercise frequency, and family history should be elicited. A review of medications, including over-the-counter medications, may identify the underlying cause. The review of systems should include questions about weight loss, fatigue, depression, and anxiety.

PHYSICAL EXAMINATION

The physical examination begins with a general assessment of nutritional status, weight, and vital signs. The thyroid gland should be examined for abnormalities and the skin assessed for pallor or signs of scleroderma. The abdominal examination should note the frequency and pitch of bowel sounds, the presence of any distention or masses, and focal tenderness. Rectal examination is useful for determining stool consistency, detecting occult blood, and ruling out rectal abnormalities such as fissure, ulcers, masses, or hemorrhoids as well as detecting impaction. A neurologic examination may detect signs of dementia, Parkinson disease, or neuropathy.

DIFFERENTIAL DIAGNOSIS

Box 11-1 lists the differential diagnosis for constipation. Causes can be related to colonic disease, structural abnormalities, anorectal disease, extracolonic disease, medications, diet, and psychological factors. In the outpatient setting, dietary factors (particularly inadequate fiber), medications, IBS, and poor fluid intake are common causes of constipation.

DIAGNOSTIC EVALUATION

The history and physical examination determine the need for further testing. In younger persons with a reasonable explanation for constipation, management can be instituted without further evaluation. Further testing

■ BOX 11-1 Causes of Constipation

| Insufficient dietary fiber |
| Inactivity |
| Medications |
| Opiates |
| Calcium channel blockers |
| Anticholinergics |
| Tricyclic antidepressants |
| Diuretics |
| Antacids |
| Clonidine |
| Levodopa |
| Laxative abuse |
| Metabolic Abnormalities |
| Hypokalemia |
| Hypercalcemia |
| Hypothyroidism |
| Scleroderma |
| Amyloidosis |
| Pregnancy |
| Neurologic Disorders |
| Parkinson disease |
| Paraplegia |
| Prior pelvic surgery |
| Diabetes mellitus |
| Irritable bowel syndrome |
| Colonic mass |
| Hirschsprung disease |
| Perianal Pathology |
| Fissure |
| Hemorrhoids |
| Rectocele |
| Rectal prolapse |
| Diverticular disease |

Abdominal x-rays are of limited value unless obstruction or fecal impaction is suspected. Further evaluation using flexible sigmoidoscopy, coupled with a barium enema or colonoscopy, may be necessary to detect strictures, masses, polyps, or diverticular disease. A full colonoscopy is indicated in patients with anemia, weight loss, heme-positive stools, or other situations in which a malignancy is suspected. During colonoscopy, biopsies of the mucosa can be performed to rule out amyloidosis, Hirschsprung disease, and cancer. The absence of neurons on a rectal biopsy demonstrates the presence of Hirschsprung disease.

TREATMENT

Disorders causing constipation such as hypothyroidism, bowel obstruction, or anal fissure should be treated accordingly. Some patients may only require education and reassurance that their bowel pattern is normal.

Increasing fluid and fiber is the cornerstone for treating cases of functional constipation. Patients should drink at least eight 8-oz glasses of water and consume large amounts of bran, fresh fruit, vegetables, beans, and whole grains. For those with limited fiber intact, dietary fiber should be increased gradually over a 2- to 3-week period in order to minimize adverse effects with a target of consuming 20 to 25 g daily. If possible, medications suspected to be causing or contributing to constipation should be discontinued or changed.

Patients may also benefit from "bowel retraining." Specifically, patients should spend 10 to 15 quiet and unhurried minutes each day on the commode. This should take place at the same time each day and occur after a meal so as to utilize the gastrocolic reflex. Bowel retraining often requires 2 to 3 weeks to become effective and should become a part of the patient's daily routine.

If these modalities fail to alleviate the patient's symptoms and bowel obstruction has been ruled out, medications may be required. Numerous medications are available to treat constipation and some have significant side effects (Table 11-1). However, with adequate knowledge of the mechanism of action and risks, most medications for constipation can be administered safely.

BULK-FORMING AGENTS

Bulk-forming agents are high in fiber and increase stool volume by absorbing water. Examples include psyllium (Metamucil), methylcellulose (Citrucel), and polycarbophil (FiberCon). Common side effects include bloating and flatulence; if these agents are not taken with enough water, they may paradoxically worsen constipation.

OSMOTIC LAXATIVES

Osmotic laxatives are nonabsorbable solutes that draw fluid into the intestinal lumen by creating an osmotic gradient. Examples include lactulose, magnesium salts

is indicated in cases refractory to treatment, in older adults with new-onset constipation, in cases where the etiology is uncertain, or if the clinical evaluation suggests an underlying disorder that merits further evaluation. Laboratory evaluation should include a CBC, serum electrolytes, TSH, and calcium level. Anoscopy is helpful if there is concern about anal pathology such as internal hemorrhoids and fissures.

TABLE 11-1 Medications for Constipation	
Medications	**Side Effects**
Bulk agents	
Psyllium (Metamucil), 1 tablespoon qd–tid	Bloating, impaction above strictures
Methylcellulose (Citrucel), 1–3 tablespoons qd	Fluid overload, impaction with insufficient fluid
Calcium polycarbophil (FiberCon), 1 tablet qd–tid	Fluid overload, impaction
Softeners	
Docusate sodium (Colace), 1–2 capsules qd	Skin rashes, hepatotoxicity
Stimulants	
Bisacodyl (Dulcolax), 1–2 tablets or suppositories qd	Gastric or rectal irritation
Senna (Senokot), 1–3 teaspoons, 2–3 tablets qd	Degeneration of myoneural plexuses
Casanthranol (Peri-Colace), 1–2 tablets qd	Degeneration of myoneural plexuses
Osmotics	
Lactulose (Cephulac), 1–2 tablespoons qd	Bloating
Magnesium (milk of magnesia, magnesium citrate)	Magnesium toxicity (with renal failure)
Sorbitol 70%, 2–4 tablespoons qd	Bloating

qd, every day; qhs, every night; tid, three times daily.

(Milk of Magnesia), and sorbitol. Side effects include bloating, excess gas, and abdominal cramping. Magnesium salts are contraindicated in patients with renal failure.

STIMULANT AGENTS

Stimulants work by altering mucosal permeability and stimulating the activity of intestinal smooth muscle. Examples include phenolphthalein (Ex-Lax) and bisacodyl (Dulcolax). Chronic abuse of these may lead to melanosis coli and constipation secondary to enteric nervous system damage.

STOOL SOFTENERS

Docusate sodium (Colace), a commonly prescribed stool softener, is often used for patients complaining of hard stools that are difficult to pass. It decreases surface tension and allows water and fat to mix in the stool. To work optimally, stool softeners must be taken with plenty of fluid.

ENEMAS AND SUPPOSITORIES

Warm tap-water enemas and suppositories work by distending and stimulating the rectum, which then leads to evacuation. These measures are especially useful in bedridden patients and those with stool impaction. In patients with severe idiopathic constipation, surgeries such as hemicolectomy with ileorectal anastomosis may be a last resort.

KEY POINTS

- Constipation is defined clinically as less than three stools per week.
- Poor fluid intake and a lack of fiber are common causes of constipation in the primary care setting.
- Indications for laboratory testing include refractory constipation, a new onset of constipation in an older individual, heme-positive stools, and situations in which the etiology is unclear or the clinical evaluation suggests underlying pathology.
- The types of laxatives include bulk-forming agents, osmotic laxatives, stimulant laxatives, stool softeners, suppositories, and enemas.

12 Cough

Cough is among the most common complaints in family practice. It is defined as a sudden reflex expulsion of air from the glottis in an attempt to clear the airways of secretions and inhaled particles. This maneuver helps to protect the lungs against aspiration and harmful irritants. Common causes of cough include viral or bacterial infections of the upper respiratory tract, irritant exposure, allergies, COPD, cancer, cardiac diseases, asthma, and psychological factors.

PATHOGENESIS

Ciliated pseudostratified columnar epithelium and mucus-producing goblet cells line the trachea and bronchi. These two types of cells are responsible for filtering particles in inspired air. Certain irritants and viral infections can damage the cilia lining the airways, impairing the filtering process and allowing microscopic particles to reach the lungs. These particles and thermal or chemical stimulants may irritate afferent receptors in the airways and trigger the cough reflex. The cough reflex is a complex interaction mediated peripherally by the vagus, trigeminal, glossopharyngeal, and phrenic nerves. Centrally, the cough center is located in the medulla.

With upper respiratory tract infections (URIs), inflammation and increased mucous secretions stimulate the cough receptors in the upper airway. Common viral causes of infection include influenza, parainfluenza, adenovirus, respiratory syncytial virus, and rhinovirus. Bacterial causes include *Streptococcus pneumoniae*, *Mycoplasma pneumoniae*, and *Haemophilus influenzae*. Cough is also a common presenting complaint in tuberculosis (TB). The most common irritant associated with cough is cigarette smoke. Cancers and foreign bodies elicit the cough reflex by direct stimulation.

CLINICAL MANIFESTATIONS

HISTORY

A complete history of cough should include the timing, quality, associated symptoms, past medical history, smoking history, and medications. Knowing when the cough started is essential, since a chronic cough is defined as lasting more than 8 weeks. Patients who have a seasonal pattern may have a cough secondary to allergic rhinitis. Nocturnal coughing may indicate asthma, GERD, postnasal drip, or CHF. If symptoms occur with meals, aspiration should be considered. Exercise- or cold-induced cough points toward asthma. Cough and dyspnea on exertion suggest a cardiac etiology.

The quality of the cough is also important. A productive cough can be seen in infections such as bronchitis and pneumonia. A dry cough is common in postnasal drip and asthma. Furthermore, patients with postnasal drip feel an itching sensation in the throat and therefore, cough in an attempt to clear the throat. Hemoptysis is often seen in TB and cancer.

Patients should also be asked about other symptoms such as fever, chills, night sweats, weight loss, and hoarseness. Patients with weight loss and a chronic cough should be investigated for cancer.

Patients who present with cough and a past medical history of CHF may have worsening CHF. Weight gain may be an associated symptom. Postnasal drip is a common cause of cough in patients with allergies or a recent URI.

Certain medications, such as an ACE inhibitor, may cause a chronic nonproductive cough. In patients with asthma, beta blockers may exacerbate the asthma and cause a cough. Chronic use of nitrofurantoin can cause a cough secondary to interstitial fibrosis.

PHYSICAL EXAMINATION

The physical examination should focus on the ears, nose, throat, neck, and chest. Ears plugged with cerumen can result in a reflex cough (Arnold reflex). Patients with allergies often have a pale, boggy nasal mucosa with swollen turbinates. A purulent discharge from the nose may indicate sinusitis. In pharyngitis, the tonsils appear swollen and hyperemic. The posterior pharynx should be checked for increased secretions, which are often seen in patients with postnasal drip. Palpable lymph nodes in the neck support the diagnosis of an infectious cause. During the chest examination, close attention should be paid to the lung and heart sounds. Murmurs and gallops suggest a possible cardiac cause. Crackles may indicate an inflammatory process or worsening CHF. Diminished or bronchial breath sounds can occur with pneumonia. Wheezing may be heard with foreign body aspiration, COPD, or asthma.

DIFFERENTIAL DIAGNOSIS

The common causes of cough include URIs, irritants, allergies, asthma, COPD, cancer, and GERD. Viral infections, the most common cause of acute cough, are more frequent in the winter months. Following a viral infection of the respiratory tract, a cough may persist for up to 8 weeks. Bacterial infections of the respiratory tract are also common causes of acute cough; they include sinusitis, pharyngitis, bronchitis, and pneumonia. Cigarette smokers often have a chronic cough due to chronic irritant exposure. Allergies may present with a chronic cough, usually due to a postnasal drip. A child who presents with a chronic cough lasting more than 8 weeks should be suspected of having asthma and/or allergies. Typically, the cough seen in asthma is dry and may worsen at night or after exercise. Cold air may also exacerbate a cough due to asthma. Patients with COPD or bronchiectasis may present with a chronic cough.

In those individuals presenting with weight loss, night sweats, hemoptysis, and chronic cough, lung cancer and TB should be considered. GERD can cause a cough that is worsened by lying down; this may be associated with substernal burning or a sour taste in the mouth. Patients who cough when eating should be evaluated for aspiration. Individuals with an acute cough, dyspnea, and a swollen leg should be evaluated for possible PE. Certain medications such as ACE inhibitors, amiodarone, and nitrofurantoin can cause a dry cough. Finally, psychogenic cough may be a possibility. However, all the organic causes should be ruled out before this disorder is diagnosed.

DIAGNOSTIC EVALUATION

The diagnostic approach to cough begins with a good history and physical examination. When viral infections of the respiratory tract are suspected, no further workup is necessary as long as the cough resolves over a period of 6 to 8 weeks. If sinusitis is suspected, a patient may be started on antibiotics and monitored for resolution of the symptoms. If a cough is due to the use of an ACE inhibitor, discontinuing it should result in improvement within 4 weeks.

A chest x-ray is necessary in most patients without an upper airway abnormality who have a new cough, persistent cough, or hemoptysis. The chest x-ray can detect pulmonary infections, masses, pleural effusion, CHF, interstitial lung disease, bronchiectasis, and hilar lymphadenopathy. It may show changes consistent with COPD. The chest x-ray may be normal in some patients with neoplasm, pulmonary embolus, and sinus disease. If these diseases are suspected, further testing with CT scanning, bronchoscopy, a ventilation/perfusion (V/Q) scan, or an echocardiogram is indicated.

In immunocompetent patients with a persistent cough and a normal chest x-ray, occult bronchospasm, allergies, GERD, or a combination of these are the most likely diagnoses. Spirometry or an empiric trial of bronchodilator therapy may be helpful. Rarely, patients may require a methacholine challenge or postexercise spirometry to confirm the diagnosis. In patients with symptoms of reflux or for those who fail therapy for bronchospasm, empiric treatment for GERD or an upper-GI series may be helpful. Chronic cough that remains undiagnosed and persists despite therapy merits consultation.

TREATMENT

Cough is a symptom; therefore, treatment should focus on the underlying disease process as outlined in the respective chapters of this book. For example, treatment of GERD, elimination of an irritant such as smoking, or discontinuation of an ACE inhibitor would be appropriate. However, if the cough is significant enough that the patient seeks medical attention, symptomatic treatment with an antitussive may be warranted. For example, the postinfectious cough from a viral illness may last up to 8 weeks, and cough suppression may provide some symptom relief. Antitussive medications may be classified as either centrally or peripherally acting medications. Centrally acting drugs include codeine and dextromethorphan. Codeine is a narcotic that binds to the opiate receptors and suppresses the medullary cough center. Sedation is a common side effect. Dextromethorphan, a nonnarcotic centrally acting agent, is available in many over-the-counter (OTC) preparations. While both codeine and dextromethorphan are commonly used, studies examining their effectiveness are often of poor quality and demonstrate conflicting results. In children younger than 2 years of age, treatment trials have not established their benefit and serious side effects may occur. In 2008, the U.S. Food and Drug Authority (FDA) recommended against the use of OTC preparations in children younger than 2 years and advised caution in prescribing to older children. For an acute cough due to a common cold, a first-generation antihistamine plus a decongestant offers some modest decrease in the severity of cough. Another limited trial showed that the anti-inflammatory drug naproxen may also favorably affect cough.

Peripherally acting drugs such as benzonatate anesthetize the respiratory passages and the pleural stretch receptors but are of questionable value. Mucolytic agents (guaifenesin) increase the volume and decrease the viscosity of secretions, which may help to clear secretions from the respiratory tract more easily.

KEY POINTS

- In immunocompetent patients with a persistent cough and a normal chest x-ray, occult bronchospasm, allergies, GERD, or a combination of these are the most likely diagnoses.

- Postnasal drip is a common cause of cough in patients with allergies or a recent viral infection of the upper respiratory tract.

- Centrally acting antitussive medications include codeine and dextromethorphan.

13 Diarrhea

Diarrhea is defined as an increase in stool weight to more than 200 g/day. Clinically, diarrhea is defined as the passage of more than three abnormally loose stools per 24 hours. Acute diarrhea lasts less than 3 weeks, while chronic diarrhea is a persistent or recurring condition that lasts more than 3 weeks.

PATHOGENESIS

Fluid balance in the GI system represents a dynamic flux between absorption and secretion. Conditions that either increase fluid secretion or decrease absorption lead to diarrhea. Inflammation, hormones, or enterotoxins may trigger increased fluid secretion. A functional or anatomic decrease in the absorptive capacity of the bowel may cause diarrhea. Osmotically active solutes that retain fluid in the intestinal lumen may also increase stool volume. Altered bowel motility can impair absorption, either by decreasing the contact time of intestinal contents with the bowel mucosa or preventing the effective mixing of intestinal contents. Although the basic mechanisms of diarrhea are straightforward, more than one mechanism may contribute to diarrhea in an individual patient. For example, in a patient with Crohn disease, an abnormal ileum may cause decreased fluid absorption and increased secretion due to diffuse inflammation.

CLINICAL MANIFESTATIONS

HISTORY

Acute diarrhea has two common clinical presentations: either a watery, noninflammatory diarrhea or an inflammatory diarrhea with the presence of either blood or white blood cells (WBCs) in the stool. Symptoms may be mild, with no change in activity; moderate, with some limitation in activity; or severe, where patients are confined to bed.

It is important to ask patients with acute diarrhea about exposure to others with similar symptoms, recent travel, and whether they are taking antibiotics or other medications. A diet history is important, since excessive caffeine or alcohol intake and sorbitol-containing foods can all cause transient diarrhea. Overindulgence in milk or milk products in a lactose-intolerant individual can cause bloating, cramps, and diarrhea. Antibiotic use within 2 weeks suggests that diarrhea may be caused by either an alteration in bowel flora or a *Clostridium difficile* infection. Severe abdominal pain in an elderly individual accompanied by acute diarrhea suggests the possibility of ischemic colitis.

Watery stools accompanied by a low-grade fever, headache, nausea or vomiting, and achiness is consistent with a viral gastroenteritis. Traveler's diarrhea, due to toxigenic *Escherichia coli*, presents similarly to viral gastroenteritis. Bacterial infections—such as those due to *Shigella*, *Salmonella*, and *Campylobacter*—present with a prodrome of fever, headache, anorexia, fatigue, and stools that may initially be watery before becoming bloody. Salmonellosis is usually a self-limited infection acquired by ingesting contaminated poultry or eggs. *Campylobacter* infection is more common than either shigellosis or salmonellosis and is usually acquired from ingesting contaminated poultry. *E. coli* O157:H7 accounts for up to one-third of cases of bloody diarrhea. Its presentation ranges from mild, crampy, nonbloody diarrhea to life-threatening hemorrhagic colitis complicated by hemolytic uremic syndrome or thrombocytopenic purpura.

Diarrhea from food poisoning usually occurs several hours after eating contaminated food. Illness in several individuals exposed to a common food source and an absence of other associated symptoms are characteristic findings. *Staphylococcus aureus* commonly contaminates custard-filled pastries, while *Clostridium perfringens* is especially common in foods warmed on a steam table.

Chronic diarrhea can be either persistent or recurrent. IBS typically affects young or middle-aged adults, with a 2:1 female-to-male predominance. It can present as diarrhea alternating with constipation or chronic recurring diarrhea. Other symptoms include abdominal pain relieved by defecation, fecal urgency, bloating, the need to strain to pass stool, and occasionally having a small amount of mucus in the stool. This condition may wax or wane over the years. Any rectal bleeding that occurs in patients with IBS is usually due to anal trauma from passing a hard stool. In the active phase, inflammatory bowel disease

(IBD), a collective term for ulcerative colitis and Crohn disease, is associated with abdominal pain, bloody stools, and fever. Extraintestinal manifestations include arthritis, liver disease, uveitis, and skin lesions. Flushing and wheezing suggest carcinoid syndrome.

Giardiasis, amoebiasis, and C. *difficile* can present with acute, intermittent, or chronic symptoms. *Giardia* is the leading cause of parasitic diarrhea. The organism is endemic to areas such as the Rocky Mountains and Russia. It is also common in areas such as third-world countries where the water supply may be contaminated. Foul, greasy, bulky stools characterize malabsorption syndromes causing diarrhea. Associated symptoms such as weight loss or neuropathy may be a function of malabsorption.

PHYSICAL EXAMINATION

Generally, the physical examination is more helpful for assessing the severity of the disease than determining a specific cause. Vital signs should be checked and the patient assessed for indications of significant dehydration. The abdomen should be carefully examined and a rectal examination performed, checking for occult blood.

DIFFERENTIAL DIAGNOSIS

Box 13-1 lists the causes of diarrhea. Viral gastroenteritis is the most common cause of acute diarrhea. Rotavirus is the most common virus in children, while the Norwalk virus is most common in adults. Food poisoning from staphylococcal toxins, clostridial toxins, and the ingestion of *Campylobacter, Salmonella, Shigella*, and enteropathogenic *E. coli* is common. *Giardia* and amoebiasis are less frequent causes of diarrhea in the United States. Traveler's diarrhea is usually due to *E. coli* but can be caused by other bacterial diseases. Dietary indiscretion, alcohol, caffeine, and drug side effects are common noninfectious causes (Box 13-2). In the outpatient setting, the most common causes for persistent diarrhea are IBS, IBD, lactose intolerance, and chronic or relapsing GI infections, such as giardiasis, amebiasis, and C. *difficile*.

Microscopic colitis is increasingly becoming recognized as a relatively common and important cause of chronic intermittent watery diarrhea in middle-aged and elderly adults. It consists of two separate but related diseases, collagenous colitis and lymphocytic colitis, which are similar clinically but differ in histologic appearance.

Celiac disease or gluten-sensitive enteropathy is another relatively common disorder, affecting about 0.5% to 1% of the population. It is a chronic disorder in which ingesting gluten damages the small intestinal mucosa in genetically susceptible individuals. Although increasing awareness of the disease and

BOX 13-1 Causes of Chronic Diarrhea

Increased Secretion
Clostridium toxin
Cholera toxin
Noninvasive microbial gastroenteritis (e.g., viral gastroenteritis, *Campylobacter*)
Carcinoid syndrome
Vasoactive intestinal peptide secreting tumors
Villous adenoma

Increased Osmotic Load
Sorbitol ingestion (dietetic candy)
Bile salt malabsorption
Pancreatic insufficiency
Lactose intolerance
Malabsorption
Postgastrectomy syndrome
Magnesium containing laxatives

Inflammation
Ulcerative colitis
Crohn disease
Radiation-induced colitis
Invasive microbial gastroenteritis (e.g., *Shigella*)

Altered Motility
Thyrotoxicosis
Irritable bowel syndrome
Autonomic neuropathy (e.g., diabetic associated enteropathy)

BOX 13-2 Common Medications Associated with Diarrhea

Alpha-glycoside inhibitors (e.g., acarbose)
Antacids
Antidepressants (SSRIs)
Antibiotics
Colchicine
Lactulose
Laxatives
Loop diuretics
Protein pump inhibitors
Quinidine
Theophylline
Thyroxine

better screening test have led to more individuals being diagnosed, it is still under-recognized. Classically, patients experience diarrhea, malabsorption, and weight loss. The diagnosis is confirmed by observing typical mucosal changes on biopsy which then improve following gluten restriction.

DIAGNOSTIC EVALUATION

Most cases of acute diarrhea are self-limited and diagnostic tests are usually not indicated. Signs of more severe disease—such as significant dehydration, more than six stools per 24 hours, bloody stools, high temperatures, severe abdominal pain, and failure to improve after 48 to 72 hours—suggest a need for a more detailed evaluation. The threshold for evaluating immunocompromised or elderly individuals should be lower.

Examination of a stool specimen for leukocytes and occult blood is a useful first test in patients with acute diarrhea. A stool specimen with less than three to four WBCs per high-power field (HPF) usually indicates a noninflammatory, self-limited process. If there is blood in the stool or an inflammatory process is suspected, a stool culture should be sent and an assay for C. *difficile* toxin ordered for those patients with recent antibiotic exposure. The acute onset of bloody stools merits testing for Shiga toxin, along with cultures specifically for *E. coli* O157:H7. Patients at risk for *Giardia* or other parasitic infections—such as those who have traveled to a high-risk area (e.g., tropical Africa, Asia, or Latin America), attend day care, are HIV-positive, or have had possible exposure to contaminated water—should have their stools evaluated for ova and parasites.

The diagnostic evaluation for chronic diarrhea should be individualized. The history should help focus the approach. Box 13-3 lists signs suggestive of a serious underlying disorder. For patients whose history and physical examination suggest a benign illness, only a limited evaluation is needed. For example, a patient with suspected lactose intolerance who responds to a lactose-free diet needs no further testing. About 5% of cases of chronic diarrhea are due to medications, and no further evaluation is needed in

individuals who respond to either stopping or decreasing a medication known to cause diarrhea. For patients with chronic diarrhea whose cause is not readily apparent, an initial evaluation may consist of a CBC, ESR, and checking stools for occult blood, leukocytes, and ova and parasites as well as an assay for C. *difficile* toxin for patients with recent antibiotic exposure. Tissue transglutimase (tTG) antibody and endymysial antibody (EMA) are blood tests that screen for celiac disease. The antigliaden antibody test is no longer recommended for screening because of its poor sensitivity and specificity. For patients with associated left-lower-quadrant pain or bloody diarrhea, a sigmoidoscopy is indicated; this can detect mucosal ulcerations, friability, and masses. A Sudan stain can detect the presence of excess stool fat in patients with suspected malabsorption.

Suspected IBD may be confirmed by biopsy. A biopsy can also detect less common diseases, such as amyloidosis and microscopic colitis, where the colon can appear normal both visually and radiographically. In individuals with suspected IBS, a limited evaluation, including sigmoidoscopy, may be sufficient to exclude more serious disorders. Often patients with chronic diarrhea of unclear etiology or suspected IBD may need referral to a gastroenterologist for evaluation.

TREATMENT

Most patients with acute diarrhea can be managed with an alteration in diet and fluid therapy. Oral rehydration is sufficient unless the patient is severely dehydrated. Commercial rehydration solutions, such as Pedialyte or Rice-Lyte, designed to replace fluids and electrolytes, are most commonly used for infants and children. Sports drinks, fruit drinks, and flat soft drinks supplemented with crackers, soup, or bland foods are usually adequate for treating older children and adults.

Boiled starches such as rice, noodles, or potatoes and avoiding milk products or caffeine-containing foods are usually recommended for patients with acute diarrhea. For children, a BRAT diet (*b*ananas, *r*ice, *a*pplesauce, and *t*oast) is traditionally used despite limited evidence demonstrating its efficacy. Preparations containing kaolin and pectate are available OTC but are of uncertain value. Bismuth subsalicylate (Pepto-Bismol) is also used for diarrhea and may have an antisecretory effect. The antimotility drugs such as loperamide are considered the drugs of choice for nonspecific treatment. They should not be used in febrile patients with inflammatory or infectious diarrhea.

Specific management depends on the cause of the diarrhea. The decision to use antibiotics in patients with bacterial diarrhea depends on the organism, health of the individual, and systemic symptoms. All cases of shigella should be treated with a fluoroquinolone or, if the organism is sensitive, with trimethoprim/

■ **BOX 13-3** Symptoms Suggestive of a Serious Underlying Etiology for Diarrhea
New onset in patients greater than age 40
Nocturnal symptoms
Aggressive course
Weight loss
Rectal fissures
Anemia
Elevated erythrocyte sedimentation rate

sulfamethoxazole (TMP/SMX). *Salmonella* infections causing mild to moderate symptoms should generally not be treated, since antibiotics may prolong the carrier state. Patients with salmonellosis who have severe symptoms or those at risk for bacteremia (easily infected individuals or elderly patients) should be treated with a fluoroquinolone.

If symptoms are still present when the culture results become available, erythromycin or a fluoroquinolone will shorten the duration of a *Campylobacter* infection. Invasive *E. coli* with bloody diarrhea should be treated with a fluoroquinolone or TMP/SMX. Traveler's diarrhea due to toxigenic *E. coli* responds to a short course of a fluoroquinolone or TMP/SMX. Azithromycin is the antibiotic of choice for traveler's diarrhea in children and pregnant women and for areas in which quinolone-resistant campylobacter is endemic.

C. difficile infections should be treated with metronidazole (an alternative is oral vancomycin). *Giardia* is treated with metronidazole.

For lactose-intolerant patients, a 1- to 2-week trial of a lactose-free diet is usually sufficient to decrease symptoms. Lactase-containing capsules taken orally before consuming dairy products are also effective. Antimotility agents such as loperamide may provide relief for IBS patients with significant diarrhea. Antispasmodics, such as dicyclomine, can benefit patients with crampy abdominal pain and antidepressants have been shown to relieve pain and may be effective in low doses. Alosetron appears to be modestly effective but is indicated only for women with severe diarrhea or resistant disease because of its risk for severe and life-threatening GI side effects.

A high-fiber diet may be helpful for IBS patients with alternating diarrhea and constipation.

Management goals for IBD are to control active disease, monitor stool frequency and amount, detect complications, and refer for surgery when appropriate. Commonly used medications are sulfasalazine and corticosteroids. Patients are generally managed conjointly with a gastroenterologist.

Microscopic colitis is usually treated stepwise, first with nonspecific therapy followed by bismuth or budesonide and either cholestyramine or 5-aminosalicylic acid. Resistant cases may require oral corticosteroids or immune modifiers. Similar to IBD, patients are generally managed conjointly with a gastroenterologist.

Celiac disease responds to diet and patients should be referred to a dietician knowledgeable about gluten-free diets.

KEY POINTS

- Most cases of diarrhea are due to infectious agents, particularly viruses.
- A bacterial infection, IBD, ischemic colitis, or malignancy can all cause bloody diarrhea.
- The most common viral pathogens causing diarrhea are the Norwalk virus, rotavirus, and enterovirus.
- Fluoroquinolones are active against *Salmonella*, *Shigella*, and *E. coli*.

14 Dizziness/Vertigo

Dizziness, or vertigo, is a sensation of movement due to disease in the central or peripheral vestibular system.

PATHOGENESIS

Patients who experience true vertigo have a problem affecting either the peripheral or the central vestibular systems. The peripheral vestibular apparatus is located bilaterally in the semicircular canals. Peripherally, inflammation, stimulation, or destruction of the hair cells of the eighth cranial nerve may cause vertigo. For example, in benign positional vertigo (BPV), particulate matter or otoliths may form in the semicircular canal (analogous to renal stone formation). When these otoliths become dislodged and stimulate the sensory hair cells in the semicircular canals, vertigo results. In acute labyrinthitis or vestibular neuronitis, viral infection of the semicircular apparatus causes vestibular dysfunction and vertigo. Ménière disease, a condition of undetermined etiology, occurs when endolymphatic hydrops results in increased pressure within the semicircular canals and damage to the sensory hair cells. Finally, direct damage to the eighth cranial nerve may result from ototoxic medications or from an acoustic neuroma. An acoustic neuroma is a tumor (schwannoma) of the eighth cranial nerve that will gradually grow and compress the eighth cranial nerve and eventually the brainstem.

Vascular insufficiency or hemorrhage, demyelination, brain tumors, or medications may affect the brainstem's vestibular pathways. Centrally, the vestibular pathways are located in the brainstem and communicate and allow coordination of position with the cerebellum and cerebral cortex. Typically, patients with central vertigo will have other brainstem or cranial nerve findings in association with the vertigo. Vertigo may rarely occur in association with migraine as a result of vascular spasm in the vertebrobasilar artery system. Multiple sclerosis (MS) is a demyelinating disease that may affect the brainstem and disrupt the vestibular pathways. Finally, medications such as phenytoin may affect the brainstem nuclei and cause vertigo.

CLINICAL MANIFESTATIONS

HISTORY

The patient's description of the symptoms helps distinguish vertigo from dizziness. True vertigo is suggested when the patient uses terms such as "spinning," "weaving," or "rocking" to describe the sensation. Vertigo is commonly associated with head movements, can occur in the supine or upright position, and is often accompanied by nausea and vomiting. Symptoms that occur only in association with change in position from the supine to upright positions suggest another etiology, such as dehydration or anemia.

BPV generally occurs as an isolated symptom and is short-lived, recurrent, and associated with particular head movements. Vertigo, tinnitus, and hearing loss are the cardinal features of Ménière disease. The vertigo and hearing loss are initially fluctuating. The vertigo may last from 30 minutes to 12 hours. If untreated, the hearing loss may become permanent.

The presence of other cranial nerve symptoms, cerebral, or cerebellar neurologic symptoms suggests vertebrobasilar insufficiency, neoplasm, stroke, MS, or acoustic neuroma as a cause. Vertebrobasilar insufficiency may present acutely as a transient ischemic attack or stroke. Vertigo from MS may present as a flare of the underlying disease. Acoustic neuromas generally have an insidious onset. Vertigo in association with a viral illness is termed vestibular neuritis and, when accompanied by hearing loss, is called labyrinthitis. However, the nomenclature for vestibular disease is ill defined and terms such as "vestibular neuronitis," "neurolabyrinthitis," and "unilateral vestibulopathy" are often used interchangeably. Vertigo in association with a viral illness generally resolves in 2 to 10 days.

Past medical history should note prior occurrence of similar symptoms, the presence of other medical diseases, and medication use. BPV recurs in up to 30% of patients in 2 to 3 years following an episode. MS patients may have symptoms that wax and wane with disease activity but typically have other symptoms in association with vertigo. Hypertensive patients and those who smoke are at risk for atherosclerotic disease, which may suggest vertebrobasilar insufficiency as a cause. Medication use may reveal a cause of vertigo. Loop diuretics and aminoglycoside antibiotics are drugs associated with vertigo from damage to the eighth cranial nerve. Diuretics and antihypertensive medications may lead to orthostatic symptoms through volume depletion or blood pressure–lowering effects. High-dose salicylates may also cause vertigo.

PHYSICAL EXAMINATION

The physical examination should include assessment of orthostatic blood pressure and pulse as well as cardiovascular, ear, and neurologic examinations. Carotid bruits should be noted. The neurologic examination should include a hearing assessment and examination of the cranial nerves. The presence and direction of nystagmus should be noted. Bidirectional or vertical nystagmus suggests a brainstem origin for the vertigo. Provocative maneuvers for the symptoms should be included in the examination. For example, true vertigo will be brought on by head movement and by the Barany maneuver. During the Barany maneuver, the patient is seated with the head turned to the right and is quickly lowered to the supine position with the head over the edge of the examination table 30 degrees below horizontal. The test is then repeated with the head turned to the left. The test is positive if symptoms are reproduced. Nystagmus is also typically seen during this maneuver. Orthostatic positional changes that bring on symptoms suggest dehydration, anemia, or cardiac causes. Symptoms brought on by hyperventilation suggest anxiety or other psychogenic causes.

DIFFERENTIAL DIAGNOSIS

The differential diagnosis of vertigo includes the many different diseases that cause dizziness. True vertigo is due to either central or peripheral vestibular disease and has a narrower differential diagnosis. In assessing for central versus peripheral causes of vertigo, important distinguishing features are the presence of isolated vertigo with or without hearing loss, which suggests peripheral disease, and associated brainstem or other neurologic symptoms, which suggest a central disease (Box 14-1).

DIAGNOSTIC EVALUATION

The history and physical examination direct any further evaluation and the treatment approach. For those patients in whom the diagnosis is unclear or if it is uncertain whether the vertigo is central or peripheral, further testing with electronystagmography and audiometry may be helpful. Audiometry is useful for diagnosing Ménière disease (low-frequency hearing loss) and may suggest the need for further evaluation for acoustic neuroma (asymmetric hearing loss).

Additional testing that may be helpful in identifying central causes of vertigo and to identify acoustic

■ **BOX 14-1** Differential Diagnosis for Vertigo
Peripheral Vestibular Disease
Benign positional vertigo (BPV)
Acute labyrinthitis
Vestibular neuronitis
Ménière disease
Acoustic neuroma
Central Vestibular Disease
Vertebrobasilar insufficiency or hemorrhage
Multiple sclerosis
Brain tumor (e.g., glioblastoma or metastatic disease)
Other Medical Diseases
Cerebellar disease (e.g., degeneration, infarcts)
Peripheral neuropathy (e.g., diabetic)
Ophthalmologic disease (e.g., cataracts, macular degeneration)
Hypoglycemia
Psychiatric disease (e.g., panic disorder, anxiety)

neuromas include MRI and brainstem auditory evoked response (BAER) testing. MRI may reveal scattered areas of demyelination, suggesting MS, or may show evidence of prior stroke or masses, suggesting vertebrobasilar insufficiency or brain tumors as causes. BAER testing can distinguish cochlear from retrocochlear hearing loss, thus helping to distinguish peripheral disease from more central disease. To identify posterior circulation atherosclerotic disease, magnetic resonance angiography (MRA) can be performed.

TREATMENT

Central causes for vertigo are generally associated with more serious underlying diseases. When a central cause is suspected, aggressive evaluation and therapy directed at the underlying disease are warranted. Peripheral causes of vertigo are usually acute and self-limited, although empiric therapy often helps control symptoms. Follow-up to assure resolution of symptoms and assess the need for further workup should be part of the care provided.

The Epley maneuver for BPV is performed by rotating the patients through a series of positions in an attempt to relocate the debris in the semicircular canal into the vestibule of the labyrinth. It is reported to have a success rate approaching 80%. Vestibular exercises where a patient performs a Barany maneuver to reproduce his or her symptoms and holds the position until the symptoms are extinguished are also useful. This exercise is repeated several times daily and the time to extinction of symptoms should progressively grow shorter the more the exercise is performed. Medications used to treat labyrinthitis, vestibular neuronitis, and BPV include meclizine, dimenhydrinate, antiemetics, and benzodiazepines. These medications do not treat the underlying cause but may help to alleviate symptoms. Drowsiness is their primary side effect. Acoustic neuroma is managed surgically and requires referral to an otolaryngologist.

Ménière disease is a chronic condition that can lead to permanent hearing loss. These patients require chronic therapy directed at the underlying disease, not just symptomatic therapy. Diuretics, in particular acetazolamide or hydrochlorothiazide, have been found to be helpful in managing Ménière disease. Salt restriction is also considered an important adjunct to the use of diuretics. Vertigo associated with central vestibular disease is also often chronic. Vestibular exercises and gait training may be beneficial to these patients, along with therapy directed at the underlying disease. For example, in patients with vertebrobasilar vascular disease, blood pressure should be controlled, lipid levels lowered, and aspirin or warfarin prescribed to help prevent additional events.

KEY POINTS

- True vertigo occurs due to disease in the central or peripheral vestibular system.

- BPV generally occurs as an isolated symptom; the vertigo is short-lived, recurrent, and associated with particular head movements.

- Vertigo, tinnitus, and hearing loss are the cardinal features of Ménière disease. The vertigo and hearing loss are initially fluctuating.

- In assessing for central versus peripheral causes for vertigo, important distinguishing features are the presence of isolated vertigo with or without hearing loss, which suggests peripheral disease, and associated brainstem or other neurologic symptoms, which suggest a central disease.

- Peripheral causes of vertigo are usually acute and self-limited.

- Medications used to treat labyrinthitis, vestibular neuronitis, and BPV include meclizine, dimenhydrinate, antiemetics, and benzodiazepines.

15 Fatigue

Fatigue is defined as the subjective complaint of tiredness or diminished energy level to the point of interfering with normal or usual activities. It is one of the top 10 chief complaints leading to family practice office visits; surveys report that between 5% and 20% of the general population suffer from persistent and troublesome fatigue. It is a constitutional symptom with many etiologies that can lead to multiple diagnoses, extensive lab testing, and repeat office visits. Thus, it is important to narrow down the vast differential diagnosis, in which organic causes comprise the minority of cases.

PATHOGENESIS

The exact pathogenesis of fatigue is ill defined and will vary depending on the underlying cause. For example, fatigue associated with psychiatric conditions is part of the symptom complex of many of these diseases and is likely psychogenic in origin. Fatigue associated with conditions such as CHF, COPD, and metabolic abnormalities may be due to altered oxygen and nutrient delivery peripherally. Fatigue associated with inflammatory conditions, such as connective tissue diseases and infectious diseases, may be due to factors released as part of the inflammatory response.

CLINICAL MANIFESTATIONS

The history is crucial in differentiating a patient's source of fatigue. Characterizing the patient's complaint in terms of time course, exacerbating and alleviating factors, stressors, variability in symptoms, and associated symptoms can help to narrow the potential causes for the fatigue and direct the initial workup. Preexisting medical conditions and medication use should be noted. Characteristic features of both psychogenic and organic disease are discussed below.

HISTORY

Psychogenic

Fatigue that has been present for more than 6 months and that fluctuates in its severity is more likely to be functional. The patient may have identifiable stressors, a stressful and nonsupportive family structure, or a primary mood disturbance that points toward psychogenic

fatigue. Frequently, patients with psychological disease have a sleep disturbance with either insomnia or early morning awakening. The fatigue associated with psychiatric causes is frequently worse in the morning and may be alleviated by activity. The patient may have multiple and nonspecific complaints along with a normal physical examination. As fatigue is strongly associated with psychiatric disorders, behavioral etiologies should be screened for accordingly.

Physiologic

Physiologic fatigue results from situations that would cause most people to be fatigued, such as not getting enough sleep. Physiologic fatigue is common in mothers of newborns, individuals who do shift work, athletes who overtrain, and in third-year medical students.

Organic Disease

In contrast to psychogenic fatigue, fatigue from organic causes will often present more abruptly and show a progressive course. Identifiable stressors are often absent and the family structure may be supportive. Sleep disturbance may be present but is often related to the underlying disease process. A reactive or secondary depression may result when the patient recognizes that something is wrong. The fatigue will be noted to be less in the morning and worsened with activity. The patient may have fewer and more specific associated symptoms and the physical examination may suggest potential underlying causes.

PHYSICAL EXAMINATION

In patients presenting with a complaint of fatigue, a complete physical examination should be performed in an attempt to determine the etiology. The patient's general appearance and vital signs should be noted. A patient with fatigue from physical illness may look pale and sickly, with slumping posture and a sagging face. Pallor suggests anemia, whereas darkening of the skin may point toward Addison disease as a potential cause. The thyroid gland should be palpated and signs of hyper- and hypothyroidism noted. Careful examination of all lymph nodes is essential, along with checking the individual's joints for signs of inflammation. Heart and lung examination may reveal the presence of murmurs, gallops, wheezing, or rales, suggesting a cardiopulmonary etiology. Stigmata of alcohol or drug abuse should be sought. A thorough neurologic exam may identify neuromuscular disease as the cause.

DIFFERENTIAL DIAGNOSIS

The differential diagnosis for fatigue is extensive and includes psychiatric, infectious, connective tissue, endocrine, neurologic, oncologic, and cardiopulmonary causes (Box 15-1). By far the most common category of diagnosis in fatigued patients is psychiatric disease, which occurs in 60% to 80% of patients with chronic fatigue. Depression accounts for the majority of cases with a psychiatric cause. Medical causes account for up to 8% of cases. The leading physical causes of fatigue are infections, metabolic disorders, and medications. Of the remainder, 4% meet criteria for chronic fatigue syndrome (CFS), a disease of unknown etiology often attributed to a persistent mononucleosis infection from the Epstein–Barr virus (EBV) (Box 15-2). Despite exhaustive workup, many patients with fatigue remain undiagnosed.

■ BOX 15-1 Common Conditions Leading to Fatigue, by System and Process

Psychogenic: depression, anxiety, adjustment reactions, situational life stress, sexual dysfunction, physical/sexual abuse, occupational stress, and professional burnout

Endocrine: DM, hypothyroidism, hyperparathyroidism, hypopituitarism, Addison disease, electrolyte disorders, malnutrition

Hematologic: anemia, lymphoma, and leukemia

Renal: acute renal failure (ARF), chronic renal failure (CRF)

Liver: hepatitis, cirrhosis

Immunologic/connective tissue: AIDS or AIDS-related complex, sarcoid, mixed connective tissue disease (MCTD), polymyalgia rheumatica

Neuromuscular: upper/lower motor neuron disease from stroke, neoplasm, demyelination, amyotrophic lateral sclerosis (ALS), poliomyelitis, disk herniation, myasthenia gravis, muscular dystrophies

Pulmonary: infectious states (TB, pneumonia), COPD, sleep apnea

Cardiovascular: CHF, cardiomyopathy, valvular heart disease

Reproductive: pregnancy

Iatrogenic: medications, alcoholism, drug abuse

■ BOX 15-2 Diagnostic Criteria for Chronic Fatigue Syndrome

The diagnosis is established by fulfilling both major criteria plus 6 or more of the minor criteria plus 2 or more of the physical criteria, or 8 or more of the 11 minor symptom criteria.

Major Criteria

1. New onset of persistent or relapsing fatigue not previously present, sufficient to reduce daily activity by 50% or more, lasting at least 6 weeks.

2. Exclusion of other conditions which may produce similar symptoms (see Box 15-1).

Minor Criteria

1. Mild fever (37.5–38.6°C) or chills

2. Sore throat

3. Painful cervical or axillary lymph nodes

4. Unexplained generalized muscle weakness

5. Muscle discomfort or myalgias

6. Prolonged (>24 hours) generalized fatigue after previously tolerated exercise

7. Generalized headaches unlike previous cephalalgia

8. Migratory arthralgias without joint swelling or redness

9. Neuropsychiatric complaints, that is, photophobia, scotomata, forgetfulness, irritability, confusion, inability to concentrate, difficulty in thinking, depression

10. Sleep disturbances

11. Onset of main symptom complex in hours or a few days

Physical Criteria

A physician must document these on at least two occasions, at least 1 month apart.

1. Low grade fever

2. Nonexudative pharyngitis

3. Palpable or tender anterior or posterior cervical or axillary nodes (<2 cm in diameter)

DIAGNOSTIC EVALUATION

The history and physical examination help to determine the likelihood of an organic versus a psychiatric etiology. In those patients with characteristics suggesting an organic cause, further evaluation should be directed at the suspected underlying cause. For example, in patients with suspected hyperparathyroidism, elevated levels of serum calcium and parathyroid hormone might confirm the diagnosis.

In patients with suspected organic disease but without an apparent diagnosis suggested by the history and physical screening, laboratory tests including a CBC, ESR, comprehensive metabolic profile, UA, and thyroid function tests are recommended. Pregnancy testing should be considered in women of childbearing age and HIV testing for individuals at risk for this disease. A drug screen can occasionally be productive. Additional laboratory or imaging tests should be ordered based on findings in the history and physical examination. Examples of tests that may be helpful include a chest x-ray to look for adenopathy, occult CHF, and primary lung tumors or metastatic disease. An ECG may detect a silent infarction or ischemia. In patients at risk, Lyme titers and TB skin testing might be of benefit. Sleep studies may be helpful in excluding sleep apnea and other sleep disorders.

TREATMENT

Psychiatric evaluation and treatment may be necessary for patients with persistent fatigue due to anxiety or depression. For patients with an identified medical condition, treatment of the underlying process is the recommended treatment for the fatigue. There is no specific therapy for CFS, although data suggest that patients with CFS may benefit from psychotherapy and exercise. Additional therapy is targeted toward associated symptoms (e.g., NSAIDs for myalgias).

In individuals with persistent fatigue of unknown causes, therapy may consist of an empiric trial of antidepressants or withdrawal of a medication known to cause fatigue. Some patients also benefit from moderate levels of exercise and efforts to reduce the stresses in their lives.

KEY POINTS

- Fatigue occurs in up to 20% of patients seeking care.
- Psychological causes should be at the top of the differential diagnosis for all patients presenting with fatigue, as the majority of cases have psychiatric causes.
- The history can help in determining a psychiatric versus organic cause and thus aid in directing the evaluation of fatigue.

16 Headache

More than 90% of adults will experience headaches over a 1-year period and over 15% of these will consult a physician. Although most headaches seen in the outpatient setting are benign, it is important to identify those rare instances when a headache may be secondary to a life-threatening illness.

PATHOGENESIS

Headache originates in either intracranial or extracranial structures. Intracranial pain-sensitive structures include the trigeminal, glossopharyngeal, vagus, and first three cervical nerves. Additionally, the dura, the arteries, and the venous sinuses are pain-sensitive; however, the brain parenchyma is not. Disease processes that cause pressure or inflammation of pain-sensitive structures, distention of blood vessels, and obstruction of cerebrospinal fluid (CSF) can cause pain. For example, a mass lesion can cause headache by displacing a pain-sensitive structure, while a ruptured aneurysm can inflame the meninges.

The neurogenic inflammatory hypothesis is the most accepted theory explaining migraine headache. This theory views migraine as a primary neuronal event with subsequent changes resulting from the effects of neurotransmitters on the vasculature and the blood flow. Neuropeptides trigger the release of kinins and bioactive substances that lead to more inflammation and vasodilation. Serotonin receptors are believed to be an important part of this process, which explains why serotonin analogs or agonists benefit patients with migraine.

Extracranial sources of headache include skin, muscles, blood vessels, periosteum of the skull, sinuses, and teeth. Clinical problems affecting the eyes, sinuses, cervical spine, temporomandibular joint, and cranial nerves can all cause headache.

Tension headaches are traditionally thought to originate from scalp muscles. However, myographic recordings show that many but not all individuals with tension headaches have muscle contraction. Recent studies suggest that migraine and tension headaches may have similar pathophysiologic mechanisms but with different expression of symptoms. This overlap explains why some patients with tension headaches experience migrainelike symptoms.

CLINICAL MANIFESTATIONS

HISTORY

The history provides the most useful diagnostic information and the physical examination helps to exclude organic pathology. Relevant history includes location (unilateral vs. bilateral), severity ("worst headache of my life"), quality (throbbing, squeezing), duration, frequency, associated neurologic symptoms, aggravating or alleviating factors (foods, rest, menstruation, OTC medications), and associated symptoms (nausea, emesis, fever, visual changes). Other relevant information includes caffeine intake, since caffeine withdrawal is a known cause of headaches, and whether the headache awakens the patient from sleep. Foods such as chocolate, alcohol, nuts, and aged cheese may trigger migraines. Reviewing medications is important because a number of drugs such as indomethacin, nifedipine, cimetidine, captopril, nitrates, and oral contraceptives can trigger headaches.

Migraine Headaches

These typically start between the ages of 15 and 45 years, with a 3:1 female predominance. Migraine headaches require at least two of the following four headache characteristics for diagnosis: unilateral location, pulsatile quality, moderate-to-severe intensity, or aggravation by movement. They must also be associated with one of the following symptoms: nausea, vomiting, or photo- or phonophobia. Migraines last between 4 and 72 hours and may be accompanied by an aura. Migraines without aura, formerly termed common migraines, are the most common form of migraine. Migraines with aura, formerly termed classic migraines, are less common. Auras include flashing lights, shimmering lines, and blind spots. Some individuals may experience paresthesias, numbness, strange odors, and speech disturbances. Aura symptoms gradually develop over more than 4 minutes and last up to 60 minutes, with headache either following or accompanying the aura within 60 minutes. A family history of migraine is present in over 80% of those who suffer from migraines and is a useful diagnostic criterion. Common triggers include lack of or irregular sleep, hunger, alcohol, certain foods, humidity, and emotional stress.

Tension Headaches

The pain due to tension headaches is typically of mild-to-moderate intensity and is located in the bilateral occipital-frontal areas. The headache is usually described as dull or bandlike, often lasts for hours, and is often associated with stress. Tension headaches usually do not awaken patients from sleep and are not generally associated with vomiting or neurologic symptoms.

Cluster Headaches

These headaches are severe, unilateral, localized to the periorbital/temporal area, and usually accompanied by one of the following symptoms: lacrimation, rhinorrhea, ptosis, miosis, nasal congestion, and eyelid edema. These headaches occur in "clusters," with one to eight daily attacks lasting 15 to 90 minutes for a period of 4 to 6 weeks. These episodes are then followed by pain-free intervals lasting 3 to 6 months. Cluster headaches are more common in men (8:1) but overall are much less frequent than tension or migraine headaches.

Analgesic Headaches

These headaches are seen in patients who chronically use analgesic or antimigraine drugs, especially those that contain caffeine. Daily use of low-dose analgesics is much riskier for analgesic headaches than occasional use of large doses. The headache initially worsens when the analgesics are discontinued but improves after a few weeks.

New-Onset Headaches

These headaches merit close attention. A subarachnoid hemorrhage (SAH) should be considered in any patient who does not usually have headaches and presents with the "worst headache of my life." An acute headache with ataxia, profuse nausea, and vomiting is consistent with a cerebral hemorrhage. Fever with frontal or maxillary tenderness is suggestive of acute sinusitis.

PHYSICAL EXAMINATION

The physical examination should include vital signs, funduscopic and cardiovascular assessment, palpation of the head and neck, and a thorough neurologic evaluation. The examination is important to help identify secondary or organic causes of headache. A neurologic examination is essential because a neurologic deficit is an important sign of intracranial pathology. Patients with muscle contraction headaches may demonstrate muscle tightness or trigger points over the posterior occiput in several areas. Temporal artery tenderness in an elderly patient raises the possibility of temporal arteritis, while sinus tenderness, congestion, and fever are most consistent with sinusitis. Headache accompanied by a stiff neck may indicate an SAH or meningitis. Headache with abnormal physical signs—such as a high blood pressure, a focal neurologic deficit, or papilledema—may indicate the presence of a mass lesion or malignant hypertension.

DIFFERENTIAL DIAGNOSIS

Headaches may be classified as primary or secondary. Primary headaches have no underlying organic disease and include migraine with aura, migraine without aura, tension headaches, and cluster headaches. Secondary headaches result from an underlying disorder such as intracranial mass, infection, cerebrovascular accident (CVA), head trauma, drug withdrawal, or metabolic disorders (Box 16-1 gives a complete list). Although primary headaches are not life-threatening, they are often very debilitating to patients.

DIAGNOSTIC EVALUATION

The objectives in evaluating a headache patient are to (1) identify patients with life-threatening conditions, (2) identify those with secondary headaches such as sinusitis, and (3) provide symptom relief to those with primary headache.

Patients presenting with an acute onset of severe headache, especially in the presence of meningeal signs, high fever, or evidence of increased intracranial pressure, need urgent evaluation. A CT scan is helpful in detecting an SAH or intracerebral bleed. If the CT scan is negative in evaluating for an SAH, a lumbar

■ BOX 16-1 Causes of Secondary Headaches
Subarachnoid hemorrhage (SAH)
Intracranial mass
Posttraumatic
Infection
Glaucoma
Sinus disease
Drug withdrawal
Benign intracranial hypertension (pseudotumor cerebri)
Hypoxia
Hypercapnia
Postlumbar puncture
Neuralgias

BOX 16-2 Indications for Neuroimaging

Headache of recent onset (<6 months)
Headache beginning after 50 years of age
Worsening headaches
Headache that does not fit primary headache pattern
Associated seizure
Focal neurologic signs or symptoms
Personality change
Severe headaches unresponsive to therapy
History of significant trauma
New headache in a cancer patient

puncture is indicated, since a CT scan will be normal in 1 of every 10 patients with SAH. A lumbar puncture can also detect the presence of significant disease in patients with meningeal signs and provide fluid for identifying the cause of meningitis. Due to the risk of brainstem herniation, a lumbar puncture is contraindicated when increased intracranial pressure is suspected. In general, blood tests play a limited role in the evaluation of headache patients. A CBC may be helpful in assessing a patient with suspected meningitis and a normal ESR is helpful for ruling out temporal arteritis.

The role of CT and MRI scans in patients with chronic headaches is controversial. The probability of finding a significant abnormality in a patient with a history of chronic headaches and a normal physical examination is extremely low. However, imaging may still be helpful in certain instances, as when there is a change in symptoms associated with chronic headaches. Box 16-2 lists indications for neuroimaging.

TREATMENT

Treatment for tension headaches includes avoidance of the stress commonly associated with these headaches or improved stress management. Biofeedback, relaxation, and deep-breathing exercises in a quiet environment are often effective. In addition, non-narcotic analgesics such as NSAIDs (e.g., ibuprofen 400 to 600 mg three times a day) or acetaminophen (650 mg four times a day) will usually alleviate symptoms and are generally the first line of therapy. Low doses of antidepressants such as amitriptyline (10 to 75 mg PO daily) can be effective for reducing the number and severity of chronic tension headaches. If these measures fail to improve the headache significantly or if the headache is associated with neurologic symptoms, the diagnosis of tension headache should be questioned and further evaluation pursued.

Primary treatment of migraine headaches includes avoiding headache triggers, withdrawal from stressful environments (often by lying down in a dark, quiet bedroom with a cool washcloth placed on the forehead), and rest. A lifestyle that encourages a regular schedule of sleep, meals, and physical activity as well as avoidance of stress, alcohol, caffeine, tyramine (found in aged cheeses and red wine), nitrates (found in cured meats), and artificial sweeteners is potentially helpful.

Serotonin receptor agonists are available in a variety of forms and are the primary medications used to abort an attack. The triptans are the most commonly used abortive agents. Triptans are available as injections, nasal sprays, and tablets and may be given in multiple doses until the patient's symptoms resolve. All the triptans have similar chemical structures and mechanisms of action. Although there are subtle differences among them, there is no clear therapeutic advantage to one over another. If one triptan is not tolerated or does not work on at least two occasions, a different triptan should be tried. Due to their vasoconstrictive properties, the triptans are contraindicated in patients with coronary artery disease (CAD), peripheral vascular disease (PVD), and uncontrolled hypertension.

Ergotamine is another serotonin receptor agonist that also has dopamine and adrenergic receptor activity. It is available as an oral, sublingual, or suppository medication and is maximally effective when given early in the course of a migraine. Because it has vasoconstrictive properties, ergotamine is contraindicated in patients with CAD or PVD. Dihydroergotamine (DHE) can be given parenterally and can be useful in the treatment of acute migraine in the emergency room setting. Table 16-1 lists medications for treatment of acute migraines.

Depending on patients' symptoms, NSAIDs, acetaminophen, antiemetics, narcotics, and caffeine are frequently prescribed. Physicians must use caution when using mild analgesics alone to treat migraines, as their limited duration of effectiveness may result in "rebound" symptoms. As a result, patients may take higher than recommended doses. In patients who suffer from migraines more than twice a week, beta blockers, calcium channel blockers, antidepressants, and antiseizure medications (e.g., divalproex sodium) can provide effective prophylactic therapy (Table 16-2). Prophylactic therapy should also be considered in patients in whom abortive agents are ineffective, poorly tolerated, or contraindicated. Patients with menstrual migraines may benefit from a brief course of NSAIDs taken for several days before and after menses. Prophylactic therapy is selected according to a patient's age and comorbidities—for

■ TABLE 16-1 Medications for Acute Treatment of Migraines

Nonspecific Medications	Dose	Adverse Reactions
Nonsteroidal anti-inflammatory drugs (NSAIDs)		
Ibuprofen Naproxen Aspirin	400–800 mg q6h 275–550 mg q2–6h 650–1000 mg q4–6h	Upset, bleeding disorder, G6PD deficiency
Analgesics plus caffeine		
Acetaminophen, aspirin, caffeine	250–500 mg acetaminophen and aspirin, 65–130 mg caffeine q4–6h	As above plus palpitations, anxiety
Isometheptene/dichloralphenazone/acetaminophen (Midrin)	Two with onset, 1qh, maximum five per episode	Hypertension, dizziness, caution renal/liver disease, hypertension, cardiac disease, or MAOI use
Narcotics		
Hydromorphone	2–4 mg PO q3–4h 0.5–2 mg IV q1–2h	Sedation, respiratory depression
Butorphanol nasal	One spray, repeat in 60–90 minutes; may repeat sequence in 3–4 hours	As above
Antiemetics		
Prochlorperazine	5–10 mg orally or 25 mg rectally as adjunct to other treatments	Sedation, hypotension dystonic reactions
Metoclopramide	10 mg as adjunct to other treatments	Sedation, dystonic reaction
Migraine-Specific Medications	**Dose**	**Adverse Reactions**
Triptans		
Sumatriptan	6 mg SC; 25–100 mg PO or 1–2 sprays nasally; may repeat SC dose in 1 hour, oral and nasal in 2 hours	Nausea, vomiting, chest pain; contraindicated with ergot or MAOI use; caution with CAD
Rizatriptan	5–20 mg orally, may repeat in 2 hours	As above
Zolmatriptan	2.5–5 mg orally, may repeat in 2 hours	As above
Ergotamine	1–2 mg orally every hour up to three doses in 24 hours	Arrhythmia, vasospasm, nausea, vomiting
Ergotamine plus caffeine	Two tablets orally, then one every 30 minutes to maximum of six per attack and 10 per week	As above plus myocardial infarct, pulmonary fibrosis
Dihydroergotamine	1 mg parenterally every hour to maximum of 2 mg IV and 3 mg SC/IM; intranasal one spray in each nostril with repeat dose in 15 minutes; maximum four sprays per day	Hypertension, CVA, cardiac ischemia, arrhythmia, nausea, vomiting

G6PD, glucose-6-phosphate dehydrogenase; MAOI, monoamine oxidase inhibitor.

■ TABLE 16-2 Medications for Migraine Prophylaxis

Class	Dose Range	Cautions
Beta blockers		
Propranolol	40–320 mg/day	Heart block greater than first degree; congestive heart failure; asthma/reactive airways
Atenolol	50–150 mg/day	As above
Metoprolol	50–300 mg/day	As above
Tricyclic antidepressants		
Amitriptyline	10–300 mg/day	Cardiac conduction abnormalities; glaucoma; urinary retention; seizure disorder
Nortriptyline	10–150 mg/day	As above
Imipramine	10–200 mg/day	As above
Calcium channel blockers		
Verapamil	120–720 mg/day	Heart block greater than first degree; congestive heart failure; hypotension
Diltiazem	90–360 mg/day	As above
Anticonvulsants		
Divalproex sodium	250–1500 mg/day	Pregnancy, liver disease
Topiramate	25–200 mg/day	Fatigue, nausea, anorexia common
Serotonin antagonists		
Cyproheptadine	4–16 mg/day	Elderly, glaucoma, MAOI use, urinary outflow obstruction
Methysergide	2–8 mg/day	Hypertension, heart disease, pulmonary disease, collagen vascular disease, vascular disease, renal or hepatic insufficiency, pregnancy
Monoamine oxidase inhibitors		
Phenelzine	30–90 mg/day	Dietary and food restrictions necessary, congestive heart failure, liver disease

example, trying an antidepressant first in someone with concomitant depression.

Patients with cluster headaches should be counseled to avoid known precipitants. Breathing 100% oxygen at 7 to 10 L/min for 10 to 15 minutes via a tight-fitting mask may abort an acute attack. If the patient has no cardiac risk factors, sumatriptan 6 mg SC with an additional 6 mg given 1 hour later is helpful. Alternatively, dihydroergotamine mesylate 1 mg IM or IV may improve symptoms. Prednisone starting with 60 to 80 mg/day followed by a 2- to 4-week taper has been shown to shorten the duration of episodes and diminish the frequency and intensity of symptoms. Other medications commonly used to treat or prevent cluster headache include verapamil, NSAIDs, propranolol, amitriptyline, and lithium. Patients in whom these therapies do not help may benefit from referral to a neurologist or major headache center.

Temporal arteritis must be considered in older patients who have pain on palpation of the temporal artery. Although these patients often have an elevated ESR, definitive diagnosis requires biopsy of the temporal artery. Patients with temporal arteritis must be started on steroids promptly as a delay in treatment may result in blindness.

KEY POINTS

- Headache originates in either intracranial or extracranial structures. Intracranial pain-sensitive structures include the trigeminal, glossopharyngeal, vagus, and the first three cervical nerves.

- The neurogenic inflammatory hypothesis is the most widely accepted theory explaining migraine headache. This theory views migraine as a primary neuronal event with subsequent changes resulting from the effects of neurotransmitters on the vasculature and blood flow.

- Headache accompanied by a stiff neck may indicate a subarachnoid hemorrhage or meningitis.

- The objectives in evaluating a headache patient are to (1) identify patients with life-threatening conditions; (2) identify those with secondary headaches, such as sinusitis; and (3) provide symptom relief to those with primary headaches.

- Serotonin receptor agonists are available in a variety of forms and are the primary medications used to abort a migraine headache.

- Temporal arteritis must be considered in older patients who have pain on palpation of the temporal artery.

The most common causes of heartburn symptoms are GERD, peptic ulcer disease, gastritis, and nonulcer dyspepsia.

EPIDEMIOLOGY

Heartburn from GERD is experienced on a daily basis by 7% of the population, on a weekly basis by 15%, and at least monthly by up to 40%. Peptic ulcer disease is present in 1.5% of the population and has a lifetime incidence of about 10%. Duodenal ulcers occur more commonly than gastric ulcers and at a younger age. Peptic ulcer disease affects men slightly more than women. Nonulcer dyspepsia occurs in up to 25% to 30% of the population at some point.

PATHOGENESIS

Gastroesophageal reflux occurs when gastric contents reflux or enter the esophagus. Decreased lower esophageal sphincter (LES) pressure or increased intra-abdominal pressure plays a significant role in this process. Exposing the esophagus to the low pH of the gastric contents can cause inflammatory changes leading to esophagitis. Long-term acid exposure may also result in the metaplastic transformation of the squamous cells lining the esophagus to adenomatous cells (Barrett esophagus). Patients with Barrett esophagus are at a higher risk (30- to 40-fold) for developing esophageal cancer. Continued inflammatory reaction can also lead to esophageal scarring, stricture formation, and dysphagia. However, the correlation of symptoms and degree of esophageal damage is poor.

Peptic ulcer disease and gastritis have similar causes and risk factors. Typically, the gastric and duodenal mucosa are resistant to any damage from acid secretion. Peptic ulcers and gastritis occur when the defense mechanisms are compromised or, rarely, when acid secretion is sufficient to overwhelm the defenses.

Helicobacter pylori infection is the most significant risk factor for peptic ulcer disease. In 10% to 20% of infected individuals, gastric or duodenal ulcers develop. Exactly why peptic ulcers occur in some individuals and not in others is unclear. Infection with *H. pylori* is also associated with an increased risk of gastric adenocarcinoma and gastric lymphoma.

NSAIDs contribute to gastritis and ulcer formation by blocking cyclooxygenase-1 production of prostaglandins that maintain mucosal blood flow, secretion of mucus, and bicarbonate. Without these protective factors, acid-induced inflammation and ulcers may result. Stress-induced gastritis and ulcers are thought to occur due to impaired mucosal defense resulting from vasoconstriction and resultant tissue hypoxia.

Nonulcer dyspepsia is a poorly understood disease with symptoms like those of GERD and peptic ulcer disease. The pathophysiology is thought to be related to altered GI motility, GI contractile patterns, and transit of food.

CLINICAL MANIFESTATIONS

HISTORY

Initial evaluation of individuals with heartburn includes the patient's detailed description of the episodes along with assessment of risk for the different diseases with heartburn as a presenting symptom.

GERD is characterized by burning pain in the epigastric, sternal, and throat regions accompanied by a sour taste in the mouth and is aggravated by lying down or bending over. Increases in abdominal pressure, as occurs with pregnancy, may worsen reflux. Burning, aching, or gnawing pain in the epigastric region or upper quadrants of the abdomen is typical of peptic ulcer disease. Chest tightness and pain brought on by exertion and relieved by rest are more typical of cardiac disease. Colicky upper abdominal pain is more consistent with cholecystitis, nephrolithiasis, IBS, or nonulcer dyspepsia as possible etiologies.

Esophageal reflux may be alleviated by antacids or food, but it frequently recurs within 1 to 2 hours. Commonly, the pain of peptic ulcer disease is more intense in the middle of the night; it is typically mid-epigastric and is relieved by eating. Eating usually aggravates cholecystitis and sometimes gastric ulcers. The pain of nephrolithiasis is independent of ingestion of food. The pain of nonulcer dyspepsia is more variable but often related to eating.

GERD can cause respiratory symptoms of cough, wheezing, sore throat, and laryngitis. GERD is a common cause of chest pain, but heartburn associated with shortness of breath or activity should raise concerns about a cardiac etiology for the patient's symptoms.

Connective tissue and neuromuscular disease can cause esophageal symptoms from associated motility disorders. Medications such as theophylline and calcium channel blockers can precipitate or exacerbate symptoms associated with GERD. NSAIDs are associated with gastric and duodenal ulcers as well as heartburn. The patient should also be asked about medications he or she is using to alleviate symptoms, particularly with availability of OTC H_2 blockers and proton pump inhibitors (PPIs).

Smoking worsens gastroesophageal reflux and is a risk factor for peptic ulcer disease. Dietary factors associated with reducing the pressure of the LES include consumption of coffee, chocolate, mints, fatty foods, and alcohol. There are no specific dietary correlates for peptic ulcer disease. However, alcohol can cause gastric irritation, with resultant gastritis.

PHYSICAL EXAMINATION

The physical examination generally cannot distinguish between gastritis, peptic ulcer disease, nonulcer dyspepsia, and GERD. All of these typically have minimal physical findings other than epigastric tenderness. A test for fecal occult blood may show evidence of blood loss, which makes the presence of peptic ulcer disease and erosive gastritis or esophagitis more likely diagnoses than simple gastroesophageal reflux.

Cardiac findings such as S_3, S_4, pulmonary rales, or an irregular rhythm signify underlying cardiac disease. Abdominal tenderness with pancreatitis is typically periumbilical, while the tenderness with cholecystitis occurs in the right upper quadrant and is associated with a positive Murphy sign. Nephrolithiasis typically presents no physical findings other than possible costovertebral angle tenderness. Palpation of a mass suggests the presence of a neoplasm.

DIFFERENTIAL DIAGNOSIS

Table 17-1 presents a comprehensive differential diagnosis for patients complaining of heartburn. The differential diagnosis also includes infections (e.g., *Candida* or herpes), pill-induced esophagitis, biliary disease, motility disorders, and CAD. No specific etiology is found for approximately 50% to 60% of patients with heartburn.

Nonulcer dyspepsia is a poorly understood disease with symptoms overlapping GERD, peptic ulcer disease, and gastritis. Patients may have symptoms consistent with GERD, peptic ulcer disease, and gastritis, or may present with dysmotility symptoms such as abdominal bloating or cramping. This is generally considered a diagnosis of exclusion. If the initial laboratory evaluation (CBC, testing of the stools for occult blood, *H. pylori* serology) is normal in patients below age 45, empiric therapy can be initiated based on the patient's predominant symptoms. Patients presenting after age 45 require more aggressive evaluation, since organic disease becomes more prevalent as patients grow older.

Regurgitation is a classic symptom of reflux in children. Almost half of healthy infants regurgitate once daily. Symptoms such as failure to gain weight, apnea, wheezing, or recurrent pneumonia should prompt further investigation.

DIAGNOSTIC EVALUATION

No single test is accepted as the standard for diagnosing GERD. However, several tests may prove useful

■ TABLE 17-1 Differential Diagnosis of Heartburn

Condition	Typical Symptoms
Gastroesophageal reflux disease (GERD)	Regurgitation, dysphagia
Peptic ulcer disease	Gnawing epigastric pain, nausea, vomiting, bloating
Gastritis	Same as peptic ulcer disease
Nonulcer dyspepsia	Upper abdominal/epigastric pain, bloating, belching, flatulence, nausea
Coronary artery disease/angina	Chest pressure, nausea, diaphoresis, palpitations
Cholelithiasis	Colicky right upper quadrant pain, with meals, radiation to scapular region
Pancreatitis	Severe constant midabdominal pain
Infectious esophagitis	Dysphagia, associated immunocompromised condition
Medication or chemical esophagitis	Dysphagia, associated ingestion
Scleroderma/polymyositis with secondary gastroesophageal reflux	Associated signs of connective tissue disease, potential risk of stricture/dysphagia

in evaluating patients with heartburn. Early diagnostic evaluation is indicated when complications such as weight loss, vomiting, or bleeding are present or when a patient fails to respond to therapy.

Esophagogastroduodenoscopy (EGD) is the diagnostic tool most frequently used in evaluating the symptoms of heartburn or dysphagia and assessing the upper GI tract in patients with GI blood loss. EGD will detect esophagitis, erosions, ulceration, malignancies, webs, diverticuli, and strictures; it can also be therapeutically useful in treating ulcer disease and strictures. EGD is indicated in patients above age 45 with new-onset heartburn; those with evidence of GI bleeding, early satiety, and vomiting; and those individuals whose symptoms persist despite therapy.

Barium studies, such as the barium swallow or upper GI series, can reveal anatomic abnormalities such as esophageal spasm and may detect reflux. However, barium studies have a lower sensitivity than EGD for detecting ulceration, erosions, and tumors, and they do not allow tissue diagnosis.

Ambulatory esophageal pH monitoring can be useful for patients with suspected GERD who have normal endoscopy and have either atypical symptoms or are refractory to therapy. A thin pH probe is placed through the patient's nose into the esophagus 5 cm above the LES. The percentage of time the esophageal pH is below 4 in conjunction with the patient's symptoms provides diagnostic information. The reported sensitivity and specificity of this test are both about 95%.

Esophageal manometry involves monitoring of LES pressures and esophageal peristalsis. Its primary role is to evaluate patients for motility disorders.

H. pylori testing can be useful in assessing patients with heartburn. Currently, there are four different tests: the rapid urease test, histologic staining, serologic tests, fecal antigen tests, and urea breath tests.

The rapid urease test analyzes tissue samples obtained during endoscopy for the presence of urease, a marker of *H. pylori* infection. This test has a sensitivity of approximately 90% and a specificity of 98%. The test itself is inexpensive and quickly performed, but obtaining samples is expensive because of the costs associated with endoscopy. If the rapid urease test is negative in a patient with ulcers or gastritis, a separate sample can be sent for histologic staining for *H. pylori*.

Histologic staining is very sensitive and specific for *H. pylori*; however, results are less readily available and this procedure is more expensive than the urease test.

Serologic and fecal antigen tests have the advantage of being noninvasive, inexpensive, and highly sensitive and specific (>90%). The disadvantages are that serology will remain indefinitely positive; a positive test indicates only prior infection, not necessarily current activity; and patients in their twenties are rarely positive whereas more than 50% of those in their sixties are positive. Serologic testing is most useful in younger populations and for diagnosing *H. pylori* in

radiographically diagnosed duodenal ulcers. Fecal antigen testing suffers from the inconvenience of collecting a stool sample, but it is inexpensive and can be used to test for cure.

Urea breath tests involve having the patient ingest urea labeled with radioactive carbon. If *H. pylori* is present, urease hydrolyzes the urea and the patient exhales labeled carbon dioxide. The test is both sensitive and specific but can be expensive and may not be readily available.

TREATMENT

Table 17-2 outlines common heartburn treatments. Typical GERD symptoms of heartburn and regurgitation can be treated empirically with lifestyle modifications, although most patients with significant reflux will require acid-suppressive therapy using H_2 blockers or PPIs. New recommendations advocate step-down therapy from a PPI to a lesser regimen that remains effective, such as a lower dose of the PPI, H_2 blocker, antacids, or lifestyle management. Lifestyle modifications include elevating the head of the patient's bed, weight loss if he or she is obese, avoiding foods that lower the tone of the LES, eliminating aspirin and other NSAIDs, and stopping tobacco use. Patients with symptoms persisting beyond 6 weeks merit referral for diagnostic evaluation such as endoscopy.

The rate of recurrence with GERD is high because the underlying pathophysiologic process is unchanged when therapy is discontinued. Moderate-to-severe esophagitis and atypical symptoms, particularly respiratory symptoms, may require long-term treatment. Nonetheless, attempts to step-down therapy should be made after 8 weeks of symptom control. Some patients may require only intermittent therapy along with continued lifestyle modifications. Severe esophagitis, Barrett esophagus, and stricture are markers of severe reflux and require long-term treatment, even in the absence of symptoms, in order to reduce the risk of esophageal carcinoma, bleeding, and stricture.

Therapy for peptic ulcer disease and gastritis depends on whether *H. pylori* is present. If it is, therapy directed against this organism is indicated. Regimens include triple therapy with combinations of omeprazole (a PPI) or an H_2 blocker, clarithromycin, and amoxicillin or metronidazole for 7 to 14 days. Triple-therapy regimens have cure rates of approximately 90%. After the antibiotic regimen has been completed, PPIs are generally continued for 4 to 8 weeks for duodenal ulcers and for 6 to 12 weeks for gastritis or gastric ulcers. EGD is recommended to document healing of gastric ulcers because they pose a higher risk of cancer.

Patients with NSAID-related ulcers are generally treated with acid-suppression therapy and discontinuance of the NSAID. If NSAIDs must be used, options include switching the patient to a nonacetylated

■ TABLE 17-2 Treatments for Common Causes of Heartburn

Disease	Treatments	Example
GERD	Behavioral changes	• Avoid fatty foods, spicy foods, chocolate, mints, citrus • Avoid alcohol, caffeine • Avoid large meals and reclining after meals
	Medications	
	• H$_2$ blockers	Cimetidine, ranitidine, famotidine, nizatidine
	• Proton pump inhibitors	Omeprazole, lansoprazole, dexlansoprazole, esomeprazole, pantoprazole, rabeprazole
Peptic ulcer disease (PUD)/gastritis		
• H. pylori-positive	Medications	
	• Antibiotics	Clarithromycin, amoxicillin, metronidazole
	• Proton pump inhibitors	Cimetidine, ranitidine, famotidine, nizatidine
• H. pylori-negative	Medications	
	• H$_2$ blockers	Cimetidine, ranitidine, famotidine, nizatidine
	• Proton pump inhibitors	Omeprazole, lansoprazole, dexlansoprazole, esomeprazole, pantoprazole, rabeprazole
Nonulcer dyspepsia	Behavioral changes	Avoid offending foods
		Reassurance
Dysmotility symptoms	Medications	Metoclopropamide
Ulcerlike or reflux	Medications	
	• H$_2$ blockers	Cimetidine, ranitidine, famotidine, nizatidine
	• Proton pump inhibitors	Omeprazole, lansoprazole, dexlansoprazole, esomeprazole, pantoprazole, rabeprazole

salicylate such as salsalate (Disalcid), or a COX-2 inhibitor, using an enterically coated preparation and prescribing the lowest effective dose. If NSAIDs must be used in patients with a history of ulcer, misoprostol (Cytotec) or a PPI can help prevent recurrence.

Therapy for nonulcer dyspepsia involves avoiding foods or medications that aggravate symptoms, reassurance regarding the absence of serious disease, and medications directed at the predominant symptoms. In patients with ulcerlike or reflux symptoms, acid-suppressing agents are helpful, while dysmotility-related symptoms—such as nausea, bloating, or early satiety—respond better to motility agents. If treatment is initially successful, 4 weeks of continuous therapy is followed by a trial off medication. Some patients need only intermittent therapy, whereas others may require continuous treatment. In such cases, periodic attempts to wean the patient off medication should be attempted to see whether symptoms recur.

KEY POINTS

- Heartburn is a common symptom, affecting 40% or more of the population every month.
- GERD, peptic ulcer disease, gastritis, and nonulcer dyspepsia are the major causes of heartburn symptoms.
- Atypical symptoms of dysphagia, early satiety, weight loss, or blood loss should trigger a GI workup.
- EGD is the most useful diagnostic tool for evaluating heartburn.
- H. pylori is a leading causative factor in peptic ulcer disease and gastritis.
- Antibiotic therapy, along with PPIs, is used to treat H. pylori-positive patients with peptic ulcer disease or gastritis.

18 Hematuria

Hematuria can be either microscopic or grossly visible. Microscopic hematuria is defined as more than three red blood cells (RBCs) per HPF. Although hematuria may be an incidental finding, it is important to evaluate the cause, since up to 10% of cases have a serious underlying etiology.

PATHOGENESIS

Normally, the number of RBCs excreted in the urine is 2000/mL, equivalent to about 1 RBC per HPF. Hematuria may be caused by systemic illnesses, intrarenal or glomerular disease, and extrarenal or structural disease. Glomerular disease will cause leakage of RBCs into the renal tubules, resulting in RBCs and RBC casts in the urine. A urinary tract neoplasm can erode into blood vessels, causing hematuria. Prostatic disease can enlarge and dilate mucosal vessels and cause bleeding if these vessels leak or rupture. Kidney or bladder infections are a common cause for hematuria and stones can irritate the mucosa and blood vessels as they move through the urinary tract.

CLINICAL MANIFESTATIONS

HISTORY

Pyelonephritis and renal infarction, or masses, can all present with flank pain. Flank pain radiating into the groin suggests a kidney stone. Urgency, frequency, and dysuria occur with inflammation of the lower urinary tract from conditions such as cystitis. Fever is common with pyelonephritis but is sometimes associated with renal cell carcinoma. Hematuria is present in 90% of patients with renal cell carcinoma, and painless hematuria may be a presenting sign of a urinary tract malignancy. It is the most common presenting symptom of bladder cancer in individuals over age 50 and is a common cause of hematuria in this age group.

In women, the menstrual history is important, since menstrual bleeding may be mistaken for hematuria. A history of trauma increases the likelihood of a renal, ureteral, or urethral injury. It is also important to inquire about recent infectious illnesses. A recent streptococcal infection may be a clue for poststreptococcal glomerulonephritis, while exposure to TB increases the risk of a TB infection. A recent URI may cause hematuria in a patient with IgA nephropathy (Berger disease). A previous history of kidney stones, nephritis, cystitis, or bladder cancer suggests recurrence as a possible cause of hematuria. Valvular heart disease in association with recent dental work or a history of intravenous drug use increases the risk of subacute bacterial endocarditis. Hemoptysis combined with hematuria is a symptom of Goodpasture syndrome.

Reviewing the patient's medications is important. Interstitial nephritis can result from a number of medications, such as NSAIDs, cephalosporins, and ciprofloxacin. Interstitial nephritis may cause hematuria accompanied by fever and a skin rash. Chemotherapeutic agents, particularly cyclophosphamide, can cause hemorrhagic cystitis. A red coloration caused by medications that discolor the urine, such as pyridium and rifampin, may be mistaken for hematuria.

Family history is valuable for recognizing risk factors for certain diseases. For example, sickle cell disease or trait is much more prevalent in African-American patients with a family history of the illness. Patients with benign familial hematuria have normal renal function and often have similarly affected relatives. Polycystic kidney disease can either be of adult onset (autosomal dominant) or found in childhood. Alport syndrome (autosomal recessive) is associated with deafness.

PHYSICAL EXAMINATION

Costovertebral angle tenderness is common with pyelonephritis and tumors that stretch the renal capsule. Kidney stones may cause pain so severe that patients find it difficult to sit still. An abdominal mass may be present with polycystic kidney disease or renal cell carcinoma. Suprapubic tenderness occurs with cystitis, while a urethral discharge suggests urethritis. In men, a rectal examination may reveal an enlarged smooth prostate gland, consistent with benign prostatic hypertrophy (BPH), or a nodular hard prostate, as is found in prostate cancer. A tender, boggy prostate is a sign of prostatitis.

The finding of a malar rash, fatigue, and joint pain suggests systemic lupus erythematosus (SLE). In children and young adults, palpable purpura, arthritis, and abdominal pain are signs of Henoch–Schönlein purpura. Hypertension and peripheral edema are common findings with glomerulonephritis. Patients with atrial fibrillation are at risk for developing emboli and renal infarction. A pelvic examination in a woman may reveal a pelvic source of the bleeding.

DIFFERENTIAL DIAGNOSIS

Lesions involving the kidney, ureters, bladder, prostate, and urethra can all present with hematuria. Gross hematuria is usually associated with infection, stones, and neoplasm. In children, benign familial hematuria, glomerular disease, hypercalciuria, infection, and perineal irritation or trauma are the most common etiologies. In young adults, the most likely causes are infection, stones, trauma, and a urinary tract tumor. In older age groups, bladder cancer and prostate disease increase in prevalence. The underlying prevalence of a serious disease such as a neoplasm or polycystic kidney disease varies, but it may be as high as 10%.

SLE may present with hematuria. Blood disorders such as sickle cell, coagulopathies, and leukemia are possible but infrequent causes of hematuria. As noted earlier, drugs may cause hematuria. Although anticoagulants can cause bleeding, those individuals on anticoagulants who have hematuria should still be evaluated because underlying lesions are frequently found. Box 18-1 lists the differential diagnosis for hematuria.

■ BOX 18-1 Differential Diagnosis of Hematuria

Hematologic

Coagulopathy, sickle cell hemoglobinopathies

Renal/Glomerular

Glomerulonephritis, benign familial hematuria, multisystem disease (systemic lupus erythematosus, Henoch–Schönlein purpura, hemolytic uremic syndrome, polyarteritis nodosa, Wegener granulomatosis, Goodpasture syndrome)

Renal/Nonglomerular

Renal vein or artery embolus, tuberculosis, pyelonephritis, polycystic kidney disease, medullary sponge kidney, acute interstitial nephritis, tumor, vascular malformation, trauma, papillary necrosis, exercise

Postrenal

Stones, tumor of ureter/bladder/urethra, cystitis, tuberculosis, prostatitis, urethritis, Foley catheter placement, exercise, benign prostatic hypertrophy

DIAGNOSTIC EVALUATION

The quantity of bleeding, the clinical setting, and other associated findings on the UA determine the extent of the evaluation. Dipstick testing may be too sensitive and lack specificity, since the presence of myoglobin or hemoglobin may lead to a false-positive result. A positive dipstick should be confirmed by microscopic examination. The presence or absence of dysmorphic RBCs, such as RBC casts or proteinuria, is important, since RBC casts or heavy proteinuria suggest bleeding from a glomerular source.

Pyuria, defined as more than four or five WBCs per HPF, points to infection as the cause. Even in asymptomatic individuals, the initial test for hematuria is a urine culture. An entirely normal repeat study after treatment of an infection in a healthy individual below 35 to 40 years of age usually requires no further evaluation other than a follow-up UA in 1 to 2 months. Similarly, a repeat UA to confirm the presence of hematuria in an individual suspected of having a benign cause, such as menstrual bleeding or vigorous exercise, is helpful before an extensive workup is begun. If interstitial nephritis is suspected, eosinophiluria may be present.

Persistent hematuria or hematuria in individuals over 40 years of age merits further investigation. In the absence of significant proteinuria (>2+ proteinuria), dysmorphic RBCs, or infection, hematuria usually indicates a structural abnormality of the urinary tract.

After obtaining routine chemistries, such as a CBC, platelet count, BUN, and creatinine, an intravenous pyelogram (IVP) is usually the initial test. This imaging procedure can detect stones, masses, cysts, and hydronephrosis. An ultrasound (US) study is an alternative for individuals who are allergic to contrast media, are at risk for contrast nephropathy, or have renal insufficiency. Suspicious lesions on IVP or US usually require further evaluation by CT or MRI and possibly biopsy. Rarely, renal arteriography is needed to evaluate a traumatic injury, a suspicious renal mass, and an arteriovenous (AV) malformation.

If imaging reveals normal upper tracts, cystoscopy is indicated in patients over 40 years of age. This procedure can detect bladder neoplasm, bladder stones, BPH, and cystitis. Since bladder cancer is rare in those under age 40, the value of cystoscopy is less certain in younger individuals. Urine cytology is a safe test that can detect some bladder cancers and may be an alternative in younger individuals. If performed on three consecutive first-voided morning urine specimens, it has a sensitivity of about 60% and a specificity of about 95%. Cystoscopy should still be considered in persistent hematuria, even in younger individuals, and in those with risk factors for bladder cancer, such as smoking or exposure to aniline dyes.

For patients with evidence of glomerular bleeding such as RBC casts or heavy proteinuria (>3 or 4+), a more extensive laboratory workup is indicated. Tests include an ESR, antinuclear antibody (ANA) test, cryoglobulin assay, antistreptococcal enzyme tests (ASO, anti-DNAse B), and an antineutrophil cytoplasmic antibody (ANCA) test to screen for Wegener granulomatosis and vasculitis. Plasma complement levels should be tested, since low levels are associated with SLE and poststreptococcal glomerulonephritis. Other useful tests include checking for eosinophiluria in patients with suspected interstitial nephritis and TB cultures in cases of persistent sterile pyuria. A hemoglobin electrophoresis can detect sickle cell disease and other hemoglobinopathies. Serum IgA levels may be helpful in patients suspected of having Berger disease or Henoch–Schönlein purpura. Serum antiglomerular basement membrane antibodies can be positive in Goodpasture syndrome, and serum and urine immunoelectrophoresis can help diagnose multiple myeloma.

TREATMENT

Management depends on the underlying cause. The presence of a defined lesion or the need to undergo cystoscopy merits referral to a urologist. Poststreptococcal glomerulonephritis therapy is generally limited to treating the associated hypertension. Rapid or progressive deterioration of renal function merits consultation. Most other patients with hematuria associated with proteinuria (>2+) or suspected glomerulonephritis warrant referral to a nephrologist for evaluation and consideration of renal biopsy.

Despite an extensive evaluation, no cause of hematuria can be found in 10% to 15% of patients. These individuals require long-term follow-up with monitoring of the urine sediment and renal function at 6-month intervals.

KEY POINTS

- Asymptomatic microscopic hematuria is defined as more than three RBCs per HPF.

- In patients below age 20, glomerulonephritis and urinary tract infection (UTI) are the most common causes of hematuria. In the age group between 20 and 40, one should consider UTI, stone, trauma, and neoplasm of the urinary tract. In the age group from 40 to 60, the most common cause of hematuria is bladder carcinoma, followed by kidney stone, UTI, renal carcinoma, and BPH.

- Familial causes of hematuria are benign familial hematuria, sickle cell disease or trait, polycystic kidney disease, Alport syndrome, and familial hypercalciuria.

Chapter 19

Jaundice in Adults

Jaundice (icterus) is yellow staining of the sclera, skin, and other tissues due to hyperbilirubinemia. Total serum bilirubin in a healthy person is normally 0.2 to 1.2 mg/dL and consists of both conjugated and unconjugated bilirubin. Jaundice becomes clinically evident when the bilirubin level reaches 2.0 to 2.5 mg/dL. Increased levels of bilirubin can be due to overproduction, impaired uptake by the liver, or impaired excretion. In adults, jaundice is most often due to liver disease or obstruction of the common bile duct.

EPIDEMIOLOGY

Hepatitis accounts for up to 75% of the cases of jaundice in young adults. Hereditary disorders such as Gilbert and Crigler–Najjar syndromes are less common causes of jaundice. Gilbert syndrome is a benign, lifelong condition and is often diagnosed early in life. It affects 3% to 5% of the population. Crigler–Najjar syndrome is a rare disorder that is also diagnosed early in life.

PATHOGENESIS

Bilirubin is the major breakdown product of hemoglobin. Bilirubin binds to albumin and is transported to the liver for conjugation with glucuronic acid to form bilirubin diglucuronide (conjugated bilirubin or direct bilirubin). After conjugation, the bilirubin is excreted through the biliary system into the small intestine. In the intestine, bacteria convert bilirubin to stercobilinogens, which give stool its brown color. Unconjugated bilirubin cannot pass the glomerular membrane; as a result, it does not appear in the urine. However, conjugated bilirubin (bilirubin diglucuronide) is water soluble and, when present in the urine, gives it a tea color. Bilirubinuria is typical of hepatocellular or cholestatic jaundice and results in a positive urine dipstick test for bilirubin.

An elevated bilirubin can either be unconjugated or conjugated. The causes of unconjugated hyperbilirubinemia are secondary to overproduction, hemolysis, or defects in bilirubin conjugation. Overproduction of bilirubin can be seen in diseases such as thalassemia, sideroblastic anemia, and vitamin B_{12} deficiency, all of which result in ineffective erythropoiesis. Gilbert and

Crigler–Najjar syndromes are characterized by a defect in the liver's ability to conjugate bilirubin, causing unconjugated hyperbilirubinemia. Decreased hepatic uptake of bilirubin, secondary to sepsis or right heart failure, can also elevate unconjugated bilirubin.

Impaired excretion of bilirubin from the liver causes conjugated hyperbilirubinemia. This can occur at the cellular level due to hepatocellular disease, in the ductule due to medication exposure (e.g., phenothiazines or estrogens), or in the septal ducts due to primary biliary cirrhosis. In addition, obstruction of the common bile duct by gallstones or pancreatic cancer can cause conjugated hyperbilirubinemia.

CLINICAL MANIFESTATIONS

HISTORY

The presence of right-upper-quadrant pain suggests a hepatobiliary cause. Nausea and vomiting accompanied by flulike symptoms preceding jaundice may indicate hepatitis. Other questions in the history of present illness should include the presence of pruritus, urine discoloration, increased abdominal girth (ascites), fever, and weight loss. Patients should be asked about intravenous drug use, alcoholism, contact with hepatitis patients, recent blood transfusions, recent travel, and prior history of immunizations. A family history of episodic jaundice in the setting of intercurrent illness is consistent with Gilbert disease. Current and past medicines and any herbal medicines should be noted. Drugs that may cause jaundice include acetaminophen, isoniazid, nitrofurantoin, methotrexate, sulfonamides, oral contraceptives, chlorpromazine, and phenytoin.

Patients with hereditary cholestatic syndromes or intrahepatic cholestasis may present with pruritus, light-colored stools, and malaise, or they may be totally asymptomatic. Patients with hepatitis may have malaise, anorexia, low-grade fever, and right-upper-quadrant pain. Also, the urine may appear tea-colored because of the excretion of conjugated bilirubin. Patients who present with right-upper-quadrant pain without fever may have an obstruction of the common bile duct, resulting in jaundice. In patients who present with Charcot triad (high fever, right-upper-quadrant pain, and jaundice), cholangitis must be ruled out.

Jaundice and weight loss are findings associated with carcinoma of the head of the pancreas.

PHYSICAL EXAMINATION

The physical examination should focus on signs of liver disease, such as spider angiomas, gynecomastia, and palmar erythema. The abdominal examination should assess for liver size, abdominal tenderness, and masses. Splenomegaly may be present, indicating hemolysis as a possible cause of jaundice. A palpable gallbladder (Courvoisier sign) indicates gallstones as a cause of jaundice. Viral hepatitis usually causes a mildly tender liver with slight to moderate enlargement. Findings such as a small liver, ascites, splenomegaly, spider angiomas, gynecomastia, palmar erythema, and other stigmata of cirrhosis suggest advanced hepatocellular disease. The eyes should be checked for Kayser–Fleischer rings, which indicate Wilson disease.

DIFFERENTIAL DIAGNOSIS

Box 19-1 lists the causes of jaundice grouped by pathophysiology. Obstruction, intrahepatic cholestasis, and hepatocellular disease cause the majority of cases of jaundice. In young patients, hepatitis is the most common cause of jaundice. In older individuals, obstruction from stones or tumors is more common.

DIAGNOSTIC EVALUATION

The diagnostic approach begins with the history and physical examination, which should provide clues as to the etiology of the patient's jaundice. Testing usually begins with a CBC, UA, and a liver panel test, including transaminases, total bilirubin, alkaline phosphatase, and albumin. An elevated conjugated bilirubin level and urine dipstick positive for bilirubin indicate obstruction, cholestasis, or hepatocellular injury. If the urine dipstick is negative for bilirubin, the cause is more likely a hemolytic process or a hereditary hyperbilirubinemia, most commonly Gilbert syndrome. Anemia with an elevated reticulocyte count, lactate dehydrogenase, fragmented RBCs on peripheral smear, and a low serum haptoglobin suggests hemolysis. Gilbert syndrome is characterized by a mild, recurrent elevation of bilirubin precipitated by fasting or mild illness without systemic symptoms or other liver test abnormalities.

In patients with elevated conjugated bilirubin, the pattern of the liver enzyme elevations provides clues to the cause of the jaundice. Transaminases elevated out of proportion (more than five times the normal) to the alkaline phosphatase suggest liver dysfunction. Conversely, an obstructive enzyme pattern is characterized by an elevated alkaline phosphatase (more than three times the normal) out of proportion to the rise in transaminases (less than four to five times the

BOX 19-1 Differential Diagnosis for Adult Jaundice
Unconjugated Hyperbilirubinemia
Increased production
Hemolytic anemia secondary to ineffective erythropoiesis
Thalassemia
Sideroblastic anemia
Pernicious anemia
Impaired uptake
Gilbert syndrome
Crigler–Najjar syndrome
Conjugated Hyperbilirubinemia
Hereditary cholestatic syndromes
Faulty excretion of bilirubin
Dubin–Johnson syndrome
Rotor syndrome
Hepatocellular dysfunction
Biliary epithelial damage
Hepatitis
Cirrhosis
Intrahepatic cholestasis
Drugs
Biliary cirrhosis
Sepsis
Biliary obstruction
Choledocholithiasis
Biliary atresia
Carcinoma of biliary duct
Sclerosing cholangitis
Pancreatic cancer

normal). Gamma glutamyl transpeptidase usually parallels the rise in alkaline phosphatase. This test is useful for confirming that an elevated alkaline phosphatase is caused by liver disease, since an increase in alkaline phosphatase can also occur in bone disease. A low serum albumin concentration suggests chronic liver disease.

If liver disease is suspected as the cause of jaundice, the following tests should be performed, as indicated by the history and physical examination:

1. Hepatitis profile to screen for hepatitis A, B, and C
2. Antimitochondrial antibody to screen for primary biliary cirrhosis

3. Serum iron, transferrin saturation, and ferritin to screen for hemochromatosis
4. Serum ceruloplasmin and urine copper levels to screen for Wilson disease
5. Antismooth muscle and antinuclear antibodies to screen for autoimmune hepatitis

Imaging tests are useful for patients with obstructive disease. US is a noninvasive test for detecting dilated bile ducts indicative of obstruction. The sensitivity and specificity of this test is in the range of 90% to 95%. Although a US can detect obstruction, it is less helpful in determining the site and cause of the obstruction. A CT scan or magnetic resonance cholangiopancreatography (MRCP) is more likely to identify the site or cause of obstruction but is more expensive than US.

If an obstruction is identified and additional anatomic detail is needed, endoscopic retrograde cholangiopancreatography (ERCP) can provide visualization. This test is also useful if obstructive jaundice is suspected despite negative imaging procedures. Complications of ERCP include infection and pancreatitis.

TREATMENT

The treatment of jaundice depends on the underlying disease process. Any drug that may cause jaundice should be discontinued. If there is complete resolution of laboratory abnormalities within 2 weeks of withdrawing the offending agent, no further workup or treatment is needed. Symptomatic pruritus can be treated with cholestyramine and antihistamines such as diphenhydramine. Pernicious anemia, which may cause a hemolytic anemia, can be treated with vitamin B_{12} replacement.

Patients with obstructive jaundice may have to be treated surgically. For patients with gallstones, either open or laparoscopic cholecystectomy is indicated.

In some cases of obstructive jaundice, an ERCP can be both diagnostic and therapeutic. Common bile duct stones may be removed via the endoscope or a stent placed to relieve the biliary obstruction, to reduce inflammation, and prepare a patient for surgery. Most patients with neoplasm require surgery. This surgery can either be palliative or intended for definitive treatment. Patients with obstructive jaundice and fever with chills must be hospitalized and treated for possible cholangitis with intravenous antibiotics.

Hepatitis can usually be treated on an outpatient basis. However, patients with severe nausea and vomiting who become dehydrated must be hospitalized.

KEY POINTS

- Jaundice becomes clinically evident when the bilirubin level is greater than 2.0 to 2.5 mg/dL.
- Hepatitis accounts for up to 75% of the cases of jaundice in younger adults.
- Biliary obstruction from gallstones or malignancy is more common in older patients.
- Drugs causing jaundice include acetaminophen, isoniazid, nitrofurantoin, methotrexate, sulfonamides, and phenytoin.
- Weight loss and painless jaundice are signs of pancreatic cancer.
- Low serum albumin in a jaundiced patient suggests a chronic process.

20 Knee Pain

Knee pain is most often due to acute trauma or overuse but can also be the result of degenerative disease, inflammatory arthritis, and crystalline arthropathies. Knowledge of the function and anatomy of the knee is essential in diagnosing and treating knee pain.

PATHOGENESIS

The knee is the largest joint in the body and performs a hingelike motion. The lateral and medial tibiofemoral articulations are the weight-bearing portions of the knee, whereas the patellofemoral articulation acts as a fulcrum for added quadriceps strength. The meniscal cartilage provides cushioning between the bones and a smooth surface for movement. The lateral and medial collateral ligaments provide lateral and medial stability to the knee joint, while the anterior and posterior cruciate ligaments, located inside the joint, provide anterior-to-posterior stability. The knee also has multiple bursae that provide lubrication for the many dynamic components of the knee and allow for fluid movement.

Injury or inflammation to either the soft tissue or the bony structures of the knee may cause pain. For example, inflammation of the bursae from either direct trauma or microtrauma associated with overuse can cause pain. Patellar tendonitis is another common cause of pain that results from overuse with activities such as running or jumping. Twisting injuries place stress on the cartilage and may result in a meniscal tear, while sprains of the medial and lateral collateral ligaments usually result from a direct blow to the knee while the foot is planted.

Patellofemoral pain syndrome occurs with overuse in combination with biomechanical factors, such as muscle imbalance. These factors cause improper tracking of the patella, which normally rests in the patellofemoral groove of the femur. Overuse and repeated impact with the knee in flexion lead to increased pressure in this groove and discomfort.

Osgood–Schlatter disease is a common cause of anterior knee pain in adolescents. The pain is located on the anterior tibial tubercle and is thought to be due to activities that increase traction on the patellar tendon. This stress leads to microavulsions of the growth plate on the tibial tubercle where the patellar tendon inserts.

CLINICAL MANIFESTATIONS

HISTORY

Depending on the cause of the knee pain, patients may also report swelling, erythema, limited range of motion, bruising, and decreased activity. If an injury caused the knee pain, the mechanism of injury (e.g., direct impact to the lateral knee during full extension), occurrence of a "popping" sensation, degree of swelling, and ability to ambulate after the event are all relevant pieces of information. The sensation of an unstable knee (the feeling of giving way) suggests damage to a ligament. Locking of the knee is more consistent with a torn meniscus or loose body that becomes trapped. Further useful history includes recent trauma, initiation of a new exercise regimen, duration of the knee pain, and a description of activities or positions that aggravate or alleviate the pain.

A sudden onset of severe knee pain and effusion in a middle-aged man without a history of trauma is most commonly due to gout. Often there is a previous history of a gout attack. Although patients with gout may have a fever, an elevated temperature with a swollen, red joint is more consistent with septic arthritis. In younger individuals, gonorrhea is the most common infection; it is, therefore, important to inquire about genitourinary symptoms, such as a vaginal or penile discharge.

Up to 10% of the population over age 65 suffers from symptomatic osteoarthritis of the knee. Obesity is a major risk factor. The pain is chronic, often starting in the anterior and medial portions of the knee, but it can involve the whole knee joint. Mild stiffness in the morning is common, which usually loosens up on moving about. Prolonged standing or walking may precipitate or worsen symptoms.

Prolonged morning stiffness and pain that is worse in the morning, improves with motion, and associated with systemic symptoms such as fever suggests an inflammatory arthritis. In rheumatoid arthritis, multiple symmetric joint involvement is the rule, although patients may develop pain only in the knee. Pain behind the kneecap that is worsened by standing up or climbing stairs is consistent with patellofemoral pain syndrome.

PHYSICAL EXAMINATION

Examination should be performed with the patient lying down in the supine position with both legs fully exposed. During general inspection, asymmetry, bruising, bony deformities, effusions, and erythema of the knee should be noted. The feet and hips should be examined for abnormalities contributing to or causing the knee pain. A key part of the examination is to determine whether the pain is intra- or extra-articular. Pain on both active and passive range of motion suggests an intra-articular problem, while pain on active but not passive motion of the joint suggests extra-articular disease. Palpation along the joint line and bony landmarks is followed by determining the degree of flexion and extension of both the healthy and injured knees. Pain during any segment of the examination provides clues as to which components of the knee may be injured. Varus and valgus stress while maneuvering the knee between full flexion and full extension are used to assess the medial and lateral collateral ligaments. Anterior-to-posterior laxity is assessed via the Lachman test. This maneuver is performed by flexing the knee at 20 to 30 degrees, holding the femur stable, and moving the tibia forward. The degree of laxity is assessed by comparison with the healthy knee and determines the competency of the cruciate ligaments. The McMurray test is used to evaluate the meniscus. This test is performed with the knee fully flexed and the foot rotated outward to test medial meniscus and inward to test lateral meniscus. The knee is then fully extended while rotating the foot in the opposite direction. A painful "click" is considered a positive test and indicates a possible meniscal injury.

DIFFERENTIAL DIAGNOSIS

Common diagnoses of knee pain include ligamentous injuries, meniscal injuries, bursitis (patellar, anserine), fractures, patellofemoral pain syndrome, Osgood–Schlatter disease, iliotibial band syndrome, Baker cyst, osteoarthritis, rheumatoid or other inflammatory arthritis, gout, pseudogout, and septic arthritis.

DIAGNOSTIC EVALUATION

Many patients can be diagnosed by history and physical examination alone. However, x-rays should be obtained in all patients who are thought to have a possible fracture and may help to determine the degree of arthritis. MRI is useful to diagnose rupture of the anterior cruciate ligament (ACL) and can often detect injury to the meniscus and collateral ligaments.

Laboratory testing may be helpful in evaluating patients with fever, rash, or involvement of other joints. An elevated ESR can be a clue to a systemic process. A rheumatoid factor and an ANA can help screen for rheumatoid arthritis and lupus. A CBC and UA level may also be helpful.

Acute isolated knee pain with an effusion should usually be evaluated with an arthrocentesis. The fluid should be sent for determination of cell count, glucose, Gram stain, culture, and examination for crystals. Uric acid crystals (negatively birefringent under polarized light) in the joint fluid are diagnostic of gout, while calcium pyrophosphate crystals (weakly positively birefringent) are seen in pseudogout. A bloody aspirate following trauma suggests a significant injury to the knee, and the rare finding of fat globules indicates a fracture. Diagnostic arthroscopy may be helpful in patients with persistent pain despite normal x-ray and laboratory testing.

TREATMENT

Rest and NSAIDs or acetaminophen are sufficient to manage the majority of patients with knee pain. In patients with mild-to-moderate degenerative joint disease (DJD), weight loss, judicious use of exercise and rest, physical therapy, and medications control most symptoms. Glucosamine sulfate may help treat symptoms of osteoarthritis in some patients. A series of intra-articular injections of hyaluronic acid for treatment of osteoarthritis can be useful for alleviating symptoms in patients with mild-to-moderate osteoarthritis. With severe DJD that is unresponsive to conservative therapy, referral to an orthopedist for possible surgery is appropriate.

Following a knee injury, acute pain usually responds to rest, ice, and NSAIDs. A knee immobilizer may provide support, reduce pain by restricting mobility, and prevent further injury. If there is suspicion of a more severe injury such as a meniscus or ligament tear, orthopaedic referral is appropriate.

Treatment of patellofemoral pain syndrome is geared toward the perceived causes. In patients with overpronation, orthotics are often beneficial. Relative rest, physical therapy, nonimpact activities, ice, and NSAIDs all benefit patients suffering from this disorder. Taping and patellar stabilizing braces may benefit those patients with obvious lateral subluxation.

NSAIDs usually improve the pain of inflammatory arthritis. Most family physicians will comanage individuals with rheumatoid arthritis along with a rheumatologist, especially those patients requiring disease-modifying medications (e.g., methotrexate). Joint infection is a medical emergency and merits hospitalization, drainage, and intravenous antibiotics. Gout usually responds to NSAIDs. Patients with multiple attacks may benefit from prophylactic therapy with allopurinol, probenecid, or colchicine. Colchicine or prednisone may be used for acute attacks in patients unable to take NSAIDs.

Osgood–Schlatter disease and soft tissue inflammatory conditions such as patellar tendonitis usually respond to treatment consisting of relative rest from activities that exacerbate the pain, application of ice, occasional use of NSAIDs, and range-of-motion and stretching exercises. Rarely, referral for surgical consultation and care is necessary.

A tear of the ACL is a more serious injury with long-term implications. Patients often report a "popping" sensation inside the knee related to a sudden change in direction or direct trauma. Patients will experience immediate pain, and a significant effusion typically develops within a few hours. In patients who want to remain active, surgical reconstruction is the preferred therapy. However, in older, less active patients, physical therapy and use of a brace may suffice.

Tears of the meniscus typically result from a twisting motion, but a clear event causing the injury may not always have occurred. Treatment of meniscal tears is symptomatic with rest, ice, compression, and elevation. Many patients with persistent symptoms benefit from arthroscopic knee surgery to remove the torn piece, thus allowing for smooth tracking between the articulated surfaces.

KEY POINTS

- The feeling of the knee giving way suggests damage to a ligament. Locking of the knee is more consistent with a torn meniscus or loose body that becomes trapped.
- A sudden onset of severe knee pain and effusion in a middle-aged man in the absence of trauma is most commonly due to gout.
- Up to 10% of the population over age 65 suffers from symptomatic osteoarthritis of the knee.
- Plain x-rays should be obtained in all patients who are thought to have a possible fracture. MRI is used to diagnose rupture of the ACL and can often detect injury to the meniscus and collateral ligaments.
- Acute isolated knee pain with an effusion should usually be evaluated with an arthrocentesis.
- A knee injury usually responds to rest, ice, and NSAIDs. A knee immobilizer may provide support, reduce pain by restricting mobility, and prevent further injury.
- NSAIDs usually improve the pain of inflammatory arthritis.

21 Lymphadenopathy

Lymphadenopathy is enlargement of the lymph glands, usually greater than 1 cm. Two exceptions are inguinal lymph nodes (LNs), which are considered normal up to 1.5 cm, and epitrochlear lymph nodes, which are considered enlarged if greater than 0.5 cm. Generalized lymphadenopathy is defined as enlargement of LNs in three or more noncontiguous areas. Regional lymphadenopathy exists when the swelling is limited to a specific region, such as the cervical lymph nodes.

PATHOGENESIS

Three mechanisms can produce enlarged LNs. First, LNs can increase in size due to reactive hyperplasia when cells within the gland respond to an antigen or inflammation. They also can increase in size if primary cells within the lymph gland transform into neoplastic cells and enlarge the gland as they proliferate. Finally, LNs may enlarge if there is an invasion of cells from outside the node, such as malignant cells from a metastatic cancer or from a benign infiltrating disorder, such as sarcoidosis.

CLINICAL MANIFESTATIONS

HISTORY

Lymphadenopathy usually causes no symptoms unless the nodes are acutely inflamed, large enough to cause lymphatic obstruction, or are pressing on a nerve or other structure. If symptoms are present, they usually relate to the underlying disease. Regional lymphadenopathy can be caused by a local infection or inflammation in the area drained by the lymph node. The history should focus on the area in question. For example, in the cases of cervical lymphadenopathy, asking about pharyngeal symptoms, dental problems, and hoarseness is appropriate.

Generalized lymphadenopathy requires a thorough history, since it is seen in a wide spectrum of diseases, including infections as well as immunologic, metabolic, and malignant disorders. Onset is important, since acute infection becomes a less likely cause as time passes. Constitutional symptoms such as fever and weight loss suggest cancer, systemic infection, or connective tissue disease. Recent rashes, arthralgias, pharyngeal symptoms, or pet exposure may suggest a specific diagnosis, such as connective tissue disease, viral illness, or cat scratch fever. Syphilis and AIDS should be considered in patients at risk for these infections. Lymphadenitis associated with lymphangitis is a common manifestation of bacterial infections in the extremities and is usually associated with pain and tenderness. Systemic symptoms such as fever and chills are common.

Risk factors for less common infections include contact with sheep (brucellosis), geographic locale (coccidioidomycosis or histoplasmosis), and animal bites (*Francisella tularensis* or *Pasteurella*).

PHYSICAL EXAMINATION

All LNs should be characterized by size, tenderness, texture, and consistency. Small, palpable cervical LNs (less than 1 cm) are common in children. Mild inguinal bilateral lymphadenopathy (less than 1.5 cm) is common throughout life. Box 21-1 lists characteristics associated with different etiologies and other clues on physical examination that may suggest a specific

---

■ **BOX 21-1** Lymphadenopathy Characteristics and Findings

Lymph Node Characteristics

Malignant: hard, matted, fixed, nontender, and usually greater than 3 cm

Infectious: warm, erythematous, fluctuant

Reactive: discrete, rubbery, and freely mobile

Key Findings of Associated Disorders

Thyromegaly: hyperthyroidism

Arthritis: connective tissue disease and leukemia

Massive splenomegaly: cancer, infectious mononucleosis, storage diseases, leukemia, and lymphoma

Skin rash: viral exanthem, connective tissue disease, and Kawasaki disease

etiology. Red streaks extending from a cellulitis toward a swollen, tender LN are consistent with lymphangitis and lymphadenitis.

Generalized lymphadenopathy is usually characterized by multiple, small, discrete LNs often associated with splenomegaly.

DIFFERENTIAL DIAGNOSIS

Generalized lymphadenopathy can be caused by infection, immunologic disorder, metabolic disease, malignancy, and miscellaneous inflammatory conditions. Common viral infections causing lymphadenopathy include infectious mononucleosis, cytomegalovirus (CMV), and HIV. Less common infections include TB, syphilis, histoplasmosis, and toxoplasmosis. Immunologic disorders include connective tissue disease such as SLE or rheumatoid arthritis and immunologic reactions such as a drug reaction or serum sickness. Metabolic disorders include hyperthyroidism and, rarely, storage diseases such as Gaucher and Niemann–Pick disease. Malignant causes of generalized lymphadenopathy include leukemia, lymphomas, metastatic carcinoma, and malignant histiocytosis. Additional causes include disorders such as Kawasaki disease and intravenous drug use.

The differential diagnosis of localized lymphadenopathy depends on the involved region. Cervical lymphadenopathy is the most commonly encountered form and is usually caused by infections, primarily URIs. Box 21-2 lists the differential diagnoses of lymphadenopathy by region.

DIAGNOSTIC EVALUATION

Lymphadenopathy is common and usually indicates benign, self-limited disease. This is particularly true in children and young adults who are prone to reactive lymphadenopathy. Localized lymphadenopathy usually represents disease from the area of drainage. For example, cervical LNs are commonly enlarged by infections involving the pharynx, salivary glands, and scalp. If it appears that the patient has a benign cause of lymphadenopathy, close observation or limited testing (e.g., a mononucleosis spot test [Monospot or strep screen]) is indicated to confirm the suspected diagnosis. In contrast, in individuals whose initial assessment suggests a malignant disorder, such as an enlarged cervical LN unassociated with an obvious infection in a patient with a history of smoking or alcohol abuse (both risk factors for head and neck squamous cell cancer), more extensive testing and consideration of an LN biopsy are indicated.

If the diagnosis is uncertain, stepwise testing with a CBC and serology is appropriate. A markedly abnormal CBC revealing a severe anemia or malignant

■ **BOX 21-2** Differential Diagnosis of Lymphadenopathy by Region
Cervical
Upper respiratory infection
Bacterial infection of head and neck
Mononucleosis
CMV
Toxoplasmosis
Mycobacterial infection
Neoplasm—primary and metastatic
Kawasaki disease
Sarcoidosis
Reactive hyperplasia
Supraclavicular Lymphadenopathy
Tuberculosis
Histoplasmosis
Sarcoid
Lymphoma
Metastatic disease, particularly lung and gastrointestinal
Axillary
Upper extremity infection
Connective tissue disease
Cat scratch disease
Neoplasm
Epitrochlear
Hand infection
Secondary syphilis
Inguinal
Local or lower extremity infection
Localized skin rash
Syphilis
Lymphogranularum venereum
Genital herpes
Chancroid
Cat scratch disease
Neoplastic disorders
Mediastinal Lymphadenopathy
Sarcoidosis
Tuberculosis
Histoplasmosis
Coccidioidomycosis
Lymphoma
Metastatic cancer

cells implies cancer and an urgent need for more complete evaluation, including bone marrow or LN biopsy. A CBC may also suggest infectious mononucleosis or a viral infection (atypical lymphocytes), pyogenic infection (granulocytes), or hypersensitivity states (eosinophilia). Serologic testing may be helpful, including a Monospot or EBV titers. Other serologic tests that may be helpful are those for CMV or toxoplasmosis titers, HIV antibodies, ANA, and rheumatoid factor. A chest x-ray is indicated in the presence of pulmonary symptoms, in severely ill patients, or in those with supraclavicular lymphadenopathy. A chest x-ray is also useful as a second level of evaluation for persistent undiagnosed lymphadenopathy. The presence of hilar lymphadenopathy suggests sarcoidosis, lymphoma, fungal infection, TB, or metastatic cancer. A positive TB skin test suggests mycobacterial infection. Urethral and cervical cultures can be helpful for determining the cause of inguinal lymphadenopathy. Culturing LN tissue or aspirated fluid may also be of value. Special stains can detect cat scratch disease and mycobacteria. Rarely, blood cultures are required in the cases of suspected bacteremia or unusual diseases such as tularemia, plague, and brucellosis.

Imaging studies such as US, CT, or MRI of the involved area may be useful to differentiate lymphadenopathy from nonlymphatic enlargement. A CT scan is used for evaluating hilar LNs or to demonstrate the presence of abdominal lymph nodes. Imaging may also identify a primary lesion that accounts for the regional lymphadenopathy. A bone marrow examination is indicated for patients with severe anemia, thrombocytopenia, or the presence of malignant cells on peripheral smear.

If there is clinical suspicion of a neoplasm or an illness such as TB or sarcoidosis and a diagnosis cannot be established, LN biopsy should be considered. Clinical factors such as LN size and irregularity, the presence of weight loss, or an enlarged liver or spleen suggest a need for an early biopsy. Enlarged supraclavicular LNs are often associated with serious underlying disease and usually require early biopsy. During follow-up for undiagnosed lymphadenopathy, LNs that remain constant in size for 4 to 8 weeks or fail to resolve in 8 to 12 weeks should be biopsied.

TREATMENT

Management is directed at the underlying cause. The treatment of viral infections is largely symptomatic. Cat scratch disease may benefit from antibiotics such as TMP/SMX. Nodes affected by atypical mycobacteria may need surgical excision combined with three antituberculosis drugs such as isoniazid, rifampin, and ethambutol. Initial therapy for acute lymphadenitis consists of antibiotics active against *Streptococcus* and *Staphylococcus*, such as a cephalosporin, erythromycin, or a semisynthetic penicillin such as dicloxacillin. Neoplastic disease should be referred to an oncologist for treatment.

KEY POINTS

- Generalized lymphadenopathy is defined as enlargement of LNs in three or more noncontiguous areas. Regional lymphadenopathy exists when the swelling is limited to a specific region, such as cervical LNs.

- Lymphadenopathy usually causes no symptoms unless the nodes are acutely inflamed, large enough to cause lymphatic obstruction, or are pressing on a nerve or other structure.

- Infection, immunologic disorder, metabolic disease, malignancy, and miscellaneous inflammatory conditions can cause generalized lymphadenopathy.

- Localized lymphadenopathy usually represents disease from the area of drainage.

Nausea and Vomiting

Nausea is the sensation of having to vomit and often precedes or accompanies vomiting. Vomiting, which can be either voluntary or involuntary, is the forceful expulsion of gastric contents through the mouth. In most instances in the family practice setting, the symptoms are caused by self-limited illness, such as viral gastroenteritis. However, vomiting can be a presenting symptom for a more serious illness.

PATHOGENESIS

Vomiting is under the control of two central nervous system (CNS) centers, the vomiting center in the medullary reticular formation and the chemoreceptor trigger zone in the fourth ventricle. Vagal nerve irritation and impulses from the sympathetic nerves in the throat, head, abdomen, and GI tract can send impulses to the vomiting centers. Vestibular disturbances, drugs, and metabolic abnormalities can activate the chemoreceptor trigger zone and cause vomiting. Efferent impulses from the CNS then travel to the effector muscles, causing a stereotypical vomiting response that varies little regardless of cause.

CLINICAL MANIFESTATIONS

HISTORY

A thorough history is critical to sorting out the many causes of nausea and vomiting effectively. It is important to characterize the duration, timing, frequency, and type of vomiting. Acute symptoms lasting less than 1 week suggest an infection, intoxication, drug effect, metabolic abnormality, or visceral disease. Early-morning nausea and vomiting are common with pregnancy but are also typical of vomiting associated with uremia and adrenal insufficiency. Symptoms precipitated by eating are common with GI disorders, such as acute gastritis, peptic ulcer disease, gastric outlet obstruction, or psychogenic factors. Vomiting several hours after eating can occur with diabetic gastroparesis, gastric outlet obstruction, or gastric malignancy, while vomiting immediately after meals suggests bulimia as a possible cause. Projectile vomiting may indicate pyloric stenosis in children or occasionally CNS disease causing increased intracranial

pressure. Characterizing the type of vomitus can be helpful. The presence of bile indicates an open pylorus, while feculent vomitus is seen in patients with a lower GI obstruction or gastrocolic fistula. Bloody or coffee-ground emesis indicates bleeding from the esophagus, stomach, or duodenum. Less commonly, bloody vomitus is seen in patients with blood swallowed from bleeding in the mouth or nose.

Nausea and vomiting accompanied by fever, watery diarrhea, and abdominal cramps are typical for viral gastroenteritis. Food poisoning usually begins within 6 hours of eating the offending substance and resolves within 24 to 48 hours. Abdominal pain may indicate a surgical problem, such as appendicitis or cholecystitis. Cramps may be caused by gastroenteritis or an early obstruction. Visceral pain syndrome—seen with MI, renal colic, and pancreatitis—can commonly cause nausea. Vestibular vertigo suggests an acute vestibular cause, such as labyrinthitis. Recurring vertigo, tinnitus, and vomiting are consistent with Ménière disease. Headache associated with vomiting is common with migraine.

The possibility of drug-induced nausea should always be considered. Common examples include macrolide antibiotics, metronidazole, opiates, NSAIDs, estrogen and other hormone preparations, digitalis, theophylline, and chemotherapeutic agents. The medical and surgical history often suggests possible causes. Diabetic ketoacidosis should always be considered in diabetic individuals with nausea and vomiting. A history of coronary artery disease or renal insufficiency raises the possibility that nausea and vomiting are caused by one of these conditions. Previous abdominal surgeries increase the risk of obstruction.

PHYSICAL EXAMINATION

The physical examination includes an overall assessment of appearance, vital signs, and volume status. Infants and elderly individuals are most prone to significant dehydration and electrolyte imbalance. The abdominal examination can provide clues to the underlying etiology in patients with abdominal pain. Localized tenderness may indicate a specific cause. For example, a large, tender liver suggests hepatitis. Tenderness with guarding, or rebound tenderness, occurs with peritoneal irritation. High-pitched bowel sounds are consistent with an early obstruction, whereas decreased or absent bowel sounds are consistent with peritonitis, ileus, or obstruction.

With vestibular disorders, head movement will reproduce the patient's symptoms of vertigo, nausea, and vomiting in association with the physical finding of nystagmus. A neurologic examination can detect signs such as papilledema, indicating increased intracranial pressure; ataxia, indicating a cerebellar disorder; or a stiff neck, suggesting meningitis.

DIFFERENTIAL DIAGNOSIS

In addition to GI diseases, the list of diseases that can cause nausea and vomiting encompasses a wide range of conditions (Table 22-1). The most common causes of acute nausea and vomiting in the family practice setting are infection, gastroenteritis, food poisoning, metabolic disorders, and medication side effects. The acute onset of nausea with severe abdominal pain suggests a more severe cause, such as obstruction, peritoneal irritation, and pancreatic or biliary disease.

Chronic nausea and vomiting are commonly related to structural lesions in the upper GI tract, such as peptic ulcer disease, gastroparesis, and gastric outlet obstruction. Other causes include metabolic abnormalities such as uremia or chronic hepatitis. Psychological causes are common in younger individuals, especially women. Persistent early-morning vomiting without another explanation such as pregnancy raises the possibility of increased intracranial pressure and an underlying neurologic disease.

DIAGNOSTIC EVALUATION

The history and physical examination may suggest a cause for nausea and vomiting, such as pregnancy, dietary indiscretion, labyrinthitis, gastroenteritis, food poisoning, or medications. In these instances, testing may be indicated only to confirm the diagnosis (e.g., pregnancy) or, in situations of more protracted vomiting, to check for electrolyte abnormalities. Significant volume depletion elevates the BUN and can cause hemoconcentration with a rise in hematocrit. Drug levels, such as a digoxin level, are useful in suspected drug toxicity. Liver function tests are useful when hepatitis is suspected. Visceral pain syndromes causing nausea, such as an MI or renal colic, usually have associated symptoms that indicate the need to investigate these possibilities. However, in diabetic individuals and the elderly, it is not uncommon for an MI to present primarily with nausea and vomiting. The threshold for obtaining an ECG in these individuals should be low.

Patients with nausea and vomiting may need imaging tests along with blood tests. Plain films can

TABLE 22-1 Differential Diagnosis for Nausea and Vomiting
Gastrointestinal
Gastroenteritis
Food poisoning
Biliary/cholecystitis
Intestinal obstruction
Pancreatitis
Appendicitis
Diverticulitis
Gastritis/peptic ulcer disease
Metabolic
Hepatitis
Renal failure
Diabetes mellitus (poorly controlled)
Adrenal insufficiency
Medications
Hormones (estrogen/OCPs)
Nonsteroidal anti-inflammatory
Macrolides
Metronidazole
Theophylline
Digitalis
Narcotics
Chemotherapy
Other
Pregnancy
Psychogenic
Migraines
Vestibular (Ménière, labyrinthitis)
Elevated intracranial pressure (e.g., pseudotumor cerebri, CNS malignancy)
Visceral
Myocardial infarction
Nephrolithiasis

help rule out an acute obstruction. A US can detect gallstones and changes compatible with pancreatitis. Testing for *Helicobacter pylori* antibodies may be helpful, since ulcer disease is a common cause of persistent nausea.

Chronic nausea and vomiting are most commonly related to structural lesions affecting the upper GI tract. Endoscopy and barium studies are helpful in identifying outlet obstruction and motility disorders. Evidence of extrinsic compression on a barium study may require a US or CT scan for further evaluation. Suspected gastoparesis can be confirmed with a nuclear study.

Persistent early-morning nausea in the absence of a pregnancy or metabolic disease raises the possibility of increased intracranial pressure; therefore, CT or MRI of the head should be considered. Recurrent vomiting of unknown cause may be due to a psychological problem. Indications of this include vomiting around mealtimes, inappropriate attention to body image, abnormal appetite, and a conflict-filled social environment.

TREATMENT

Management should be directed at the underlying cause. For most individuals with self-limited illnesses, simple dietary measures are sufficient. Typical dietary advice consists of advising clear liquids followed by small quantities of dry foods such as crackers. Nausea and vomiting resulting from medications are usually resolved by discontinuing the medication. If the drug is essential, decreasing the dosage of the medication or changing to an alternative medication may help reduce nausea.

Phenothiazines such as prochlorperazine (Compazine) and promethazine (Phenergan) are among the most commonly used drugs to treat nausea and vomiting; they are centrally acting agents that can control symptoms due to drugs, metabolic diseases, or gastroenteritis. Their most common side effects include sedation, but they can also cause extrapyramidal symptoms, especially in children. Trimethobenzamide (Tigan) is a nonphenothiazine centrally acting agent. The serotonin antagonists, such as ondansetron, are another useful category of medication that are commonly used with chemotherapy-related nausea and vomiting. In patients with vestibular symptoms, the antihistamine meclizine (Antivert) is helpful. Other antihistamines such as dimenhydrinate (Dramamine) or diphenolate are also effective. Antihistamines can cause drowsiness; thus, patients should be cautioned

about driving or operating machinery when taking these drugs.

Patients with motility disorders may benefit from a prokinetic agent such as metoclopramide (Reglan). Side effects include anxiety, extrapyramidal reactions, and, rarely, tardive dyskinesia. Scopolamine, an anticholinergic, is used primarily for the prophylaxis of motion sickness. It comes in the form of both a pill and a patch. Psychogenic vomiting is best managed with a psychiatric consultation.

Treatment of the nausea and vomiting of pregnancy depends on the severity of disease. Dietary manipulation, such as eating small, frequent meals that are bland, high in carbohydrates, and low in fat, may be helpful. Ginger, pyridoxine (vitamin B_6), and doxylamine may be useful in patients failing dietary therapy. If these treatments are ineffective, a trial of one of the phenothiazines (e.g., Compazine) is warranted.

Patients with evidence of significant dehydration or with a significant laboratory abnormality warrant intravenous fluids. Patients failing to benefit from intravenous fluids and medication may benefit from nasogastric suction to decompress the stomach.

KEY POINTS

- In most instances, patients seen in the family practice setting with nausea and vomiting have a self-limiting illness.

- Nausea and vomiting accompanied by fever, watery diarrhea, and abdominal cramps are typical of viral gastroenteritis.

- Common medications causing nausea include the macrolide antibiotics, metronidazole, opiates, NSAIDs, estrogen, digitalis, theophylline, and chemotherapeutic agents.

- Phenothiazines are commonly used centrally acting agents that help control nausea. Side effects include sedation and extrapyramidal symptoms, especially in children.

23 Painful Joints

The key to evaluating joint pain involves three issues: (1) Are the symptoms related to the joint or the periarticular structures? (2) Is the problem monoarticular or polyarticular? (3) Is the process inflammatory or noninflammatory?

PATHOGENESIS

Arthritis can result from degenerative processes or inflammatory disease. A noninflammatory disease, such as osteoarthritis, usually stems from the breakdown of cartilage and can eventually cause mechanical joint problems.

Inflammatory disease is mediated by cellular and humoral factors, such as prostaglandins, leukotrienes, interleukin-1, and tumor necrosis factor (TNF). Neutrophils, macrophages, lymphocytes, and other cellular mediators of inflammation are involved. Infection, crystalline arthritis, and the autoimmune diseases (e.g., rheumatoid arthritis [RA]) are examples of inflammatory arthritis. Periarticular symptoms involve tendons and muscles but may also present as joint pain.

CLINICAL MANIFESTATIONS

HISTORY

The number and location of joints involved are important. Monoarticular complaints make infection, gout, pseudogout, trauma, or toxic synovitis more likely. Multiple joint involvement suggests a connective tissue disease, osteoarthritis, or RA. Symmetric polyarthritis is consistent with RA. An acute onset of joint pain is most consistent with trauma, infection, or crystalline arthropathy, while a more prolonged course suggests osteoarthritis, RA, connective tissue disease, or fibromyalgia. RA and other connective tissue diseases are systemic diseases and symptoms such as fatigue and malaise are common associated complaints.

Factors affecting the pain are also important. Nocturnal pain in a single joint in a younger individual raises the possibility of a tumor. Pain that increases with use is consistent with osteoarthritis and tendonitis. Pain that decreases with use is more consistent with RA. Morning stiffness that lasts more

than 45 minutes suggests an inflammatory arthritis. Migratory patterns raise the possibility of rheumatic fever, disseminated gonococcemia, Reiter syndrome, and Lyme disease. Nonarticular pain usually does not produce loss of joint function and may cause pain only with movement in certain directions. In contrast, arthritic pain usually causes discomfort with all joint motions. Gout is characterized by the sudden onset of pain, erythema, limited range of motion, and swelling. The attack may be triggered by trauma, dietary or alcohol excess, or surgery.

Medications such as procainamide and isoniazid can cause a lupus-like syndrome. Clinical features such as fever, rash, oral ulcers, renal disease, and serositis suggest systemic lupus erythematosus (SLE). A complete review of systems is helpful to avoid overlooking symptoms such as dry eyes and dry mouth, which might suggest Sjögren syndrome, or urethritis, which is associated with Reiter syndrome. Table 23-1 lists clues from the history that suggest certain diagnoses.

PHYSICAL EXAMINATION

Many causes of arthritis have systemic manifestations. Skin manifestations of SLE include malar rash or mouth ulcers. Other skin lesions and associated illnesses include nail pitting and psoriatic arthritis, erythema migrans and Lyme disease, papulovesicular pustular lesions and disseminated gonococcemia, tophi and gout, heliotropic eyelid rash with dermatomyositis and SLE, and rheumatoid nodules with RA. Fingertip atrophy or ulcers along with calcinosis and telangiectasia are signs of scleroderma. Keratoderma blennorrhagia, a hyperkeratotic lesion on the palms and soles, and balanitis circinate, a shallow, painless ulcer on the penis, are signs of Reiter syndrome. Conjunctivitis and uveitis are suggestive of joint diseases associated with inflammatory bowel disease (IBD). The cardiopulmonary examination may reveal signs of an effusion, pleuritis, or pericarditis, which can be seen in RA and SLE. Splenomegaly can also be found in individuals with RA and SLE.

An inflamed joint is usually diffusely tender and there is often increased warmth, redness, and joint effusion. Noninflammatory joint disease usually has more focal tenderness and few signs of inflammation. Range of motion and joint deformity should

■ **TABLE 23-1** Diagnostic Clues for Arthritis	
Historical Clues	**Associated Disease**
Recent URI	Toxic synovitis
Recent sore throat	Rheumatic fever
Deer tick bite	Lyme disease
Recent Rubella immunization	Immunologic-related arthritis
Diarrhea	Inflammatory bowel disease
Podagra	Gout
Urethral discharge	Reiter disease or gono-coccal arthritis
Dry mouth/dry eyes	Sjörgren syndrome
Muscle weakness	Myositis
Photosensitivity	SLE
Heliotropic rash	Polymyositis/dermato-myositis
Low back pain	Ankylosing spondylitis
Conjunctivitis	Reiter syndrome
Uveitis	Inflammatory bowel disease
Older age	Gout, pseudogout
Younger age	Rheumatoid arthritis, SLE
Male	Gout, ankylosing spondylitis, Reiter disease, and hemochromatosis

■ **TABLE 23-2** Differential Diagnosis of Polyarthritis	
Inflammatory	**Noninflammatory**
Rheumatoid arthritis	Osteoarthritis
SLE	Amyloidosis
Gout	Sickle cell disease
Pseudogout	Hypertrophic pulmonary osteoarthropathy
Septic arthritis	Myxedema
Reiter syndrome	Hemochromatosis
Sarcoidosis	Paget disease
Lyme disease	
Gonococcemia	
Viremia	
Subacute bacterial endocarditis	
Psoriatic arthritis	
Scleroderma	

be noted. Irregular bony enlargements in the proximal and distal interphalangeal joints (Bouchard and Heberden nodes) are signs of osteoarthritis. A tender bony mass near a joint may be a sign of a tumor.

Examination of the periarticular tissues is important, since tendonitis, bursitis, and myositis can mimic joint pain.

DIFFERENTIAL DIAGNOSIS

The differential diagnosis can be approached by the number of joints involved and whether the process is inflammatory or not. Table 23-2 lists the differential diagnosis of polyarticular arthritis.

The differential diagnosis of monoarthritis includes infection, crystal-induced arthropathies (gout and pseudogout), trauma, and osteoarthritis. Gonorrhea is the most common infection causing septic arthritis. Another cause of monoarticular arthritis is solitary joint involvement of polyarticular arthritis, such as RA presenting in a single joint. Reiter syndrome, ankylosing spondylitis, psoriatic arthritis, colitis-associated arthritis, and viral synovitis often present with monoarticular arthritis.

DIAGNOSTIC EVALUATION

Arthrocentesis is the definitive diagnostic procedure for patients with monoarticular arthritis and joint effusion. Cloudy fluid suggests infection or crystalline disease, while bloody joint fluid following trauma suggests internal derangement. Joint fluid examination should include leukocyte count, Gram stain, culture, glucose, and an examination for crystals using polarized microscopy. Calcium pyrophosphate crystals, which cause pseudogout, are positively birefringent, while uric acid crystals, which cause gout, are negatively birefringent. Table 23-3 shows guidelines for determining whether or not the fluid is inflammatory.

Early in the course of arthritis, x-rays may be normal. Radiographic changes in osteoarthritis include nonuniform joint space narrowing, changes in the subchondral bone, and osteophytes. Osteoarthritic changes may be seen in the absence of symptoms, and the severity of the x-ray does not correlate with the degree of symptoms. RA usually affects the hands and wrists; x-rays of these joints can assist in establishing the diagnosis and assessing disease progression. Radiographic evidence of RA includes periarticular soft tissue swelling, periarticular osteopenia, uniform

TABLE 23-3 Joint Fluid Analysis

WBC (cells/mm³)	Interpretation
<2000	Noninflammatory (e.g., osteoarthritis)
2000–50,000	Mild to moderate inflammation (rheumatoid arthritis, crystalline arthritis)
50,000–100,000	Severe inflammation (sepsis or gout)
>100,000	Septic joint until proven otherwise

loss of joint space (nonuniform loss is more consistent with osteoarthritis), and bony erosions, which generally occur only after several months of active disease. Bony erosions can also be seen in septic arthritis and gout. MRI scanning is useful for diagnosing periarticular soft tissue injury.

In suspected inflammatory disease, an ESR is a useful but nonspecific measure of inflammation. A leukocytosis is common in patients with septic arthritis. RA is a clinical diagnosis and there are no laboratory tests, histologic findings, or radiologic findings that confirm the diagnosis of RA. However, a rheumatoid factor is positive in about 85% of the patients and helps establish the diagnosis in a patient with polyarthritis. Generally, the higher the rheumatoid factor titer, the more likely it is that the patient has RA. Up to 5% to 15% of normals are rheumatoid factor-positive, but usually in lower titers. Box 23-1 lists the criteria for diagnosing RA.

ANA testing is sensitive for SLE but lacks specificity, and low titers are often falsely positive. Titers greater than 1:160 or more are falsely negative in only about 5% of individuals. If an ANA is positive,

BOX 23-1 Diagnostic Criteria for Rheumatoid Arthritis

Morning stiffness greater than 1 hour
Arthritis in three or more joints
Involvement of the wrist, metacarpophalangeal (MCP), or proximal interphalangeal (PIP) joints
Symmetric arthritis
Rheumatoid nodules
Positive rheumatoid factor
Bony erosions on hand or wrist films
(Four or more criteria are needed for diagnosing rheumatoid arthritis)

testing for antibodies to double-stranded DNA (dsDNA) and for extractable nuclear antigens is indicated. Antibodies to dsDNA are present in about 70% of SLE patients and are very specific. Antibodies to the Smith antigen are also very specific for SLE but positive in only 30% of patients.

Routine chemistries are useful in assessing renal function and uric acid. A UA can screen for glomerular injury associated with connective tissue disease.

TREATMENT

Management depends on the underlying cause. The goals of treating arthritis are to alleviate pain, control inflammation, and prevent joint destruction. Regardless of the cause, physical therapy is often helpful for maintaining joint function, muscle strength, and mobility. In acute flares, it is important to protect the joint (e.g., splinting) to reduce pain and prevent future damage.

Septic arthritis requires appropriate antibiotics and drainage. The first line of pharmacologic therapy of osteoarthritis is acetaminophen. NSAIDs are effective but have more side effects. The symptoms of RA are treated with NSAIDs. Studies suggest that much of the

TABLE 23-4 Disease-Modifying Drugs for RA

Drugs	Side Effects
Nonbiologic disease-modifying drugs	
Methotrexate	Bone marrow toxicity, hepatitis, and stomatitis
Sulfasalazine	Rash
Hydroxychloroquine	Retinopathy
Gold	Glomerular toxicity, proteinuria, rash
Penicillamine	Bone marrow toxicity, proteinuria, rash
Azathioprine	Immunosuppression
Leflunomide	Bone marrow toxicity, immunosuppression, hepatitis
Biologic disease-modifying drugs	
Etanercept, infliximab, adalimumab	Immunosuppression
Anakinra	Immunosuppression
Abatacept	Immunosuppression
Rituximab	Bone marrow suppression; arrhythmias, renal failure, hepatitis

joint damage seen in RA occurs early in the course of the disease, and most experts recommend consulting with a rheumatologist and starting disease-modifying drugs (Table 23-4) such as methotrexate early in the course of RA. Corticosteroids in RA may be used as bridge therapy until other medicines take effect and may be given orally or in the form of a single joint injection. Biologic disease-modifying drugs have been recently approved for severe RA and are directed at interfering with cytokines. These drugs break the inflammation cascade by affecting the activity of TNF, interleukin-1, or other cytokines. Examples of biologic disease-modifying agents include Infliximab, a monoclonal antibody against TNF, and entanercept, a soluble receptor for TNF. SLE is treated with NSAIDs, corticosteroids, antimalarials, or azathioprine. Gout may be treated with NSAIDs, colchicine, or corticosteroids. NSAIDs are first-line agents and are given in high doses and then tapered over several days. If NSAIDs are contraindicated, either a short course of oral prednisone or an intra-articular injection of a corticosteroid is usually very effective. Colchicine exerts its effect by inhibiting the leukocyte phagocytosis of urate crystals. It is less favored than NSAIDs because of its slower onset and GI side effects. For patients with frequent attacks, allopurinol, which inhibits the formation of uric acid, or a uricosuric agent, such as probenecid, may be helpful.

KEY POINTS

- The key to evaluating joint pain involves three issues: (1) Are the symptoms related to the joint or to the periarticular structures? (2) Is the problem monoarticular or polyarticular? (3) Is the process inflammatory or noninflammatory?

- Morning stiffness that lasts more than 45 minutes suggests an inflammatory arthritis.

- The differential diagnosis of monoarthritis includes infection, crystal-induced arthropathies (gout and pseudogout), trauma, and osteoarthritis.

- Although RA is a clinical diagnosis, a rheumatoid factor is positive in about 85% of patients. Generally, the higher the rheumatoid factor titer, the more likely the patient has RA.

- Regardless of the cause, physical therapy is often helpful for maintaining joint function, muscle strength, and mobility.

- The first line of pharmacologic therapy of osteoarthritis is acetaminophen. NSAIDs are effective but may have more side effects.

24 Palpitations

The patient with palpitations has an abnormal awareness of the heartbeat. He or she may describe the palpitations as a fluttering, skipping, pounding, or racing sensation. Most palpitations are benign, but it is essential to identify those that are life-threatening.

PATHOGENESIS

Normally, individuals are unaware of the 60 to 100 heartbeats that occur each minute. Awareness of the heartbeat may occur when there are changes in the rate, rhythm, or contractility of the heart. Palpitations may occur as a result of cardiac or endocrine disease, an increase in sympathetic tone, or medications. Patients with underlying cardiac disease, such as valvular heart disease or a cardiomyopathy, may have altered conduction within the cardiac chambers or an increased automaticity of foci within the heart, leading to tachycardias such as atrial fibrillation or flutter. Disease within the conduction system may alter conduction of the cardiac impulses, resulting in either bradycardia or tachycardia. If impulses are blocked, a bradycardia will result. If a re-entrant circuit is present, then a tachycardia may result.

Hyperthyroidism causes a hyperkinetic state, and palpitations or tachycardias are associated with this disease. Pheochromocytoma is a rare adrenal disorder in which there are excess circulating catecholamines. These can cause sympathetic overstimulation, resulting in tachycardia and palpitations. Psychiatric conditions—such as anxiety, panic disorder, and depression—are also associated with increased sympathetic tone. Other noncardiac medical causes of palpitations include anemia and dehydration or hypovolemia.

Medications can affect cardiac conduction. Common medications associated with palpitations include theophylline, digoxin, beta agonists, antiarrhythmic medications, and OTC stimulants such as pseudoephedrine. Alcohol, tobacco, and illicit drugs such as cocaine can also cause palpitations.

CLINICAL MANIFESTATIONS

HISTORY

The patient's description of symptoms and associated complaints such as lightheadedness, dizziness, or syncope is important. Patients with palpitations and dizziness, near-syncope, or syncope may warrant hospitalization, monitoring, and aggressive evaluation. The onset and duration of symptoms may give clues to the cause. Paroxysmal episodes that begin and resolve abruptly are characteristic of paroxysmal arrythmias such as atrial fibrillation or supraventricular tachycardia. Isolated extra or pounding beats are characteristic of premature ventricular contractions (PVCs) or premature atrial contractions (PACs). The duration of symptoms as well as provocative or palliative factors may help in determining the cause. For example, sinus tachycardia and supraventricular tachycardias may be associated with exertion or emotional upset, whereas benign PACs or PVCs will often disappear with exertion. Medication use should be reviewed for possible toxicity or side effects. Diabetics may experience palpitations with hypoglycemic reactions. Patients taking stimulants by prescription or illicitly may experience palpitations as side effects. Alcohol use is associated with supraventricular tachycardia and atrial fibrillation. A review of systems should include assessment for other cardiac symptoms, pulmonary disease, abnormal bleeding, and symptoms suggestive of either thyroid or adrenal disease.

PHYSICAL EXAMINATION

The physical examination should include assessment of orthostatic changes. The pulse rate and any heart rhythm irregularity or extra beats should be noted. Pallor suggests anemia and exophthalmos or goiter may indicate hyperthyroidism. Special attention should be paid to the cardiopulmonary examination, including not only the rhythm but also the presence of rubs, murmurs, clicks, and gallops. A mental status examination—looking for signs of anxiety disorders, depression, or substance abuse—may provide clues to noncardiac etiologies.

DIFFERENTIAL DIAGNOSIS

Box 24-1 lists the differential diagnosis for palpitations and includes both cardiac and noncardiac etiologies. The majority of patients seen in the family practice setting will not have a cardiac etiology. Generalized anxiety disorder and panic disorder are the psychiatric disturbances most commonly associated

■ **BOX 24-1** Causes for Palpitations
Cardiac
PVCs
PACs
Paroxysmal supraventricular tachycardia/atrial fibrillation
Multifocal atrial tachycardia
Frequent PVCs/PACs
Ventricular tachycardia
Mitral valve prolapse
Sick sinus syndrome (tachycardia–bradycardia syndrome)
Cardiomyopathy
Prolonged QT interval syndrome
Ischemic heart disease
Wolff–Parkinson–White syndrome
Noncardiac
Exertion
Anxiety
Medications:
Theophylline
Beta agonists
Pseudoephedrine
Antiarrhythmic drugs
Tricyclic antidepressants
Phenothiazines
Stimulants/cocaine
Alcohol
Tobacco
Caffeine
Hypoglycemia
Hyperthyroidism
Pheochromocytoma
Anemia
Electrolyte imbalance
Dehydration
Fever
Pregnancy
Panic disorder
Anxiety
Somatization
Hyperventilation

with palpitations. Panic disorders are frequently associated with other psychiatric disorders such as agoraphobia, major depression, and substance abuse. Predictors of a cardiac etiology include male sex, report of irregular heartbeat symptom duration of greater than 5 minutes, and a history of heart disease. Isolated extra heartbeats or skipping of heartbeats suggest PACs or PVCs as the cause. Sudden onset and cessation of palpitations suggest paroxysmal supraventricular tachycardia. A less abrupt onset and cessation of palpitations are more common with stimulant or medication use. Sustained symptoms are associated with fever, dehydration, hyperthyroidism, or anemia. Some patients experience an exaggerated perception of sinus rhythm or palpitations. These patients are more likely to be female, have a fast heart rate, report palpitations during normal examination, and engage in lesser amounts of physical activity.

DIAGNOSTIC EVALUATION

Initial laboratory testing should include a hemoglobin, electrolytes, and TSH. Patients on medications such as digoxin should have levels checked. Blood glucose should be checked in diabetic patients. In selected patients, screening for a pheochromocytoma by measuring urine and serum catecholamines may be warranted.

Cardiac evaluation begins with a 12-lead ECG, which may detect an arrhythmia or abnormalities associated with arrhythmias. For example, a short PR interval and a delta wave occur with Wolff–Parkinson–White syndrome, which is associated with paroxysmal supraventricular tachycardias. Abnormalities in atrial or ventricular voltages and Q waves may signify the presence of underlying cardiac disease.

Further, cardiac evaluation often includes echocardiography to assess cardiac anatomy. Information can be gained about atrial and ventricular size, valvular abnormalities, ventricular systolic function, and whether hypertrophic subaortic stenosis or wall motion abnormalities are present. A 24-hour Holter monitor records the cardiac rhythm for 24 hours and can detect an arrhythmia. During this period, the patient keeps a log of symptoms, and correlation with the monitor recording will show the heart's rhythm at the time of symptoms. For patients who do not have daily symptoms or those who did not have symptoms while the monitor is being worn, an event monitor may be an effective tool. Event monitors can be carried for 30 days or more and are patient-activated at the time of symptoms. The event recording can be transmitted by telephone to a monitoring station.

Stress testing should be considered for patients who have symptoms in association with exercise or who describe chest pain or pressure. Finally, invasive electrophysiologic study should be considered in syncopal or near-syncopal patients with heart disease and those with suspected ventricular tachycardia or heart block. Electrophysiologic study may document the abnormality and direct therapy.

TREATMENT

Therapy will be directed by the underlying cause of the palpitations. Patients with panic disorder may benefit from treatment with tricyclic antidepressants or selective serotonin reuptake inhibitors (SSRIs). SSRIs have a slow onset of action and bridge therapy with either anxiolytics or beta blockers may be needed for 4 to 6 weeks until antidepressant therapy becomes effective. Patients with anemia will need further evaluation for its cause. Treatment of underlying hyperthyroidism, anxiety, infection, and dehydration will resolve symptoms in patients affected with these diseases. For many patients, adjustment of medication or insulin dosages and avoidance of stimulants such as caffeine may resolve symptoms.

Treatment of supraventricular tachycardias may include use of medications (beta blockers or calcium channel blockers) or catheter ablation of any identified bypass tracts. Patients with chronic or intermittent atrial fibrillation usually merit anticoagulation with warfarin to prevent thromboembolism. Younger, low-risk patients with atrial fibrillation and no history of hypertension, CHF, coronary artery disease, or history of transient ischemic attacks (TIAs) or a CVA

may be treated with aspirin. Malignant ventricular arrhythmias may be treated with antiarrhythmics along with implantation of an automatic implantable cardiac defibrillator. Isolated PVCs or PACs do not require treatment but may be treated for symptom relief with medications such as beta blockers. If an antiarrhythmic drug is used, consultation with a cardiologist is often helpful, since therapy can be complex and arrhythmia is a side effect of many of these drugs. Angioplasty or bypass surgery may be required for individuals with severe coronary artery disease.

KEY POINTS

- The patient with palpitations has an abnormal awareness of the heartbeat, in terms of either the rate or intensity of the perceived heartbeat.

- Palpitations may occur due to the presence of cardiac or endocrine disease, increase in sympathetic tone, fever, dehydration, or medications.

- Cardiac evaluation should include a 12-lead ECG, echocardiography, monitoring (Holter, event monitor), and, in selected patients, stress testing or electrophysiologic study.

- Therapy is directed by the identified underlying cause.

25 Pharyngitis

Sore throat, or pharyngitis, is a common reason for visits to family physicians' offices. There are many potential causes for pharyngitis, including viral and bacterial infections, allergies, gastroesophagal reflux, thyroiditis, smoking, and other irritants. A careful history and physical examination can help determine which patients need further evaluation. Appropriate laboratory investigations can help identify the cause of these symptoms.

PATHOGENESIS

Bacteria and viruses are responsible for causing most cases of infectious pharyngitis and are spread from person to person either by inhalation of airborne particles or by exposure to respiratory or oral secretions. Winter and early spring are peak seasons for sore throat. The incubation period for symptoms to develop may be as short as 24 to 72 hours.

The most common etiologic viral agents are respiratory viruses, such as adenovirus, parainfluenza virus, and rhinovirus. Pharyngitis associated with infections with these agents is usually part of a broader upper respiratory tract infection causing rhinorrhea, cough, and often conjunctivitis. Herpangina, characterized by tonsillar and palatal ulcerations, is caused by Coxsackievirus. Infectious mononucleosis caused by EBV may present with pharyngitis alone or with fever, posterior cervical lymphadenopathy, and malaise. The herpesvirus can also cause a pharyngitis or stomatitis.

Streptococcus pyogenes (group A strep) pharyngitis accounts for about 10% of infectious cases in adults and as many as 35% in children. It typically presents with fever and sore throat that is self-limited. Immunologically mediated complications of streptococcal infection include acute rheumatic fever and glomerulonephritis. Rheumatic fever can lead to long-term valvular heart disease, such as mitral stenosis, unless treated within 10 days of onset. Acute glomerulonephritis is self-limited and prompt antibiotic therapy does not prevent this complication. Serious local complications include peritonsillar and retropharyngeal abscesses that result from tissue invasion by group A strep. These infections may lead to deeper infections and airway compromise.

Other bacteria that may lead to self-limited pharyngitis, either alone or as part of a respiratory infection, include *Mycoplasma*, *Chlamydia*, *Haemophilus*, and *Corynebacterium*. Pharyngitis may occur in association with sinusitis. Fungal pharyngitis may occur in immunocompromised patients, and gonococcal pharyngitis may occur as a sexually transmitted disease with oral sex.

Noninfectious causes of pharyngitis include sleep apnea, GERD, and cigarette smoke through primary irritant effects. Allergies may cause lymphoid hyperplasia, nasal obstruction, and postnasal drip, which can lead to pharyngeal irritation.

CLINICAL MANIFESTATIONS

HISTORY

Streptococcal infection most commonly occurs in children from 5 to 15 years of age and is rare in children below age 3. Mononucleosis is classically a disease of teenagers. The history should include associated symptoms and known exposures to illness. For example, only 25% of patients with positive strep cultures will have rhinorrhea and cough. The presence of these symptoms and a low-grade fever suggests a viral etiology. The classic symptoms for streptococcal infection are fever over 101°F (38.3°C) in association with a sore throat but few other respiratory symptoms. The chronicity of the disease is also helpful in determining its cause. Viral and uncomplicated bacterial infections resolve in about 1 week, whereas noninfectious causes are more persistent. Early-morning sore throat without fever or other associated symptoms suggests a noninfectious cause such as GERD.

Past medical history may suggest potential causes or lead to consideration of less common ones. For example, patients with a history of allergies may be experiencing a sore throat related to the allergies. Immunocompromised patients may develop fungal infection or complications with bacterial infection (e.g., peritonsillar abscess). Greenish exudates and dysuria with pharyngitis are present in gonococcal pharyngitis. Patients with sandpaper-like exanthems with a "strawberry tongue" may have scarlet fever, which is associated with group A beta-hemolytic streptococci. A past history of rheumatic fever with or without carditis warrants evaluation for recurrence of streptococcal disease.

Group A streptococcus may lead to rheumatic fever. A rare complication is poststreptococcal glomerulonephritis. Other complications are peritonsillar abscess, retropharyngeal abscess, meningitis, pneumonia, bacteremia, otitis media, sinusitis, cervical lymphadenitis, and scarlet fever.

PHYSICAL EXAMINATION

Vital signs and an examination of the ears, nose, and throat are essential parts of the evaluation. The throat in classic group A strep infection is erythematous with tonsillar exudates. There are often palatal petechiae and there may be a "strawberry tongue," with prominent red papillae on a white-coated tongue. Tender cervical lymphadenopathy is often present. The physical examination should also include a lung examination, since many patients also have respiratory symptoms. Patients with a history of a previous streptococcal infection may present with symptoms and signs of rheumatic fever. They may present with joint swelling, pain, subcutaneous nodules, erythema marginatum, or a heart murmur. Mononucleosis, gonococcal infection, and on occasion other bacterial or viral infections may, on pharyngeal examination, be indistinguishable from streptococcal pharyngitis. About half of the patients with mononucleosis have splenic enlargement on abdominal examination. Vesicular lesions suggest either herpesvirus or Coxsackievirus infection, while adenovirus often causes an accompanying conjunctivitis. Diphtheria is characterized by an adherent gray membrane, low-grade fever, tonsillitis, and tender cervical lymphadenopathy. Kawasaki disease affects children who are below 5 years of age. Signs and symptoms include conjunctivitis, a strawberry tongue, fever, and a rash involving the hands and feet. The rash leads to desquamation of the palms.

DIFFERENTIAL DIAGNOSIS

Most patients with an acute pharyngitis have either a viral or a bacterial infection. Table 25-1 lists differentiating features of viral versus bacterial pharyngitis. Common viruses include adenovirus, parainfluenza virus, rhinovirus, Coxsackievirus, herpes, CMV, and EBV. In addition to group A strep, other streptococcal bacteria (groups C and G) may cause pharyngitis but are not associated with the complications of group A. Other bacteria including *Gonococcus*, *Chlamydia*, *Mycoplasma*, *Corynebacterium*, and less commonly pneumococci, staphylococci, fusobacteria, and *Yersinia* can also cause pharyngitis. Fungi may cause infection in immunosuppressed patients. An unusual but important cause of pharyngitis is the retroviral syndrome (HIV).

■ TABLE 25-1 Characteristics of Viral versus Bacterial Pharyngitis

Signs and Symptoms	Viral	Bacterial
Conjunctivitis	More common	Less common
Malaise and fatigue	More common	Less common
Hoarseness of voice	More common	Less common
Low-grade fever	More common	Less common
High-grade fever	Less common	More common
Diarrhea	More common	Less common
Abdominal pain	More common	Less common
Rhinorrhea	More common	Less common
Cough	More common	Less common

Noninfectious causes of pharyngitis should be suspected in patients without fever and with persistent or recurring symptoms. Common noninfectious causes of pharyngitis include sleep apnea, gastroesophageal reflux, allergies, and referred pain from primary otologic or dental disease. Uncommon but important noninfectious causes include malignancy, aplastic anemia, lymphoma, and leukemia.

DIAGNOSTIC EVALUATION

Physical examination alone cannot accurately determine whether a bacterial infection is present. Options in testing for group A strep include rapid antigen detection assays, used in many offices, and throat culture. Throat culture is the "gold standard" test and is considered definitive. Rapid tests are reported to have a sensitivity of 80% to 90% and a specificity of over 90%. Testing for gonococcal pharyngitis requires a throat swab inoculated in Thayer–Martin media. Fungal infection may be identified by use of a slide prepared with potassium hydroxide (KOH) stain or may be detected on routine throat cultures.

Testing is also commonly performed for mononucleosis. Heterophile antibody testing, commonly known as the **Monospot test**, is available in many offices. Although the Monospot test may be positive as early as 5 days into the infection, it can take up to 3 weeks to convert to positive. Alternatively, EBV IgM antibodies may be elevated as early as 2 weeks after infection. In patients presenting with suspected mononucleosis and an initial negative test, repeat testing may be necessary.

TREATMENT

Streptococcal pharyngitis should be treated in order to prevent rheumatic fever, prevent suppurative complications, and decrease person-to-person spread of the infection. The treatment of choice for strep throat is penicillin, either as a 10-day oral course or a single intramuscular injection. For patients allergic to penicillin, clindamycin, erythromycin, or a newer macrolide such as azithromycin may be used. For treatment failures, amoxicillin-clavulanic acid or clindamycin is commonly used.

Treatment for viral pharyngitis is largely supportive and symptomatic. Lozenges and warm saltwater gargles may provide topical relief. Analgesic drugs such as acetaminophen or ibuprofen can help reduce pain. The treatment of gonococcal infections is covered in Chapter 52.

KEY POINTS

- There are many potential causes of pharyngitis, including viral and bacterial infections, allergies, and irritants.
- Evaluation and testing for infectious etiologies is largely targeted toward identification of group A strep infection because of its association with complications such as rheumatic fever.
- The treatment of choice for strep throat is penicillin, whereas treatment for the other causes of pharyngitis is largely symptomatic.

26 Proteinuria

Proteinuria in adults is defined as protein excretion greater than 150 mg per 24 hours; in children, proteinuria varies with the child's age and size. Nephrotic-range proteinuria is defined as the daily excretion of more than 3.5 g of protein over 24 hours. The causes of proteinuria range from benign conditions such as orthostatic proteinuria to life-threatening conditions such as glomerular nephritis and rapidly progressive renal failure. Proteinuria is often first identified as an incidental finding on UA during a routine office visit.

PATHOGENESIS

The glomerulus allows the easy passage of water while providing a barrier to protein excretion. Each day the normal glomerular filtrate contains between 500 and 1500 mg of low-molecular-weight proteins. Most of these proteins are resorbed and metabolized by the renal tubular cells. Since urine testing may turn positive at 100 mg/mL, normal individuals may test trace-positive for proteinuria on an office dipstick.

Significant proteinuria can occur from glomerular damage and increased filtration of normal plasma proteins, renal tubular diseases that affect resorption, and overflow proteinuria. Glomerular disease can be either primary or secondary. Primary glomerular diseases include minimal change disease, focal glomerular sclerosis, membranous glomerular nephropathy, and IgA nephropathy. Secondary causes include infections such as poststreptococcal glomerular nephritis and systemic diseases such as SLE or a drug-related effect on the glomerulus. Overflow proteinuria occurs when there is production of abnormal proteins, such as Bence–Jones proteins as seen in multiple myeloma, which easily pass through the glomerulus. The type of protein found in the urine differs depending on the cause. Glomerular disease usually results in excess albumin excretion, while tubular disease is associated with an array of low-molecular-weight proteins. Plasma proteins are found in multiple myeloma or monoclonal gammopathy.

Functional proteinuria may occur in association with fever, strenuous exercise, seizures, abdominal surgery, epinephrine administration, and CHF without evidence of intrinsic renal disease. The proteinuria is related to changes in renal hemodynamics that result in increased glomerular filtration of plasma proteins. The proteinuria usually resolves within several days of the inciting event and is not associated with progressive disease.

CLINICAL MANIFESTATIONS

HISTORY

Proteinuria can be either transient or persistent. Persistent proteinuria is defined as the presence of proteinuria on at least two separate occasions. Orthostatic or postural proteinuria accounts for 60% of patients with asymptomatic proteinuria. Typically, patients are less than 30 years old and have protein secretion of less than 2 g/day; and the proteinuria occurs when the patient is in the upright position but normalizes in the supine position. Nephrotic-range proteinuria (>3.5 g/24 hours) is usually the consequence of glomerular damage.

Proteinuria can either be primary or occur in the setting of renal or systemic diseases. Patients with glomerular nephritis usually present with hematuria, RBC casts, and mild-to-moderate hypertension. These patients typically have proteinuria and edema, but not as severely as patients with nephrotic syndrome. Nephrotic syndrome consists of massive proteinuria, hypoalbuminemia, hyperlipidemia, lipiduria, and edema.

The focus of the history is to determine the possible causes of proteinuria and assess the severity of the condition. Edema suggests nephrotic-range proteinuria, and hypertension indicates the possibility of significant renal disease. The history may reveal the presence of systemic illnesses that are associated with proteinuria, such as long-standing diabetes mellitus, SLE, CHF, multiple myeloma, and amyloidosis. A detailed review of medications is important, since medications such as penicillin and cephalosporins may cause proteinuria. Other medications causing proteinuria include ACE inhibitors, cyclosporines, NSAIDs, heavy metals, aminoglycosides, and sulfonamides. Heroin abuse is also a cause. Chronic renal disease suggests possible polycystic disease. Dysuria and frequency along with a fever indicate a possible urinary tract infection (UTI).

PHYSICAL EXAMINATION

Skin changes such as malar rashes, vasculitis, and purpura can be signs of a connective tissue disease. Diabetic retinopathy is strongly associated with proteinuria and the fundi should be carefully examined. Looking for lymphadenopathy, heart failure, abdominal masses, hepatosplenomegaly, and peripheral edema as well as measuring blood pressure are important parts of the physical examination. Fever may be present in infectious causes.

DIFFERENTIAL DIAGNOSIS

The differential diagnosis for proteinuria is extensive. Benign transient proteinuria is a common problem that resolves spontaneously and is most often seen in children or young adults. Exercise, CHF, fever, UTI, and orthostatic proteinuria are common causes of transient proteinuria in patients without significant renal disease.

Although individuals may have isolated proteinuria without other urinary symptoms or disease, persistent isolated proteinuria suggests underlying glomerular or tubular disease. Primary renal diseases include acute renal failure, acute tubular necrosis, acute glomerular nephritis, and polycystic disease. The systemic illnesses listed in Box 26-1 can all cause proteinuria. Diabetes, in particular, is an important cause of proteinuria. About one-third of type 1 and one-fourth of type 2 diabetics have persistent proteinuria. Drugs and toxins that cause proteinuria include

■ **BOX 26-1** Systemic Illnesses Causing Proteinuria
Amyloidosis
Carcinoma
Cyroglobulinemia
Diabetes mellitus
Drugs/toxins
Goodpasture syndrome
Henoch–Schönlein purpura
HIV-associated nephropathy
Leukemia
Lymphoma
Multiple myeloma
Polyarteritis nodosa
Pre-eclampsia
Sarcoidosis
SLE
Transplant nephropathy

antibiotics, analgesics, anticonvulsants, ACE inhibitors, and heavy metals. Infectious causes include bacterial (subacute bacterial endocarditis [SBE], syphilis, post-streptococcal glomerular nephritis), viral (CMV, EBV, HIV, and hepatitis B), and parasitic diseases (malaria and toxoplasmosis). About 50% to 75% of the cases of nephrotic-range proteinuria are due to intrinsic renal disease. The remainder are due to systemic illnesses such as diabetes, SLE, amyloidosis, and other diseases that cause glomerular injury.

DIAGNOSTIC EVALUATION

A urine dipstick is a simple, readily available screening tool for proteinuria. A 1+ protein level usually represents approximately 300 mg/dL of protein excreted per 24 hours. A 4+ usually indicates over 1 g/dL per day. A urine dipstick reacts to albumin and can fail to detect abnormal proteins such as Bence–Jones proteins. A sulfosalicylic acid test measures the total concentration of proteins, including Bence–Jones proteins. False-positive dipstick results can be seen with dehydration, gross hematuria, or highly alkaline urine.

If the patient has two or more positive dipstick tests, a 24-hour urine protein collection is indicated, along with a urine creatinine clearance determination. If orthostatic proteinuria is suspected, an orthostatic test should be performed. The patient is instructed to urinate and discard the first morning urine before a collection. A 16-hour daytime collection should stop before bedtime, followed by an overnight specimen collection. Patients with true orthostatic proteinuria have elevated proteinuria during the day that returns to normal at night.

A total 24-hour protein excretion exceeding 1 g suggests significant renal impairment. A qualitative urine protein electrophoresis to rule out a monoclonal component is indicated. Further evaluation includes a complete UA, a chemistry panel (including a BUN, creatinine, albumin, and total protein), lipid profile, ESR, antistreptolysin O (ASO) titer, and a C3-C4 complement level. The presence of RBC casts in the urine indicates glomerular disease. WBC casts may be seen in pyelonephritis and interstitial nephritis. Oval fat bodies, if present, are due to lipiduria, as seen in nephrotic syndrome. A chemistry panel will identify electrolyte imbalances and assess renal function. The CBC identifies a normocytic normochromic anemia, as seen in chronic renal insufficiency or multiple myeloma. Serum complement levels are low in acute glomerulonephritis and lupus nephritis. An ESR screens for connective tissue diseases and other inflammatory states. ASO titers indicate whether there has been a recent streptococcal infection. An ANA, hepatitis panel, rapid plasma reagin (RPR) test, HIV testing, and serum protein electrophoresis should be ordered selectively based on the history, physical examination, or previous laboratory results. An ultrasound is helpful in determining kidney size, ruling out polycystic kidney disease or masses, and detecting an obstructive nephropathy.

TREATMENT

Treatments for proteinuria depend on the underlying cause. Transient proteinuria is very common in children and young adults and disappears with repeat testing. Long-term studies indicate that both transient proteinuria and orthostatic proteinuria are benign conditions that require no treatment.

Those with renal insufficiency, nephrotic-range proteinuria, hematuria or RBC casts, or an uncertain underlying cause should be referred to a nephrologist. Patients with nephrotic syndrome also are more susceptible to atherosclerosis, thrombotic processes, and infection by encapsulated bacteria. They require pneumococcal vaccine (Pneumovax) and treatment for dyslipidemia. A nephrologist may perform a renal biopsy to rule out treatable forms of glomerulonephritis, such as membranous glomerulonephropathy, which may respond to steroids or immunosuppressive therapy. ACE inhibitors benefit patients with diabetes and proteinuria. Asymptomatic patients with low-range proteinuria may be observed with periodic blood pressure monitoring and an annual assessment of renal function. Referral to a nephrologist should be considered if renal insufficiency or hypertension develops.

KEY POINTS

- Proteinuria in adults is protein excretion greater than 150 mg per 24 hours. Nephrotic-range proteinuria is the excretion of more than 3.5 g of protein over 24 hours.

- Patients who have glomerular nephritis generally present with hematuria or RBC casts, and mild-to-moderate hypertension. Nephrotic syndrome consists of massive proteinuria, hypoalbuminemia, hyperlipidemia, lipiduria, and edema.

- Diabetes is an important cause of proteinuria. About one-third of those with type 1 and one-fourth of those with type 2 diabetes have persistent proteinuria.

- A total 24-hour protein excretion exceeding 1 g suggests significant renal impairment.

- Patients with renal insufficiency, nephrotic-range proteinuria, hematuria or RBC casts, or proteinuria of uncertain etiology should be referred to a nephrologist.

Red Eye

A red eye is the most common ophthalmologic complaint encountered by family physicians. Most cases are benign, self-limited conditions that can be treated by the family physician. However, a few conditions that cause red eye are sight-threatening, such as corneal ulceration, iritis, and glaucoma. The family physician must recognize these and, if necessary, refer the patient to an ophthalmologist.

PATHOGENESIS

Redness of the skin around the eye may result from diseases that can affect the skin elsewhere or from inflammation of structures unique to the eye. Infection or occlusion of glandular structures—namely, the meibomian glands, glands of Zeis, or nasolacrimal duct—can cause swelling and redness of the eyelid or periorbital structures. Infection of the meibomian glands is termed internal hordeolum, whereas an external hordeolum or sty is an infection of the gland of Zeis. Sterile inflammation of the meibomian gland due to glandular occlusion is termed a chalazion. Blepharitis is infection, inflammation, and scaling of the eyelid margins. Occlusion of the nasolacrimal duct with secondary infection is referred to as dacryocystitis. Infection may also spread to the orbital or periorbital region from sinus infections, leading to orbital or periorbital cellulitis.

The conjunctiva is a thin, transparent vascular tissue that lines the inner aspect of the eyelids (palpebral conjunctiva) and extends over the sclera (bulbar conjunctiva) before terminating at the limbus, where it is continuous with the corneal epithelium. A healthy conjunctiva is the first barrier to infection from the outside, which is why external infections of the eye commonly cause an inflammation or hyperemia of the subconjunctival vessels. This causes the conjunctiva to appear erythematous and injected, hence the term "red eye." Other ocular inflammatory conditions, such as iritis or glaucoma, can also manifest as a red eye due to hyperemia of the ciliary vessels of the sclera through the transparent conjunctiva. Another cause of red eye is a subconjunctival hemorrhage, which is a benign condition that results from bleeding in the small fragile vessels of the conjunctiva, usually in response to minor trauma or straining. However, conjunctivitis is by far the most common cause of red eye.

CLINICAL MANIFESTATIONS

HISTORY

A careful history should include a thorough ocular, medical, and medication history. The ocular history should focus on the type of discomfort, changes in vision, presence of discharge, duration of symptoms (acute, subacute, or chronic), unilateral or bilateral involvement, contact with anyone having similar ocular symptoms, and any specific environmental or work-related exposure. In addition, particular attention should be given to the following ocular symptoms: pain, visual changes (blurred vision/photophobia), and the type of discharge.

The type of discomfort helps determine the need for urgent referral to an ophthalmologist. Pain suggests a more serious ocular pathology, such as acute angle-closure glaucoma, iritis, keratitis, scleritis, uveitis, corneal ulceration, or orbital cellulitis. Discomfort associated with conjunctivitis is often described as burning, tearing, or irritating. Itching is the hallmark of allergic conjunctivitis, but it can also be present in viral or bacterial conjunctivitis. Visual changes suggest serious ocular disease and are not seen with conjunctivitis or subconjunctival hemorrhage. Discharge is a common finding in patients with conjunctivitis and the type of discharge, purulent or mucoid, may help in distinguishing bacterial from viral or allergic causes of conjunctivitis. A history of trauma or a gritty feeling in one eye associated with pain may suggest a foreign body or corneal abrasion.

PHYSICAL EXAMINATION

The eyelids and periorbital region should be checked for erythema and inflammation. Next, examine the conjunctiva for a pattern of any redness detected. Conjunctival erythema may be due to subconjunctival hemorrhage, conjunctival hyperemia, or the presence of a "**ciliary flush**." Subconjunctival hemorrhage is a collection of blood under the conjunctiva and is bright red, with distinct borders. Conjunctival hyperemia is diffuse erythema of the conjunctival lining with no borders and involves both the bulbar and palpebral conjunctiva. The term "ciliary flush" refers to a violaceous hyperemia of the vessels surrounding the cornea; along with photophobia and a sluggishly reactive pupil, this flush is a sign of iritis.

Note the presence, quality, and quantity of any discharge. Examine each pupil, looking for any irregularities in shape or size in comparison to the other pupil and its reactivity to light. Evaluate the intraocular movement and then, with the ophthalmoscope, inspect the cornea for opacities, surface irregularities, or foreign bodies. Assess the optic disk for an increase in the cup-disk ratio, which may signify the presence of glaucoma. An important part of the examination is checking visual acuity with a Snellen eye chart.

DIFFERENTIAL DIAGNOSIS

The most common causes for red eye include hordeolum, chalazion, blepharitis, corneal abrasion, subconjunctival hemorrhage, and conjunctivitis. One should also be familiar with the signs and symptoms of glaucoma and iritis, so that a prompt referral for therapy can be provided. These diseases are described in Table 27-1. Other less common causes of red eye include scleritis, episcleritis, anterior uveitis, and keratitis, all of which require ophthalmologic referrals.

DIAGNOSTIC EVALUATION

Initial assessment involves a thorough physical examination, including ophthalmoscopic examination. When a patient presents with ocular pain, corneal ulceration or laceration must be ruled out by a fluorescein dye test. To perform this test, apply fluorescein dye to the lower eyelid (drops or impregnated strip) and view the cornea under a cobalt-blue light searching for disruptions of the corneal epithelium (ulcers or lacerations).

Most cases of conjunctivitis are self-limited and the cost–benefit ratio for culturing the eye discharge precludes its routine use. The conjunctiva has a bacterial flora composed of many species, including *Staphylococcus aureus* and, less commonly, *Corynebacterium* and *Streptococcus* species. Some healthy patients may also harbor *Pseudomonas* and fungi as a part of their normal conjunctival flora. Infectious conjunctivitis is usually due to a viral

■ TABLE 27-1 Differential Diagnosis of Red Eye

Disease	Description	Other
Blepharitis	Chronic lid margin erythema, scaling, loss of eyelashes	Associated with staphylococcal infection, seborrheic dermatitis
Hordeola/chalazion	Painful nodules on or along lids	Hordeola associated with staphylococcal infection; chalazion-sterile
Conjunctivitis	Burning, itching, discharge, lid edema	
Viral	Clear, mucoid discharge	Associated with upper respiratory infection; very contagious
Hyperacute bacterial	Copious purulent discharge	Potentially sight-threatening; associated with gonorrhea, sexually transmitted disease (STDs), neonates
Acute bacterial	Moderate purulent discharge	*Haemophilus influenza*, staphylococcal, *Streptococcus pneumoniae*
Inclusion conjunctivitis	Persistent watery discharge	Chlamydia; neonates and young adults, associated with STDs
Allergic	Itching, tearing	Associated with other allergy symptoms
Subconjunctival hemorrhage	Nonblanching red "spot," painless without visual changes or discharge	Associated with trauma, cough, or Valsalva (e.g., straining)
Corneal abrasion/foreign body	Pain, "foreign body" sensation	Abrupt, associated with incident or work exposure
Iritis	Pain, photophobia, papillary constriction, cloudy cornea, and anterior chamber	Associated with connective tissue diseases, ocular injury
Acute angle-closure glaucoma	Pain, tearing, dilated pupil, shallow anterior chamber, halos around lights	Ocular emergency, more common over age 50

infection, but about 5% of the time it is bacterial. In severe cases, in the very young, or in patients who do not respond to therapy, cultures may be useful. A Gram stain of the discharge may help to identify a bacterial agent. Multinucleated giant cells are suggestive of a herpes infection. Tonometry to measure intraocular pressure is useful in a suspected case of acute glaucoma. In a patient with suspected serious orbital or periorbital cellulitis, a CBC and imaging, such as an orbital CT scan, may be indicated.

TREATMENT

Therapy for blepharitis generally involves measures aimed at eyelid hygiene. Specifically, use of a mild soap, such as a baby shampoo, diluted with water to scrub the lids, is recommended. Additional measures may include the use of warm compresses and a topical antibiotic ointment.

The inflammation and pain from a hordeolum or chalazion may respond to the use of warm compresses. A hordeolum may also respond to topical antibiotic therapy. If an associated cellulitis is present, systemic antibiotics that are active against *S. aureus*, the most common pathogen, are indicated. A chronic chalazion may require intralesional steroid injections or surgical drainage for resolution. Hordeola rarely require incision and drainage for treatment.

Treatment recommendations for conjunctivitis are presented in Table 27-2. For hyperacute bacterial conjunctivitis, prompt, aggressive treatment is necessary to avoid sight-threatening complications. Viral conjunctivitis is self-limited, lasting 7 to 10 days. Although many clinicians prescribe antibiotic drops for these infections, there is only modest evidence that this practice shortens the duration of symptoms. Ninety-five percent of patients shed the virus for up to 10 days after the onset of symptoms. All patients should receive advice regarding hygiene, such as avoiding eye–hand contact, good hand-washing habits, and using a personal face cloth and towel in order to limit the spread of the infection.

Subconjunctival hemorrhage requires no treatment and will usually resolve over several days. Treatment for a foreign body includes removal with the help of a topical anesthetic for the eye and a moistened cotton swab. If the foreign body cannot be removed, an ophthalmology referral is indicated.

Patients with iritis and acute glaucoma need urgent referral to an ophthalmologist. After thorough ophthalmologic examination, therapy for iritis often involves use of cycloplegic and anti-inflammatory (e.g., topical steroids) medications. Acute medical treatment for glaucoma usually involves acetazolamide 500 mg and topical 4% pilocarpine ophthalmic solution to constrict the pupil. Patients with apparent benign conditions whose symptoms persist or recur should also be referred to an ophthalmologist.

TABLE 27-2 Therapy for Conjunctivitis

Etiology	Treatment
Viral	Local measures: cool compresses
Herpes	+/– Oral antiviral, topical antiviral (e.g., acyclovir) ophthalmology referral
Bacterial	Local measures Gonococcal conjunctivitis requires systemic antibiotics (e.g., IV or IM ceftriaxone) Chlamydial conjunctivitis requires 2–3 weeks of oral therapy (e.g., erythromycin or doxycycline)
Allergic	Local measures Allergen avoidance Topical or systemic antihistamines (e.g., loratadine, levocabastine)

KEY POINTS

- The most common cause of red eye is conjunctivitis.
- The most common etiology of conjunctivitis is viral; this is a self-limited but extremely contagious condition.
- In conjunctivitis, a purulent discharge usually indicates a bacterial infection, while a watery discharge is more consistent with an allergic or viral etiology.
- Itching is the hallmark of allergic conjunctivitis.
- Acute angle-closure glaucoma must be considered in patients over 50 years of age with a painful red eye.
- Suspected corneal ulceration, iritis, and glaucoma are sight-threatening and should be referred to an ophthalmologist.

28 Respiratory Infections

Respiratory tract infections are the leading cause of illness among children and adults. Clinically, it is useful to distinguish between upper and lower respiratory tract infections. URIs consist of infections affecting the respiratory structures above the larynx. Lower respiratory tract infections (LRIs) encompass the trachea, bronchi, and pulmonary structures.

EPIDEMIOLOGY

URIs include the common cold, sinusitis, and pharyngitis. Adults average two to four colds per year. Although most individuals with these conditions do not seek medical care, they are still among the most common reasons for family physician visits. Rhinoviruses account for 30% to 50% of the cases of the common cold; coronaviruses represent another 10% to 20%. The remaining cases are either due to an unidentifiable virus or a host of viruses including influenza, parainfluenza, respiratory syncytial virus, and adenovirus. Laryngitis is viral in origin in 90% of the cases, most commonly due to influenza, rhinovirus, adenovirus, or parainfluenza virus. The etiologic agents of pharyngitis and otitis media are described in Chapters 25 and 72, respectively.

LRIs include bronchitis and pneumonia. Bronchitis is an inflammation of the lining of the bronchial tube. Viral infections cause approximately 95% of bronchitis cases in healthy adults. Nonviral causes include chemical irritation, *Mycoplasma*, and *Chlamydia*.

Pneumonia is defined as inflammation of the lung parenchyma. In the United States, there are over 4.5 million cases of community-acquired pneumonia (CAP) each year; about one-third of these require hospitalization. Pneumonia is the sixth leading cause of death.

PATHOGENESIS

Most URIs are caused by viruses, which replicate in the nasopharynx and cause inflammation as well as edema, erythema, and nasal discharge. Transmission occurs primarily by hand contact with the infecting agent.

Sinusitis is an infection that occurs when inflammation and swelling of the mucosal membranes block the ostia draining the sinuses, thus allowing pooling of mucus and bacterial proliferation. Sinusitis may also occur if anatomic abnormalities such as polyps obstruct the ostia. Occasionally, sinusitis results from a dental abscess. Bronchitis is characterized by edematous mucosal membranes, increased bronchial secretions, and diminished mucociliary function. Acute exacerbations of chronic bronchitis are frequently precipitated by a viral infection, but bacteria colonizing the airway appear to play a role in the infection.

Pneumonia is an inflammation of the terminal airways, alveoli, and lung interstitium, usually from infection. The primary mechanism by which pneumonia occurs is through the aspiration of oropharyngeal secretions colonized by respiratory pathogens. Aspiration of gastric contents and hematogenous spread are less common. Factors that predispose an individual to develop pneumonia are abnormal host defenses (e.g., malnutrition, immunocompromise), altered consciousness (which can lead to aspiration), ineffective cough (as is seen in patients with neuromuscular diseases or following surgery), and abnormal mucociliary transport (which is seen in smokers, COPD patients, and following a viral bronchitis).

CLINICAL MANIFESTATIONS

HISTORY

The clinical symptoms of a cold are well known and typically begin with a scratchy sore throat followed by sneezing, nasal congestion, and rhinorrhea. General malaise, fever, hoarseness, cough, low-grade fever, and headache are also frequent symptoms. The acute syndrome usually resolves in about 1 week; however, a cough may persist for several weeks.

Persistent purulent nasal discharge, facial pain exacerbated by leaning forward, and a maxillary toothache are symptoms of sinusitis. Many patients with acute sinusitis may experience "double sickening," with improvement in their cold symptoms followed by a relapse with increased pain and nasal discharge.

Acute bronchitis usually presents with a productive cough and is often accompanied by URI symptoms. Low-grade fever and fatigue are common.

Pneumonia may present with symptoms very similar to those of bronchitis. However, patients with pneumonia are more likely to have a high fever, experience dyspnea and chills, have chest pain, and develop complications such as hypoxia or cardiopulmonary failure. Common organisms for CAP in previously healthy adults are *Streptococcus pneumoniae, Haemophilus influenzae, Mycoplasma pneumoniae,* and *Chlamydia pneumoniae.*

In patients with suspected pneumonia, it is important to obtain a history of underlying diseases such as diabetes mellitus, COPD, asthma, alcohol abuse, and HIV. It is also important to inquire about recent travel, seizures, and environmental or occupational exposures. HIV positivity increases the likelihood of an opportunistic infection, as by *Pneumocystis carinii,* CMV, fungus, or *Mycobacterium tuberculosis.*

PHYSICAL EXAMINATION

The history and physical examination are often sufficient to make the diagnosis. Important examination elements include measuring vital signs, an ear, nose and throat (ENT) examination, palpation of the neck and sinuses, and a thorough cardiopulmonary examination.

Patients with URIs usually have a swollen, red nasal mucosa. Fever accompanied by purulent nasal discharge, facial tenderness, and a loss of maxillary transillumination suggest sinusitis. Although most patients with bronchitis will have clear lungs, some may have rhonchi, hoarse rales, or wheezing. Patients with pneumonia are more likely to have abnormal vital signs such as fever, tachypnea, tachycardia; they tend to look more ill. The vital signs and general appearance are also important in assessing the degree of illness. Marked abnormalities of the vital signs and poor general appearance suggest the need for hospitalization. Although the lungs may be clear in patients with pneumonia, usually there are abnormalities such as localized rales, bronchial breath sounds, wheezing, or signs of consolidation such as dullness to percussion.

DIFFERENTIAL DIAGNOSIS

The diagnosis of a cold is usually self-evident. Occasionally, allergic or vasomotor rhinitis can be confused with a URI. Influenza should be differentiated from the common cold, since specific treatment may be effective. The differential diagnosis of acute sinus pain includes dental disease, nasal foreign body, and migraine or cluster headache. Table 28-1 lists some clinical features that help to distinguish between pneumonia and bronchitis.

TABLE 28-1 Distinguishing Features of Lower Respiratory Tract Infections

Bronchitis	Pneumonia
Antecedent URI	Acute onset of cough, fever, and tachypnea
Cough	
No or low-grade fever	Chest pain
Clear lungs or coarse rhonchi	Leukocytosis
Normal chest x-ray	Pulmonary infiltrate on chest x-ray

Although most patients with fever, cough, and an infiltrate on chest x-ray have an infection, noninfectious causes should also be considered. These include cardiac disease, pulmonary embolus, atelectasis, and malignancy. Generally, the presentation of noninfectious causes tends to be more insidious and the patient is afebrile.

DIAGNOSTIC EVALUATION

Most patients with URIs are diagnosed clinically. Blood testing or imaging is not required for patients with acute sinusitis unless they appear toxic or have a complication of sinusitis, such as orbital cellulitis or cavernous thrombosis. CT is the imaging procedure of choice and is also indicated in patients with chronic sinusitis, recurrent sinusitis, poor response to therapy, those with a possible tumor, and those planning to undergo surgery.

If pneumonia is suspected by history and physical, a chest x-ray is indicated. This can distinguish between bronchitis and pneumonia, assess the extent of disease, detect pleural effusions, and help distinguish between infectious and noninfectious causes. Laboratory tests for suspected pneumonia include a CBC, electrolytes, BUN, creatinine, pulse oximetry, sputum for Gram stain and culture, and liver function tests. Patients admitted to the hospital should have blood cultures and—based on the clinical evaluation—HIV and serology testing (e.g., *Legionella* testing) may be indicated. Urinary antigen testing (e.g., *S. pneumoniae* and *Legionella*) can help guide treatment decisions.

TREATMENT

URIs

Fluids, rest, and either NSAIDs or acetaminophen to relieve pain and fever help to relieve URI symptoms.

■ BOX 28-1 Initial Treatment of Rhinosinusitis

Hydration with increased fluid intake, saline nasal spray
Over-the-counter decongestants, analgesics
Topical nasal decongestants for no more than 3–4 days
Guaifenesin may provide some benefit
For symptoms persisting longer than 7–10 days or other signs or symptoms of bacterial infection, consider antibiotics.
First-line: amoxicillin, cefuroxime
Penicillin allergy: clarithromycin, azithromycin, trimethoprim/sulfamethoxazole
Second-line: amoxicillin/clavulanic acid, levofloxacin, gatifloxacin

Sympathomimetics such as pseudoephedrine can reduce nasal congestion. Topical decongestants (e.g., phenylephrine) have fewer side effects than oral decongestants, but their use must be limited to 3 to 4 days to avoid tolerance and rebound congestion. Ipratropium bromide nasal spray is an anticholinergic agent that reduces rhinorrhea but is of limited benefit in reducing congestion. Vitamin C and zinc supplementation may shorten the duration of symptoms. The treatment of sinusitis should be directed toward improving drainage and eradicating pathogens. Decongestants, hydration, analgesics, warm facial packs, humidification, and sleeping with the head of the bed elevated are useful adjunctive measures. Mucolytics such as guaifenesin may be of benefit. Most patients with a URI have some element of sinusitis that is self-limited and will resolve with symptomatic care. If symptoms persist for more than a week, antibiotics are usually started and administered for 10 to 14 days. Amoxicillin or TMP/SMX is suitable for initial therapy. For patients allergic to these medications, cephalosporins, macrolides, or quinolones may be substituted. Most individuals respond within 5 days of initiating treatment. Box 28-1 summarizes the initial treatment of rhinosinusitis.

For patients who fail to respond, a broader-spectrum antibiotic is indicated. For individuals whose symptoms persist despite therapy, a CT scan and ENT referral is appropriate. In toxic-appearing patients or those with suspected complications such as osteomyelitis, orbital cellulitis, or intracranial disease, urgent hospitalization and consultation are indicated.

LRIs

Treatment for bronchitis includes symptomatic care with fluids, decongestants, smoking cessation, and cough suppressants. Although controversial, some authorities advocate using antibiotics for severe or persistent cases of bronchitis.

In patients with pneumonia, an important consideration is the locus of care. Box 28-2 lists some indications for hospitalization. For those patients suitable for outpatient therapy, antibiotics are started and close monitoring is begun. If possible, therapy is guided by the sputum Gram stain results. However, these stains are often impractical or unobtainable in the outpatient setting, so that most family physicians start empiric antibiotic therapy. For healthy adults less than 60 years old, erythromycin or a newer extended-spectrum macrolide such as azithromycin is a suitable choice. Doxycycline is an acceptable, less expensive alternative. For patients over age 60, a fluoroquinolone with good activity against *Pneumococcus* (e.g., levofloxacin), a newer macrolide, or a second-generation cephalosporin is a good choice for empiric therapy. Since infection with an atypical pathogen is unlikely in children 2 months to 5 years of age, the recommended outpatient treatment for them is high-dose amoxicillin (80 to 90 mg/kg/day) for 7 to 10 days. Older children should be treated with a macrolide because of the increased incidence among them of *Mycoplasma* and *C. pneumoniae* infections.

■ BOX 28-2 Indications for Hospitalization

Systolic blood pressure less than 90
Pulse rate greater than 140
PO_2 less than 90% or 60 mmHg
Presence of abscess or pleural effusion
Marked metabolic abnormality
Concomitant disease such as CHF Renal failure Malignancy Diabetes mellitus COPD
Age greater than 65
Unreliable social situation

KEY POINTS

- Adults average two to four colds per year. Rhinoviruses account for 30% to 50% of the cases of the common cold; coronaviruses for another 10% to 20%.

- Common organisms for CAP in previously healthy adults are *Streptococcus pneumoniae*, *Haemophilus influenzae*, *Mycoplasma pneumoniae*, or *Chlamydia pneumoniae*.

- A chest x-ray can distinguish between bronchitis and pneumonia, assess the extent of disease, detect pleural effusions, and help distinguish between infectious and noninfectious causes.

- Blood tests or imaging is not required for patients with acute sinusitis unless they appear toxic or have a complication of sinusitis, such as orbital cellulitis or cavernous thrombosis.

- Erythromycin or a newer extended-spectrum macrolide (e.g., azithromycin) or doxycycline is a suitable choice for healthy adults less than 60 years old with pneumonia. For patients over age 60, a fluoroquinolone with good activity against *Pneumococcus* (e.g., levofloxacin), a newer macrolide, or a second-generation cephalosporin is suitable for empiric pneumonia therapy.

Shortness of Breath

Dyspnea, defined as a sensation of difficult or uncomfortable breathing, is a common complaint associated with a variety of different underlying causes. Presentations may vary from acute dyspnea, associated with MI or PE, to a chronic dyspnea, associated with CHF or COPD. The manner and location in which a patient may present will likewise vary. For example, the patient with acute dyspnea is more likely to present to an acute care setting, such as the emergency room. Patients with chronic dyspnea will more likely present to an office setting for evaluation and care. This chapter discusses acute dyspnea briefly and focuses more on chronic causes.

PATHOGENESIS

Dyspnea may be caused by one of several different mechanisms. In general, dyspnea occurs when the perceived demand for oxygen or respiration is not being met or when the work of breathing is increased. For example, with a pneumonia or PE, the lungs' ability to provide sufficient oxygen to the peripheral and central chemoreceptors is diminished and the patient experiences the sensation of dyspnea. Other causes associated with limitations in respiration or oxygen delivery include CHF, interstitial lung disease, pulmonary hypertension, and severe anemia. With obstructive lung disease, such as asthma, the patient may have a normal or near-normal PO_2 and decreased PCO_2 and yet experience dyspnea due to the increased work of breathing. Other mechanical causes for dyspnea include obesity, pleural effusion, ascites, and kyphoscoliosis. Finally, anxiety may cause the patient to hyperventilate and perceive this increased respiratory effort as dyspnea.

CLINICAL MANIFESTATIONS

HISTORY

The onset, progression, associated diseases, and symptoms of dyspnea direct the evaluation of the patient. Patients presenting with acute and rapidly progressive symptoms should be questioned about chest pain, history of cardiopulmonary disease, fever, and recent surgery or travel. These patients should, in general, be directed or sent to the emergency room setting, where they can be monitored and promptly evaluated for cardiopulmonary causes such as pneumonia, MI, and PE.

Patients with chronic dyspnea, a gradually developing course, or episodic dyspnea may be evaluated in the outpatient setting. The patient should be asked about any past history of cardiac or respiratory disease. Patients with a history of asthma, COPD, or CHF may be experiencing exacerbations of their underlying disease. Associated symptoms should be noted. For example, substernal chest pressure in association with dyspnea occurs with angina. A patient who complains of a swollen leg in association with dyspnea may be experiencing a PE. Patients with a history of melena or dysfunctional uterine bleeding may be experiencing dyspnea due to severe anemia. Inquiries about stress and symptoms of perioral numbness and paresthesias help assess whether anxiety is the cause of symptoms.

PHYSICAL EXAMINATION

The physical examination should focus on the heart and lungs. Heart examination should note the rate and rhythm of the heart in search of arrhythmias, such as atrial fibrillation, that may trigger dyspneic symptoms. The presence of murmurs along with an S_3 may indicate CHF as the cause. Peripheral edema may be a sign that fluid overload is contributing to the patient's symptoms.

The lung examination should note respiratory rate and effort as indicated by the use of the accessory muscles. Inspection should note the chest and abdominal contours, looking for the barrel-chested appearance of COPD or the stigmata of cirrhosis and ascites. Percussion should be performed to assess for possible pleural effusions. Auscultation for the presence of rales, wheezing, rubs, or diminished breath sounds should be performed in the assessment for cardiopulmonary causes.

DIFFERENTIAL DIAGNOSIS

The differential diagnosis can be divided into acute and chronic dyspnea. Box 29-1 presents some of the common causes for dyspnea. Anxiety or cardiopulmonary causes account for the majority of patients

■ **BOX 29-1** Common Causes for Dyspnea

Acute Dyspnea
Bronchospasm
Pulmonary edema
Pulmonary embolism
Pneumothorax
Pneumonia
Myocardial infarction
Acute anxiety attack/panic disorder
Anemia
Upper airway obstruction
Chronic Dyspnea
Congestive heart failure
Chronic obstructive pulmonary disease
Asthma
Interstitial lung disease
Pulmonary hypertension
Pleural effusion
Obesity
Ascites
Kyphoscoliosis
Anemia
Anxiety
Lung mass

with dyspnea; asthma, COPD, pneumonia, and CHF are the most frequent cardiopulmonary causes.

DIAGNOSTIC EVALUATION

The critical initial factor in evaluating the patient with dyspnea is to assess its severity and whether the patient requires immediate intervention. Pulse oximetry is available in many offices and, along with the history and physical examination, can assess oxygenation and help to determine where and how to further evaluate the patient. Unstable patients require evaluation in the emergency room setting. A chest x-ray should be obtained for most patients with a complaint of dyspnea. X-ray findings may show an infiltrate typical of pneumonia, vascular engorgement, or pulmonary edema (characteristic of CHF), or it may reflect the hyperinflation characteristic of obstructive lung disease. A chest x-ray can also demonstrate pleural effusions, a pneumothorax, a lung mass, or increased interstitial lung markings and

the characteristic honeycomb appearance of interstitial lung disease. Patients with MI, PE, and acute anxiety may have normal chest x-rays.

For patients with suspected pulmonary disease, pulmonary function testing may be helpful in diagnosing obstructive or restrictive disease as the cause. In addition, arterial blood gases may be indicated to document respiratory status.

An ECG can help to assess those with acute presentations of dyspnea. In addition to detecting arrhythmia, acute ST-segment changes may suggest angina or MI and the need for hospitalization. An echocardiogram can assess systolic function and detect the systolic or diastolic dysfunction that may underlie pulmonary congestion and CHF. The echocardiogram can also be helpful in detection of pulmonary hypertension. Exercise stress testing may be helpful in the evaluation of cardiac abnormalities as well as exercise-induced asthma.

A CBC is indicated to determine the WBC and hemoglobin. An elevated WBC may suggest an underlying infectious process, such as pneumonia, as the cause for dyspnea. Anemia, especially acute anemia, may be a cause of dyspnea. If it is detected, further workup to determine its cause is indicated (see Chapter 36). Blood levels of **brain natriuretic peptide** (BNP) are sometimes helpful for distinguishing CHF from a pulmonary cause of dyspnea in the acute setting. BNP is a neurohormone originating in the cardiac ventricles and is elevated in the CHF.

In patients with episodic symptoms and a normal cardiopulmonary evaluation, GERD with secondary bronchospasm should be considered. Empiric therapy may be diagnostic if symptoms are relieved. For still undiagnosed patients, pulmonary referral should be considered. Finally, consideration of psychiatric causes such as anxiety and panic disorder is warranted for those patients with a normal cardiopulmonary evaluation.

In pediatric patients, CAD and pulmonary embolism are rare, while foreign-body aspiration or upper airway obstruction is more common than in adults. Other common conditions in the pediatric population include asthma and respiratory tract infections such as pneumonia and bronchiolitis.

TREATMENT

Management of dyspnea depends on the underlying cause. For example, patients with PE require hospitalization and anticoagulation. Patients diagnosed with pneumonia may be treated with antibiotics on an inpatient or outpatient basis, depending on the severity of the disease. Those with bronchospasm require bronchodilators. CHF should be treated acutely with diuretics and over the long term, as outlined in Chapter 41. Therapies for COPD, asthma, obesity, anxiety, anemia, and pneumonia are outlined in their respective chapters.

KEY POINTS

- The most common causes for dyspnea are cardiopulmonary diseases.
- Chest x-rays should be obtained in most patients with dyspnea.
- Anemia, anxiety, obesity, ascites, and kyphoscoliosis are other potential causes of dyspnea.
- Asthma and respiratory tract infections such as pneumonia and bronchiolitis are common causes of dyspnea in the pediatric population.

30 Shoulder Pain

Shoulder pain affects people of almost all ages but is most prevalent in individuals of middle to older age.

PATHOGENESIS

Normal shoulder motion requires smooth articulations between the glenohumeral, acromioclavicular (AC), sternoclavicular, and scapulothoracic joints. The head of the humerus articulates with the glenoid labrum in a "ball and saucer" fashion (vs. the "ball and socket" articulation of the hip). The shallow articulation allows for a wide range of shoulder motion and also explains why the shoulder is the most commonly dislocated joint. The four muscles of the rotator cuff (supraspinatus, infraspinatus, teres minor, and subscapularis) help stabilize the joint by holding the head of the humerus firmly against the glenoid. The subdeltoid and subacromial bursae are located above the muscles and tendons of the rotator cuff and facilitate fluid movement. Superficial to these bursae are the trapezius, serratus anterior, and rhomboid muscles, which provide scapular stability. All of these structures must function in concert to create smooth motion. Trauma or chronic stress to any single structure can lead to global dysfunction and pain.

The degenerative process that results in bursitis, tendonitis, and shoulder impingement often begins in the supraspinatus or bicipital tendons, which have a poor blood supply and are often under stress. The rotator cuff tendons can become inflamed from being compressed between the humeral head and the acromion. Degenerative changes usually occur in individuals over 50 to 60 years of age and can ultimately involve other tendons, bursae, and sometimes the entire capsule.

CLINICAL MANIFESTATIONS

HISTORY

A complete history includes age, dominant hand, medications, past medical history, type of work, and activity level. It is important to determine whether the pain is acute or chronic and to inquire about associated trauma, swelling, redness, laxity, catching, and decreased range of motion.

Patients with rotator cuff problems usually present with an aching shoulder, which becomes acutely painful with overhead activity. Discomfort while abducting the arm past 90 degrees is characteristic of rotator cuff tendonitis. Complete tears of the rotator cuff usually follow trauma, such as a fall, and rarely occur before middle age. Bicipital tendonitis often occurs in combination with rotator cuff tendonitis and is less common as an isolated condition. The pain can be severe and often radiates down the anterior aspect of the humerus.

Determining what activities increase pain provides clues to the underlying problem. For example, pain with activities such as throwing, swimming, or serving a tennis ball suggests rotator cuff tendonitis, whereas chronic pain and stiffness with limited motion suggests adhesive capsulitis (frozen shoulder). A frozen shoulder is most common in middle age and more prevalent in women than in men. It generally follows a period of immobilization from injury or some other medical condition.

Most dislocations and subluxations occur secondary to trauma. Patients often complain of a popping sensation in their shoulder, along with weakness and intermittent pain. Pain from cervical radiculopathy may result in shoulder pain and often radiates to the elbow. Referred pain to the shoulder can occur in a variety of conditions, such as gallbladder disease, subdiaphragmatic inflammation, pulmonary infarction, and intra-abdominal perforation.

PHYSICAL EXAMINATION

The physical examination should include inspection of the shoulder for asymmetry, surgical scars, deformity, or muscle atrophy. Palpation should be performed to pinpoint the areas of tenderness, as in the AC joint or the bicipital groove. A deformity may be evident in AC separations, fractures, and dislocations. If a fracture or an AC separation is not visually evident, palpation may reveal it.

Range-of-motion testing is critical in evaluating shoulder pain and should be done for both shoulders to allow for comparison. Pain with both active range of motion (AROM) and passive range of motion (PROM) suggests joint or ligament involvement, whereas pain with AROM but not PROM suggests muscular and/or tendon injury. The performance of range-of-motion movements against resistance helps to determine the etiology of the pain. For example, patients with rotator cuff injuries often have pain accompanied by weakness when they abduct the fully extended arm against resistance with the thumbs pointing down. This maneuver compresses the tendons of the rotator cuff against the coracoacromial arch and elicits pain when there is inflammation of the rotator cuff or subacromial bursa. Pain with this maneuver is often called a positive "empty can" sign and indicates inflammation of the compressed structures.

Another method for examining the rotator cuff is via the "**drop-off**" test. This test is performed by passively abducting the patient's shoulder and then observing him or her lower the hand to the waist level. A sudden drop of the arm towards the waist indicates a rotator cuff tear.

Cross-arm testing is performed by having the patient raise the arm to 90 degrees and then actively adducting the arm (thus bringing the tested arm across the body). Pain with this maneuver at the AC joint suggests pathology in that region and is therefore useful in differentiating between impingement and AC joint pathology.

Patients with a suspected shoulder dislocation or subluxation should have **stability testing** of the shoulder performed. The apprehension test measures anterior instability; it is performed by abducting the arm to 90 degrees, rotating it externally, and then applying anterior traction to the humerus. Any pain or apprehension evinced by the patient indicates anterior glenohumeral instability. Pushing the humeral head posteriorly and feeling for increased laxity when the arm is abducted to 90 degrees and the elbow flexed to 90 degrees assesses posterior instability of the glenohumeral joint.

Tenderness just lateral to the acromion suggests subacromial bursitis. Cervical root compression can sometimes be differentiated from intrinsic shoulder pain by reproducing the pain with the neck movement.

DIFFERENTIAL DIAGNOSIS

Extrinsic disease can sometimes present as shoulder pain. Examples include cervical radiculopathy, diaphragmatic irritation, and MI. Box 30-1 lists causes of shoulder pain.

Intrinsic shoulder pain is far more common than extrinsic shoulder pain and includes disorders such as osteoarthritis, fracture, dislocation, rheumatoid arthritis, gout, and osteonecrosis. In the absence of trauma, soft tissue diseases such as rotator cuff tendonitis, bursitis, and bicipital tendonitis are the most common causes of shoulder pain. Less common are rotator cuff tears, biceps tendon rupture, and adhesive capsulitis.

■ BOX 30-1 Causes of Shoulder Pain
Extrinsic
Cervical disk disease
Thoracic outlet syndrome
Gallbladder disease
Myocardial infarction
Diaphragmatic irritation
Intrinsic
Bone/joint abnormalities
Dislocation/subluxation
Arthritis
Infection
AC joint sprain
Fractures
Osteonecrosis
Soft tissue abnormalities
Bicipital tendonitis
Impingement syndrome
Bursitis (subacromial)
Rotator cuff tendonitis/tear
Adhesive capsulitis (frozen shoulder)
Subdeltoid bursitis

DIAGNOSTIC EVALUATION

The history and physical examination are often sufficient to suggest the diagnosis. In patients with bursitis, tendonitis, and rotator cuff syndromes, no diagnostic workup is indicated unless the pain persists for more than 4 to 6 weeks. If the clinical evaluation suggests cervical disease, x-ray films of the cervical spine and possibly a CT or MRI scan are indicated. The history and physical examination are usually sufficient to indicate whether or not evaluation is necessary to rule out conditions causing referred pain.

In patients with trauma or persistent shoulder pain, x-rays can detect conditions such as fracture, dislocation, arthritis, metastatic disease, or avascular necrosis. In soft tissue syndromes, x-rays are usually unremarkable except in cases with calcific tendonitis. Calcium deposits in the areas of the bicipital tendon or in the supraspinatus tendon where it inserts in the greater tuberosity of the humerus may be present. MRI is a useful and noninvasive means of assessing the presence of rotator cuff tendonitis or complete tears of the rotator cuff.

TREATMENT

The mainstay of treatment for soft tissue inflammation is NSAIDs, combined with ice or heat, and brief periods of rest followed by physical therapy. Physical therapy helps preserve normal motor function before severe weakness and decreased range of motion compound the problem. Basic principles of physical therapy include maintaining range of motion, flexibility, and strength. Treatment progresses from passive range-of-motion exercises to assisted active exercises, isometrics, and finally active strength building. Most inflammatory conditions resolve with conservative care in 6 to 8 weeks. In cases where the inflammation of the tendons is very severe or in acute calcific tendonitis, a cortisone injection is often helpful.

A completely torn rotator cuff does not heal spontaneously and may require surgery. However, many people with partial or small tears respond to symptomatic care and an exercise program.

Adhesive capsulitis may be difficult and frustrating to treat. Active exercise to increase range of motion is the cornerstone of nonoperative therapy. Occasionally, surgery may be indicated. Therapy for arthritis consists primarily of NSAIDs and exercise. Cortisone injections may also provide some relief. AC sprains are treated with NSAIDs and a sling until the pain resolves. Third-degree separations or those involving significant displacement of the clavicle should be referred to an orthopaedist. Fractures, rotator cuff tears, advanced arthritis, dislocations, or joint instability and persistent symptoms without improvement are other common indications for orthopaedic referral.

KEY POINTS

- Rotator cuff tendonitis, bursitis, and bicipital tendonitis are the most common causes of shoulder pain.
- Traumatic causes of shoulder pain include AC separation, shoulder dislocation, and fractures.
- X-ray testing should be reserved for patients with a history of traumatic injury or persistent pain despite therapy.
- Management for soft tissue etiologies of shoulder pain commonly involves use of NSAIDs and physical therapy.

Somatization is broadly defined as emotional or psychological distress that is experienced and expressed as physical complaints. Somatization can occur in the presence of physical illness, with symptoms either unrelated to the illness or out of proportion to objective findings. Somatization is an important problem in family medicine. Approximately one-third of all family practice patients have ill-defined symptoms not attributable to physical disease, and 70% of those patients with emotional disorders present with a somatic complaint as the reason for their office visit. Patients often view these physical symptoms as a more acceptable entry into the medical care system than an emotional complaint.

PATHOGENESIS

The pathophysiology of somatization is not well understood. Multiple theories have been proposed, but no single underlying theory explains somatization. Genetic factors may play a role since somatization is much more common in females and familial patterns have been reported. One theory is that the CNS regulates sensory information abnormally, resulting in symptoms. Behavioral theories suggest that somatization is a learned behavior in which the environment reinforces the illness behavior. Somatization is also thought by some to be a defense mechanism.

Precipitating factors include stressful life events, which can either be positive (such as marriage) or negative (such as a death in the family). Interpersonal conflict either at work or home is a common risk factor. Somatization can lead to symptoms in several ways. Patients may amplify symptoms of an acute or chronic problem or alternatively give several physical complaints while de-emphasizing psychological problems such as depression. Some patients experience physiologic disturbances, such as palpitations or an irritable bowel, which may be mediated through the autonomic nervous system. On rare occasions, patients can experience conversion symptoms that may serve a symbolic function, such as "hysterical blindness." Conversion symptoms typically do not conform to any known physiologic mechanisms.

CLINICAL MANIFESTATIONS

HISTORY

The symptoms of somatization range from occasional functional complaints to a full-blown syndrome that meets the criteria of the *Diagnostic and Statistical Manual of Mental Disorders*, fourth edition (DSM-IV), for a somatiform disorder. The most common of these entities is somatization disorder, which is characterized by multiple unexplained symptoms in multiple organs beginning before age 30. DSM-IV criteria require the presence of four pain symptoms, two GI symptoms, one sexual symptom, and one pseudoneurologic symptom drawn from an extended list of symptoms. Other somatiform disorders include hypochondriasis and conversion disorders. The prevalence of somatization disorder is less than 0.2% in males, 2% in the general female population, 6% in the general medical clinical population, 9% among tertiary hospital inpatients, and up to 20% of first-degree female relatives of affected patients.

A thorough history is helpful in determining the possibility of somatization. Unfortunately, the presence of a physical illness or abnormalities discovered on physical examination does not eliminate somatization. Clues that should raise suspicion for somatization disorder are listed in Box 31-1. Pain is the most frequent complaint. Symptoms often cluster around the cardiovascular system, such as atypical chest pain, palpitations, racing heart, and shortness of breath; the nervous system, such as headache, dizziness, light-headedness, and paresthesias; or the GI system, with complaints such as heartburn, gas, and indigestion.

PHYSICAL EXAMINATION

A careful and thorough physical examination is useful for eliminating organic disease. Several diseases, such as hyperparathyroidism and lupus erythematosis, can present with what appear to be somatization complaints.

DIFFERENTIAL DIAGNOSIS

The differential diagnosis includes anxiety, depression, postconcussion syndrome, hypochondriasis, schizophrenia, and malingering.

■ BOX 31-1 Clues to Somatization

Multiple and vague symptoms: description of symptoms can be inconsistent or bizarre
Symptoms persist despite adequate medical treatment
Illness begins with a stressful event
The patient "doctor shops"
History of numerous workups with insignificant findings
The patient refuses to consider psychological factors or discuss issues other than medical concepts
There is evidence of an associated psychiatric disorder
The patient has a hysterical personality
Demanding yet disparaging of the physician
Unreasonable demands for treatment and drugs
Dwelling on symptoms and proud of suffering

Medical disorders that affect multiple systems or produce nonspecific symptoms that are either transient or recurring can be confused with somatization. Box 31-2 lists some illnesses that masquerade as somatization.

DIAGNOSTIC EVALUATION

A thorough history and physical examination are essential. Not only may an unsuspected illness be diagnosed, but a normal examination is also critical for providing effective reassurance and avoiding

■ BOX 31-2 Differential Diagnosis of Somatization

Complaints that are inconsistent with known pathophysiology
Chronic fatigue syndrome
Dementia
Fibromyalgia
HIV
Hyperparathyroidism
Hyperthyroidism
Lyme disease
Systemic lupus erythematosus
Substance abuse

unnecessary testing. Unless there is evidence suggesting a specific disorder, extensive testing should be avoided.

TREATMENT

An important step is to legitimize and acknowledge the complaints, share the patient's frustrations, and express continued interest and hope. The treatment should focus mainly on restoring and maintaining function. An explanation of symptoms should be presented in functional or physiologic terms, if possible. If you cannot explain a symptom, share this with the patient.

A well-defined program should be initiated and presented to the patient. Even if the treatment consists of reassurance and symptom control, definitive information about what to expect and instructions for follow-up can help reduce anxiety. Treatments should be time-limited and expectations set. For example, a physician might say, "We will try this medicine for four weeks. Although it may not relieve your symptoms entirely, you should improve enough to participate in your weekly book club meeting. We will know how this is working by whether you miss any meeting dates. I will see you in four weeks so we can see how you are managing." Often, engaging the patient in behavioral methods, such as keeping a diary, helps. Consultation with a psychologist or a mental health counselor can help by confirming the diagnosis and recommending effective treatments. Pharmaceuticals can benefit patients with major depression or an anxiety disorder that presents with somatic symptoms. Medication should be used sparingly and in low doses. Patients with somatization often have a poor tolerance for side effects. There is rarely an indication for using narcotics in this population.

KEY POINTS

- Somatization is defined as emotional or psychological distress that is experienced and expressed as physical complaints.

- A thorough history and physical examination are essential in order to eliminate the possibility of organic disease.

- Unless there is evidence suggesting a specific disorder, extensive testing should be avoided.

- An important step in management is to legitimize and acknowledge the complaints, share the patient's frustrations, and express continued interest and hope.

- Pharmaceuticals can benefit patients with major depression or an anxiety disorder that presents with somatic symptoms.

Edema is swelling; it may be localized or generalized and is most common in dependent parts of the body, such as the legs. Leg edema is a common problem in family practice, occurring in about 15% of healthy subjects over age 65. The importance of leg edema is its frequent association with illnesses such as deep vein thrombosis, CHF, or renal failure, which can cause significant morbidity and mortality.

PATHOGENESIS

Edema results from an imbalance of factors affecting the distribution of fluid between the intravascular and extravascular spaces. Edema forms when the production of interstitial fluid exceeds its removal through the venous or lymphatic system. Factors contributing to edema are:

1. Increased capillary hydrostatic pressure
2. Reduced intravascular oncotic pressure
3. Increased capillary permeability
4. Reduced lymphatic drainage from the interstitial space

As a result of gravity, edema occurs most commonly in the lower extremities.

CLINICAL MANIFESTATIONS

HISTORY

Most patients with edema complain of leg swelling, but other symptoms include weight gain, tightness of shoes or clothing, puffiness in the eyes or face—especially in the morning—and an increase in abdominal girth. Patients with associated pulmonary edema may complain of exertional dyspnea, orthopnea, and paroxysmal nocturnal dyspnea. It is important to review the patient's medications, since NSAIDs and vasodilators, such as nifedipine or prazosin, can cause fluid retention, and ACE inhibitors can cause localized facial edema. A history of diurnal variations of 4 to 5 lb/day in healthy young women suggests idiopathic cyclic edema.

PHYSICAL EXAMINATION

A rapid increase in weight over a short period of time is one of the cardinal signs of edema. Generalized edema suggests renal disease or hepatic disease. The examination should focus on the cardiopulmonary, abdominal, and pelvic examinations. Neck vein distention along with peripheral edema and rales suggests CHF or pulmonary hypertension. Findings such as palmar erythema, spider telangiectasia, and ascites point to cirrhosis. The presence of a prostatic or pelvic mass and inguinal adenopathy suggests the possibility of lymphatic obstruction. Obesity, previous episodes of phlebitis, and peripheral neuropathy all predispose individuals to chronic edema. Chronic venous insufficiency can cause leg edema and is associated with the physical examination findings of stasis dermatitis and venous varicosities.

The degree of edema and whether it is unilateral or bilateral should be noted. The edema should be tested to see how easily it pits and whether the area is tender. Nonpitting leg edema may be a sign of hypothyroidism. Localized swelling that is not pitting is common in patients with lymphedema.

DIFFERENTIAL DIAGNOSIS

The most common causes of generalized edema are hypoalbuminemia, CHF, cirrhosis, nephritic syndrome, and renal insufficiency. Although bilateral leg edema is associated with systemic diseases, in the family practice setting it is more commonly due to chronic venous insufficiency. Regional edema is usually due to increased capillary pressure from causes such as venous insufficiency or obstruction. Venous obstruction can be due to infection, trauma, thrombophlebitis, or immobility. It can also be a result of external obstruction due to fibrosis, radiation, surgery, neoplasm, or lymph nodes. Box 32-1 lists the causes of leg edema.

DIAGNOSTIC EVALUATION

Routine laboratory tests for patients with generalized edema include a chemistry panel, a CBC, a UA, and a chest x-ray. The chemistry panel assesses renal function, albumin levels, and electrolytes. A UA provides important information about the presence of renal disease and can detect nephrotic-range proteinuria. Hypoalbuminemia occurs with malnutrition or liver disease. The chest x-ray can detect pulmonary congestion and effusions, assess heart size, and provide clues

■ BOX 32-1 Causes of Leg Edema

Bilateral or Generalized Edema
CHF
Pulmonary hypertension from lung disease
Cirrhosis
Hypoalbuminemia
Renal disease
Chronic renal failure
Glomerulonephritis
Nephrotic syndrome
Medications
Myxedema (hypothyroidism)
Idiopathic edema
Allergic reaction
Unilateral Leg Edema
Acute
Cellulitis
Deep vein thrombosis
Hematoma or soft tissue tear
Baker cyst
Chronic
Venous insufficiency
Lymphedema
Extrinsic compression
Neoplasm
Lymphoma

to the presence of pericardial disease. A TSH can rule out hypothyroidism in cases of suspected myxedema. Further cardiac testing such as an ECG and echocardiogram is indicated for patients with CHF.

For patients with unilateral leg edema, an US can test for a DVT. Failure of the vein to compress and impaired venous flow correlate with the presence of a DVT. A CT scan of the abdomen and pelvis is indicated in cases of suspected obstruction from a mass.

TREATMENT

Treatment of the underlying cause is important. For example, lymphedema may resolve with treatment of an underlying malignancy. Nephrotic syndrome may respond to corticosteroids. Diuretics and ACE inhibitors can relieve edema associated with CHF. Edema due to a medication usually responds to withdrawal of the medication.

Nonpharmacologic measures such as leg elevation, compression stockings, and salt restriction are useful. Patients with leg edema should routinely avoid prolonged sitting with their knees bent and may benefit from sleeping with a pillow under their legs. Support stockings or custom-made pressure gradient hose can reduce dependent edema. Stockings above the knee may work better but are often poorly tolerated. Compressive stockings are contraindicated in patients with arterial insufficiency. Initial salt restriction consists of eliminating added salt and avoiding high-sodium foods.

Diuretics should be used cautiously as an adjunct to nonpharmacologic therapy. Lymphedema and edema due to chronic venous insufficiency do not typically respond to diuretics. Patients receiving diuretics should be monitored to avoid overdiuresis. Symptoms of excessive diuresis are nonspecific and may include weakness, fatigue, lethargy, and confusion. Monitoring includes following the patient's weight, checking orthostatic blood pressure, and measuring electrolytes and renal function periodically to detect common metabolic abnormalities—such as hyponatremia, hypokalemia, metabolic alkalosis, and prerenal azotemia—associated with diuretics.

 KEY POINTS

- Leg edema is a common problem in family practice, occurring in about 15% of healthy subjects over age 65. The importance of leg edema is its frequent association with illnesses such as CHF or renal failure, which can cause significant morbidity and mortality.

- Generalized edema is usually a result of hypoalbuminemia or cardiac, renal, or hepatic disease.

- Nonpharmacologic measures for treating edema—such as leg elevation, compression stockings, and salt restriction—are useful.

- Diuretics should be used cautiously as an adjunct to nonpharmacologic therapy. Lymphedema and edema due to chronic venous insufficiency do not typically respond to diuretics.

Chapter

33 Weight Loss

Unintended weight loss is a worrisome finding that may indicate the presence of a significant underlying physical or psychological illness. It can occur in people of all ages and there are many potential causes.

PATHOGENESIS

Unintended weight loss results when caloric intake is less than caloric expenditure. This may be the result of diminished intake, malabsorption, excessive loss of nutrients, or increased caloric expenditure.

Diminished caloric intake may be the result of decreased interest in food, inability to obtain food, attenuated awareness of hunger, pain associated with the ingestion of food, and early satiety. Malabsorption of calories can occur with hepatic, pancreatic, and intestinal disorders. Loss of nutrients may result in the body being unable to maintain caloric homeostasis. Examples include recurrent vomiting or diarrhea, glycosuria, and significant proteinuria. Increased nutrient demand is the result of any process that increases basal metabolic rate. Chronic infection, hyperthyroidism, excessive exercise, and malignancy are common causes of increased metabolic rate.

CLINICAL MANIFESTATIONS

HISTORY

The first step in evaluating a patient with weight loss is to determine the amount of weight loss and the period of time over which it has occurred. Because many older patients may not recognize a significant weight loss, a decline in serial weight measurements is often the presenting sign. If a previous weight measurement is not available, asking about changes in waist size or how clothing fits may be helpful. Once significant weight loss is confirmed, a thorough review of systems should help direct the physical examination and laboratory testing.

Questions about daily food intake, alterations in appetite, pain with swallowing, early satiety, episodes of emesis, and changes in bowel habits are important. Foul-smelling, greasy, bulky stools suggest malabsorption. Especially in young women, attitudes toward food and body image should be assessed. A distorted body image may be a clue to the presence of an eating disorder.

Patients should be asked about fever, cough, shortness of breath, alterations in patterns of urination, abdominal pain, melena, hematochezia, rash, headaches, and other neurologic symptoms. Signs of depression—such as difficulty concentrating, changes in sleeping patterns, social isolation, and recent losses—should be elicited. In the case of cognitively impaired patients, family members and caregivers should be interviewed. The past medical history, previous surgeries, medications, tobacco use, alcohol intake, family history, and HIV risk factors should be reviewed. A social history is important in order to identify issues such as poverty, isolation, or an inability to shop or cook, which may lead to weight loss.

PHYSICAL EXAMINATION

The physical examination should begin with height and weight as well as vital signs to detect the presence of fever or tachycardia. General inspection should note stigmata of systemic disease, including hair loss, temporal wasting, pallor, poor hygiene, bruising, jaundice, and diminished orientation.

Evaluation of the oropharynx should assess dentition, presence of oral thrush, and petechiae, while the neck examination should note any thyromegaly or lymphadenopathy. The lungs should be examined for decreased breath sounds, crackles, wheezing, and evidence of consolidation, while the heart should be examined for irregular rhythm, murmurs, gallops, and the presence of a pericardial effusion. Abdominal examination should note any surgical scars, the quality of bowel sounds, and the presence of organomegaly, ascites, tenderness, or masses. The rectal examination is important for evaluating the prostate and to check for occult blood and stool consistency. In women, breast and pelvic examinations should be performed to evaluate for malignancy. Neurologic examination should assess memory, concentration, posterior column function, and focal abnormalities. Psychiatric evaluation may provide evidence of a mood disorder or anorexia nervosa.

DIFFERENTIAL DIAGNOSIS

Box 33-1 lists some important causes of weight loss. It is useful to organize the differential diagnosis by the categories of decreased intake, impaired absorption, nutrient loss, and increased demand. For many conditions, such as cancer or end-stage CHF, weight

BOX 33-1 Differential Diagnosis of Weight Loss
Decreased Intake
Alcohol/substance abuse
Anorexia nervosa
Congestive heart failure
Depression
Dementia
Hepatitis
Medications (e.g., digitoxin toxicity)
Ulcer disease
Uremia
Splenomegaly
Bowel obstruction
Poverty/social isolation
Malabsorption
Gastric bypass
Pancreatic insufficiency
Inflammatory bowel disease
Celiac sprue
Cholestasis
Protein wasting enteropathy
Nutrient Loss
Significant proteinuria
Diabetes (uncontrolled)
Chronic emesis
Fistula
Chronic diarrhea
Increased Demand
Chronic infection (e.g., tuberculosis)
Malignancy
Hyperthyroidism
Excessive exercise
Poor dentition
Infection (e.g., parasites)

loss occurs long after the diagnosis is known. However, anorexia nervosa, pancreatic cancer, early malabsorption, apathetic hyperthyroidism, diabetes, Alzheimer disease, and HIV are examples of illnesses that may cause weight loss early in their presentation. A physical cause for weight loss can be found in about 65% of patients and a psychiatric cause in another 10%. Depression is the most common psychiatric cause, and along with substance abuse may present with profound weight loss. Anorexia nervosa is seen primarily in adolescent females and young adults. The diagnosis is based on weight loss leading to a body weight 15% below that expected combined with a distorted body image, fear of weight gain, and, in females, the absence of at least three consecutive menstrual cycles. Other psychiatric and medical illness must be excluded. In approximately 25% of individuals, no identifiable cause is found.

DIAGNOSTIC EVALUATION

Unintended weight loss exceeding 5% in 1 month or 10% in 6 months deserves evaluation. Since weight loss is usually a late symptom of disease, the cause may be identified through the information gathered by the history and physical examination combined with conventional laboratory testing, such as a CBC, serum electrolytes, BUN, creatinine, calcium, glucose, liver function tests, lipase, amylase, albumin, TSH, UA, chest x-ray, and selected cancer screening tests such as a mammogram, Pap smear, prostate-specific antigen (PSA), and stool test for occult blood. In patients with GI symptoms, upper endoscopy, colonoscopy, abdominal US, abdominal CT, and stool analysis may be warranted. HIV antibody testing and TB skin testing should be performed in all individuals with risk factors. Although not specific, an ESR may be useful in determining the likelihood of occult malignancy or infection. Serum levels of medications such as quinidine or digoxin should be checked if appropriate. In patients in whom malabsorption is suspected, use of the D-xylose test may further distinguish between pancreatic and small bowel disease. Antigliadin antibodies should be measured if there is concern about celiac sprue. In alcoholics and those with a macrocytic anemia, vitamin B_{12} and folate levels should be measured.

TREATMENT

Patients with an obvious cause for weight loss—such as peptic ulcer disease, gallstones, infection, diabetes, hyperthyroidism, or cancer—should be treated accordingly. Weight loss associated with depression typically responds well to antidepressant therapy. In patients with dementia, caregivers providing one-to-one feeding support during each meal along with nutritional supplements such as Ensure can often help weight loss. Use of instant breakfast powder in whole milk is a less costly alternative in lactose-tolerant individuals. Megestrol acetate and dronabinol are sometimes used as an appetite stimulant in patients with cancer or acquired immune deficiency syndrome (AIDS).

Patients with anorexia nervosa need psychiatric referral and very close followup. The goal is restoration of normal body weight and resolution of psychological difficulties. Treatment programs conducted by experienced teams in the outpatient setting are often helpful; but in severe cases or recalcitrant cases, admission to the hospital for bed rest, supervised meals, and intense behavioral and psychotherapy is indicated, since between 2% and 6% of patients die from complications of the disorder or commit suicide. Patients with severe malnutrition may require enteral or parenteral feeding.

In the setting of pancreatic insufficiency, oral pancreatic enzyme preparations and fat-soluble vitamin supplements (vitamins A, D, E, and K) should be instituted. Alcoholics and those suffering from malabsorption should have vitamin B_{12} and folate supplementation. Finally, observation along with frequent followup is considered appropriate management in patients with a normal history, physical examination, and laboratory evaluation.

KEY POINTS

- A weight loss greater than 5% of total body weight over a period of 6 months is generally considered abnormal and warrants further investigation.

- Unintended weight loss may be the result of diminished intake, malabsorption, excessive loss of nutrients, or increased caloric expenditure. Cancer and chronic disease are common causes for both decreased intake and increased caloric expenditure.

- A physical cause for weight loss can be found in about 65% of patients and a psychiatric cause in another 10%.

Chapter

34 Acne

Acne is the most common chronic skin condition treated by physicians; it affects more than 85% of adolescents and young adults. Although most commonly seen in teenagers, acne may occur transiently in neonates and may persist beyond puberty into the third and fourth decades of life. Acne can cause physical pain in addition to psychosocial distress, especially in the teenage population.

PATHOGENESIS

The pathogenesis of acne is multifactorial. It includes hyperkeratosis with resulting blockage of the pilosebaceous canal, increased growth of *Propionibacterium acnes*, overproduction of sebum, and inflammation. Androgen production stimulates the sebaceous gland, causing an increase in cell turnover, an increase in sebum production, and cohesiveness of keratinocytes at the pilosebaceous canal. This alteration in keratinization allows/leads the keratinous material in the follicle to become more "sticky," causing a blockage of the canal. The blocked pilosebaceous gland produces a small cystic swelling resulting in a raised area of the follicular duct just below the epidermis, referred to as a microcomedone. If the duct dilates with stratum corneum cells, causing an opening of the follicular mouth, it is referred to as an open comedone or "blackhead"; if the mouth remains closed, it is referred to as a closed comedone or "whitehead."

The combination of sebum, desquamated cells, and obstruction of the follicular opening creates an environment conducive to the overgrowth of the gram-negative anaerobic diphtheroid bacteria, *P. acnes*. This bacteria is part of the normal skin flora and secretes a low-molecular-weight chemotactic factor and lipase enzymes that break down the triglycerides of sebum into free fatty acids. This breakdown results in irritation of the follicular wall which leads to the formation of an erythematous papule on the skin. Neutrophils release hydrolases, which may further disrupt the integrity of the follicular wall, causing rupture and leakage into the underlying dermis and thus leading to the formation of a pustule. If this inflammatory process continues, it will eventually lead to the formation of a nodule and subsequently a cyst.

Androgens are a primary stimulus of sebaceous gland proliferation and increased sebum production, which explains why acne often develops during puberty. Since girls reach puberty at an earlier age than boys, the peak of acne in girls is reached between 14 and 17 years of age, compared to ages 16 to 19 in boys. Neonatal acne is caused by maternal androgens that stimulate the sebaceous glands, which have not yet involuted to their childhood state of immaturity. Neonatal acne is usually mild and can be observed during the second to fifth months of life, after which the pilosebaceous units involute, only to re-emerge again near puberty.

CLINICAL MANIFESTATIONS

HISTORY

The history should include onset and distribution of skin lesions and any associated aggravating or alleviating factors. The patient should be asked about aggravating foods, whether temperature affects the skin, and if there are seasons of the year during which the lesions are worse. Cosmetics, topical skin preparations, or exposure to heavy oils or greases may contribute to follicular plugging. Medications such as corticosteroids, androgens, anticonvulsants, and lithium may contribute to acne. Patients should be asked about other symptoms of androgen excess, such as voice change and change in hair growth and distribution. The sudden onset of widely distributed, severe acne may be associated with androgen excess, either from an androgen-secreting tumor or from the ingestion of exogenous androgens.

PHYSICAL EXAMINATION

The physical examination focuses on characterizing the skin lesions. Acne lesions usually develop in areas with the greatest density and size of sebaceous glands. The face is almost always involved. Other common areas of involvement are the chest, shoulders, and upper back. Additional note should be made of hair pattern, and in cases of suspected virilization, a genital examination should be performed to assess for pelvic masses or clitoromegaly.

The prime focus of the examination is to characterize and classify the acne. Acne lesions can be classified into either **comedonal** (whiteheads, blackheads) or **inflammatory** (papules/pustules, nodules/cysts). Most cases of acne are pleomorphic and include comedones, papules, pustules, and nodules. Patients with mild acne usually have whiteheads and blackheads, a few papules, and some pustules. Moderate acne consists of many papules and pustules and a few nodules. Severe acne, also referred to as nodulocystic acne, consists of many papules, pustules, and nodules or cysts.

DIFFERENTIAL DIAGNOSIS

Common conditions that mimic the lesions of acne vulgaris include acne rosacea, folliculitis, and perioral dermatitis. Acne rosacea is a chronic vascular inflammatory disorder affecting mainly adults between the ages of 30 and 50. It is characterized by a vascular component (redness, telangiectasia, flushing, blushing) and an eruptive component (papules and pustules) affecting only the face. Patients are extremely sensitive to facial vasodilatory factors such as exposure to extreme heat or cold, excessive sunlight, and ingestion of alcohol, spicy foods, hot liquids, and highly seasoned food. Folliculitis is the infection of hair follicles from the epidermal surface by *Staphylococcus*, often from shaving. Perioral dermatitis is an eruption around the mouth, nose, and eyes affecting young women; it is thought to have a bacterial etiology. These patients have papules and pustules resembling folliculitis, there are no whiteheads or blackheads, and there is a clear zone around the vermilion border. Androgen excess and medications can be causes of acne.

DIAGNOSTIC EVALUATION

No special tests are required in the evaluation of acne other than skin examination. In those women with suspected androgen excess, serum testosterone and dehydroepiandrosterone sulfate levels may help in guiding further evaluation and therapy.

TREATMENT

The principle of acne therapy is to disrupt the cycle of follicular plugging and increased sebum production and to reduce bacterial colonization and inflammation.

Evidence suggests that diet rarely affects acne; however, if patients report that certain foods aggravate their acne, they should be avoided. Cleaning products such as Neutrogena, Dove, and Cetaphil may be helpful.

Topical agents such as tretinoin (Retin-A) are often the first line of therapy. Tretinoin increases cell turnover and reduces the cohesion between keratinocytes, helping to unplug the follicle. The medication usually causes some redness, burning, and peeling of the skin within the first 3 to 4 weeks of treatment. This may make the comedones more visible, causing many patients to believe that they are worsening and to stop using their medication prematurely. However, with continued use of tretinoin, most patients improve after the sixth week, with best results seen at 9 to 12 weeks of treatment. Retin-A also causes the skin to become much more sensitive to irritants such as sun exposure, wind, dryness, and cold temperatures. Other, milder comedolytics include salicylic acid, sulfur preparations, and azelaic acid. Azelaic acid has antibacterial and keratolytic properties and is useful in patients with mild to moderate acne who cannot tolerate tretinoin.

The goal of treatment for mild to moderate acne is to reduce the follicular bacterial population by using topical antibiotics (erythromycin or clindamycin) and keratolytics. Benzoyl peroxide has bacteriostatic properties, which make it an effective treatment for mild inflammatory acne. Patients should be advised that this medication can dry the skin and can bleach clothes and pillowcases. There are topical preparations that combine benzoyl peroxide with a topical antibiotic (Benzaclin, Benzomycin), which should be applied to the affected areas once or twice a day. There are new reports of increasing resistance of *P. acnes* to topical erythromycin and even some cross-resistance to topical clindamycin. However, combination topical preparations, such as Benzomycin, do not appear to promote resistant strains of *P. acnes*. With resistance to antibiotics increasing in this age of medicine, the regimen of topical preparations such as Benzomycin should be kept in mind in our patients who develop resistance strains of *P. acnes* and need to remain on topical treatments.

If topical retinoids are used in conjunction with topical antibacterials, they should be applied at different times (i.e., antibacterial in the morning and retinoid in the evening). If lesions do not improve after 6 weeks of treatment, an oral antibiotic is usually added to the regimen. The antibiotics that have proven most efficacious are tetracycline, doxycycline, minocycline, and erythromycin. In adolescent girls, an oral contraceptive can be an effective second-line medication. The main effect of oral contraceptives is to suppress ovarian androgen production and thus reduce sebum production.

If the combination of oral and topical antibiotics is insufficient, prescribing isotretinoin (Accutane) is often helpful in treating moderate to severe acne. Accutane is associated with significant toxicity and requires close monitoring under the direction of an experienced clinician. It is extremely teratogenic and severe malformations occur in 25% to 30% of fetuses exposed to the drug. Female patients must commit to two forms of birth control for at least 1 month prior to therapy, during therapy, and 1 month after therapy. Other adverse affects include dry skin, elevated triglycerides, and depression. Acne therapy is summarized in Table 34-1.

TABLE 34-1 Acne Treatment	
Severity	**Treatment**
Mild, noninflammatory	Topical retinoid at low strength, increase as needed or tolerated
Mild, minimal inflammation	Topical retinoid at night plus benzoyl peroxide plus/minus topical antibiotic
Moderate, pustules, some nodules	Topical retinoid and oral antibiotic
Severe, numerous cysts, nodules, and inflammation	Isotretinoin alone or topical retinoid, oral antibiotic, and isotretinoin

KEY POINTS

- Acne vulgaris affects approximately 85% of adolescents.
- Overproduction of sebum and *P. acnes* are etiologic agents leading to the development of acne.
- Comedonal acne is treated with topical keratolytics (retinoids) and/or benzoyl peroxide.
- Inflammatory acne is treated with either topical or oral antibiotics.
- Isotretinoin (Accutane) is reserved for severe acne or moderate acne that is unresponsive to treatment.

Alcohol and Substance Abuse

Substance problems encompass a wide range of severity. Consequences can include legal problems, health problems, and recurrent social, work-related, or interpersonal problems.

EPIDEMIOLOGY

Alcohol and substance abuse are among the most serious social and medical problems in the United States. Substance abuse affects all age groups, and each year there are approximately 100,000 deaths resulting from alcohol abuse and another 20,000 deaths from the use of illicit substances. An estimated 20% of adults in the United States are at risk for alcohol- and substance-related problems, with 13% meeting diagnostic criteria for substance abuse or dependence during their lifetimes. Societal costs stem from lost productivity, costs of alcohol-related illness, premature death, motor vehicle accidents (MVAs), and crime. Alcohol is associated with the three leading causes of death in adolescents (homicide, suicide, and MVAs). Fetal alcohol syndrome is the most common birth defect among newborns in the United States. Among the elderly, up to 10% may be abusing alcohol at any given time.

PATHOGENESIS

At-risk behavior occurs when an individual drinks or occasionally uses substances to the level of intoxication. The concern is the risk of progression to more frequent drinking, trauma, and accidents. A person who abuses substances is one who engages in intermittent, repetitive, and planned drinking or usage to levels of intoxication. Abuse becomes dependence when the patient loses control over his or her use despite persistent social, physiologic, occupational, and physical problems. Tolerance arises when a person requires more drugs to achieve the same "high" effect. These individuals experience withdrawal symptoms if use stops abruptly. The etiology of substance abuse is not completely understood but is most likely multifactorial. Genetic factors appear to play a role. Individuals with an alcoholic parent have a three to four times greater risk of becoming dependent on alcohol, and identical

twins have a greater concordance of alcoholism than fraternal twins.

Nongenetic factors also appear to play a role. Emotional or interpersonal stress may serve as an initiator and maintainer of alcohol abuse. Parental and peer values can contribute to substance abuse. Adults who grew up in dysfunctional families and/or are in dysfunctional family situations are at increased risk for alcohol abuse. Patients who have an underlying psychopathology, such as depression or anxiety, often abuse alcohol and other drugs as a form of self-medication.

CLINICAL MANIFESTATIONS

HISTORY

Symptoms of substance abuse vary greatly. Box 35-1 lists concerns or complaints that may be presenting symptoms of alcoholism or illicit drug use. Early diagnosis and treatment, before irreversible health problems or major psychosocial consequences arise, should be the goal of every family physician. Symptoms such as anxiety, depression, and insomnia may be related to alcohol use.

Inquiry into a patient's use of substances is best approached in a nonjudgmental, supportive manner. A useful starting point is the social history, looking for "red flags" such as marital or work problems, trauma, arrests, traffic tickets for "driving under the influence" (DUI), and financial problems, especially those related to spending on drugs. It is important to elicit the substance of choice, frequency and pattern of use, and amount ingested. Patients are more likely to be deceptive about the amount they drink or how many drugs they use rather than how often they do so. The best quantitative data are obtained in asking about a specific time, "Tell me what you drank yesterday." Patients commonly use denial as a defense mechanism; it may therefore be necessary to interview family members to obtain accurate information.

When abuse is suspected, the "Cage Test" (Box 35-2) is a useful tool. In the family practice setting, two "yes" answers have a sensitivity that ranges from 70% to 85% and specificity from 85% to 95%. Also useful is the Two-Item Conjoint Screen, which has nearly an

BOX 35-1 Alcohol-Related Symptoms

Psychosocial Complaints	Physical Complaints
Absenteeism from work	Blackouts
Antisocial behavior	Falls
Anxiety	Gastrointestinal problems
Child abuse	Gout
Depression	Headache
Domestic violence	History of trauma
Financial problems	Motor vehicle accident injuries
Interpersonal relationship problems	Muscle cramps
Irritability	Nasal congestion
Job-related problems	Nocturia
Legal problems	Palpitations or chest pains
School-related problems	Peripheral neuropathy
Suicidal ideation	Poor memory Recurrent infections Sleep disturbances Weight changes

80% sensitivity and specificity. This involves asking two questions:
1. In the past year, have you ever had more to drink or used drugs more than you meant to?
2. Have you ever felt a need to cut down on your drinking or drug use?

PHYSICAL EXAMINATION

The physical examination should be thorough and detailed. However, physical complications of substance abuse may not be evident early in the disease.

BOX 35-2 Cage Questions

Have you ever felt the need to Cut down on your drinking?
Are you Annoyed by people criticizing your drinking?
Have you ever felt Guilty about your drinking?
Do you ever need a drink in the morning to steady your nerves or help a hangover? (Eye-opener)

High blood pressure may be a sign of withdrawal or cocaine abuse. Cirrhosis, ascites, edema, palmar erythema, testicular atrophy, rosacea, cardiomegaly, and peripheral neuropathy characterize end-stage alcoholism and are usually associated with heavy drinking for at least 10 years. Binge drinking can sometimes precipitate cardiac arrhythmias or the "holiday heart" syndrome. Nasal irritation, septal perforation, tachycardia, chest pain, and paranoia are associated with cocaine. Marijuana smoking can cause cough and dark-colored or bloody sputum. Dilated pupils can be a sign of stimulant abuse, while constricted pupils in combination with sedation suggest opioid use.

DIFFERENTIAL DIAGNOSIS

The psychosocial and physical problems outlined in Boxes 35-1 and 35-3 also form the differential diagnosis for substance abuse. In evaluating patients presenting with these various complaints, consideration of underlying substance abuse is very important. Clinical and laboratory evidence of substance abuse may not be evident in early stages; hence the diagnosis depends on a constellation of medical, social, and psychological clues. Substance abuse is often complicated by anxiety, depression, chronic pain, or marital distress, and these must be considered in evaluating the patient.

DIAGNOSTIC EVALUATION

Although laboratory tests are not diagnostic of substance abuse, they can be helpful. Liver enzyme abnormalities can provide objective evidence of problem drinking. Serum gamma-glutamyl transferase (GGT) is the most sensitive indicator of alcohol-induced liver damage; however, it is not specific. Elevation of the liver enzyme aspartate aminotransferase (AST) to alanine aminotransferase (ALT) in a ratio greater than 1 is typical of alcohol-related hepatitis. In cases of alcoholism, a CBC may reveal an elevated mean corpuscular volume (MCV) or anemia. Hyperlipidemia and elevated uric acid levels are also often present.

TREATMENT

The goal of treatment is to reduce the consequences of the patient's substance abuse and prevent further abuse. For at-risk individuals or those with a short history of abusing alcohol, evidence suggests that even brief interactions may be of benefit. These may consist of short counseling sessions in which the physician educates the patient about the consequences of continued use and recommends quitting or cutting down. Setting specific goals and making a follow-up appointment to review the patient's progress are also important parts of such intervention.

■ BOX 35-3 Alcohol-Related Health Problems

Cardiovascular
Hypertension
Cardiomyopathy
Arrhythmias
Endocrine
Testicular atrophy
Feminization
Amenorrhea
Gastrointestinal
Hepatitis
Cirrhosis
Esophagitis
Gastritis
Diarrhea
Pancreatitis
Gastrointestinal bleeding
Pregnancy
Low birth weight
Fetal alcohol syndrome
Hematopoietic System
Anemia
Thrombocytopenia
Neurologic System
Cognitive impairment
Dementia
Korsakoff psychosis
Wernicke encephalopathy
Peripheral neuropathy
Musculoskeletal
Cramps
Osteoporosis
Skin
Rosacea
Telangiectasia
Palmar erythema

Self-help groups, such as Alcoholics Anonymous or Narcotics Anonymous, are a mainstay of treatment for patients willing to participate. Programs such as Al-Anon are also available for relatives and friends of individuals with substance-abuse problems. Referral to an outpatient treatment center or an addiction specialist is another treatment option. Counseling sessions may comprise individuals, groups, or families. Inpatient programs are usually reserved for those who fail outpatient therapy.

The treatment of alcohol withdrawal is aimed at reducing the patient's discomfort and preventing the progression of symptoms. Symptoms can range from minor manifestations such as tachycardia, elevated blood pressure, shakiness, and irritability to life-threatening problems such as seizures, delirium tremens (DTs), and coma. Normalization of vital signs and moderate sedation are two of the end points for managing withdrawal. Long-acting benzodiazepines (BZDs), such as diazepam or chlordiazepoxide, either given as a loading dose until the patient is sedated or using symptom-adjusted dosing, are effective for managing withdrawal. Short-acting BZDs, such as lorazepam, are preferred in patients with severe liver disease. Beta blockers, such as atenolol, can help to reduce adrenergic symptoms and control blood pressure and tachycardia. Although beta blockers may reduce BZD requirements, they should not be used as monotherapy because they do not prevent seizures, hallucinations, or DTs. Clonidine, a central-acting antihypertensive medication, can also be used to help control blood pressure and withdrawal symptoms. Thiamine and magnesium should be given to patients at risk for alcohol withdrawal.

Outpatient therapy is appropriate for patients with mild withdrawal symptoms and a supportive social structure. A family member should be available around the clock and always in control of any medications. Inpatient care is needed for those with more severe symptoms, a history of severe withdrawal, or a poor social support network. Withdrawal from BZDs is best accomplished with a long-acting BZD or phenobarbital over a period of 8 to 12 weeks. Withdrawal of other sedative hypnotic drugs is usually managed using phenobarbital. Opiate withdrawal can be treated with either propoxyphene or methadone. Clonidine is useful as an adjunctive therapy. No drug is currently indicated for managing cocaine withdrawal, although tricyclic antidepressants, SSRIs, and dopamine agonists such as bromocriptine may reduce cravings.

Some patients seeking total abstinence from alcohol may request disulfiram. Disulfiram therapy sensitizes patients to alcohol and causes reactions such as flushing, palpitations, headache, nausea, and vomiting if alcohol is consumed. Naltrexone, an opioid antagonist, is also useful in alcohol abuse. It appears to inhibit the pleasurable effects of alcohol and to reduce cravings. Contraindications include opiate use and hepatocellular disease.

It is important to remember that alcoholics and addicts have a lifelong condition even if they are abstinent. Therefore, the family physician should be cautious about prescribing narcotic- or stimulant-containing medications to these patients at any time during their medical care.

KEY POINTS

- The estimated prevalence of substance abuse disorders ranges from 10% to 20%, with an estimated 5% of the adult population using illicit substances.

- Liver enzyme abnormalities can provide objective evidence of problem drinking. Serum GGT is the most sensitive indicator of alcohol-induced liver damage; however, it is not specific.

- The goal of treatment is to reduce the consequences of the patient's substance abuse and prevent further substance abuse.

- Outpatient therapy is appropriate for patients with mild withdrawal symptoms and a supportive social structure. Inpatient care is needed for those with more severe symptoms, a history of severe withdrawal, or a poor social support network.

36 Anemia

In adults, anemia is defined as a hematocrit (Hct) of less than 41% (hemoglobin <13.5 g/dL) in males or 37% (hemoglobin <12 g/dL) in females. In the United States, the most common cause of anemia in elderly individuals is anemia of chronic disease, whereas in females of reproductive age, the most common cause is iron deficiency. The most common cause of anemia worldwide is iron deficiency.

PATHOGENESIS

Anemia can result from blood loss, increased destruction of red blood cells (RBCs), or inadequate RBC production. Individuals with anemia may experience tissue hypoxia, which is detected by the oxygen-sensing cells in the area of the juxtaglomerular apparatus of the kidney. As a result, the kidney increases erythropoietin production, the primary regulatory hormone for erythropoiesis. In chronic renal disease, anemia may result from a decrease in renal production of erythropoietin. In chronic illnesses, impaired incorporation of iron into hemoglobin can cause anemia of chronic disease. Malnutrition, inflammatory states, or bone marrow suppression by infection or drugs may also contribute to the pathogenesis of anemia of chronic disease.

For normal erythropoiesis, an adequate supply of iron is needed. Normally, the circulating RBC (erythrocyte) has a life span of approximately 120 days, and iron is primarily supplied by the recycling of iron from senescent red cells destroyed by the reticuloendothelial system. In a healthy, nonmenstruating person, the daily loss of iron is minimal; as a result, only 1 to 2 mg of iron is required per day. Iron is primarily absorbed from the duodenum, transported to the bone marrow, and used to form hemoglobin. Excess iron is converted to ferritin and stored in the liver and bone marrow. When the stores of iron are inadequate due to blood loss or chronic dietary deficiency, normal hemoglobin synthesis is disrupted and a microcytic, hypochromic anemia results.

Deficiencies in vitamins B_{12} (cobalamine) and folate impair deoxyribonucleic acid (DNA) synthesis. Although DNA synthesis is slowed, cytoplasmic development continues and there is more cytoplasm than normal, resulting in larger cells or a megaloblastic anemia. Folate deficiency generally results from inadequate dietary intake. In addition to inadequate intake, causes of B_{12} deficiency include malabsorption and lack of intrinsic factor (IF). In order for vitamin B_{12} to be absorbed, it must first bind with IF, which is secreted by the parietal cells of the stomach. Conditions such as gastric atrophy or gastrectomy can result in a vitamin B_{12} deficiency due to lack of IF. Since the cobalamine–IF complex is absorbed in the ileum, intestinal disease involving the terminal ileum, such as Crohn disease, may also lead to lack of absorption of the cobalamine–IF complex.

Genetic factors can cause abnormal hemoglobin synthesis. The normal hemoglobin molecule consists of two alpha chains and two beta chains. An abnormality in the synthesis of alpha or beta chains can result in low hemoglobin or abnormal hemoglobin consisting of only alpha or beta chains. The abnormal hemoglobin may aggregate and form insoluble cytoplasmic inclusion bodies that damage the cells, leading to premature destruction of these cells by the spleen and liver.

CLINICAL MANIFESTATIONS

HISTORY

Anemia can lead to an inadequate supply of oxygen to the tissues, which may cause symptoms in vulnerable organ systems. For example, patients with heart disease may present with angina pectoris or decompensated CHF. However, many patients are asymptomatic until their hemoglobin level falls below 8 g/dL. General symptoms include dizziness and fatigue or weakness, either at rest or brought on by exertion.

The history should focus on potential sources of blood loss. The GI tract is the most common source of blood loss, and the presence of melena, hematochezia, or hematemesis indicates GI bleeding. Premenopausal women should be assessed for abnormal vaginal bleeding, since this is a common cause of iron deficiency anemia. In the elderly population, it is important to inquire about chronic illnesses such as hepatic, renal, inflammatory, neoplastic, and infectious diseases, since these conditions are associated with anemia of chronic disease. A family history of anemia may point to an inherited cause, such as thalassemia. Alcohol consumption should be assessed, since excess alcohol can suppress the bone marrow, cause chronic liver disease, and is associated with deficiencies of folate and other vitamins. If the patient reports a history of jaundice, pruritus, and a history of gallstones, hemolytic anemia should be suspected.

PHYSICAL EXAMINATION

Physical findings include pallor, tachycardia, and dyspnea. A systolic ejection murmur may be heard due to hyperdynamic circulation. Abdominal and rectal examinations can detect organomegaly and occult blood. Signs of iron deficiency include cheilosis (scaling at the corner of the mouth), koilonychia (spoon-shaped nails), and brittle nails.

Patients with B_{12} deficiency may have neurologic deficits such as abnormal reflexes, ataxia, Babinski sign, and poor position and vibration sense. These neurologic findings are not found with folate deficiency.

DIFFERENTIAL DIAGNOSIS

Anemias can be classified on the basis of the MCV into three categories: microcytic, macrocytic, or normocytic. **Microcytic anemia** is defined as an MCV below 80 fL, a **macrocytic anemia** with an MCV greater than 100 fL, and **normocytic anemias** with MCVs between 80 and 100 fL. The differential diagnosis varies by cell size. For example, the three major causes of microcytic anemia are iron deficiency, thalassemia, and anemia of chronic disease, whereas the most common causes of macrocytic anemia are B_{12} and folate deficiency.

Most iron deficiency is caused by GI or menstrual blood loss. Iron deficiency due to a nutritional deficiency is common in children, most commonly seen with excessive intake of cow milk. Anemia of chronic disease is associated with chronic infections, neoplastic diseases, renal disease, connective tissue disease, or endocrine disorders.

Macrocytic anemia from B_{12} and folate deficiency may be secondary to autoimmune disease, nutritional deficits, infections, gastrectomy, or ileal resection surgery. Since B_{12} is found only in foods of animal origin, vegetarians are at increased risk of developing B_{12} deficiency. The most common cause of B_{12} deficiency is **pernicious anemia**, an autoimmune disease in which the parietal cells that make IF are destroyed.

The most common cause of **folate deficiency** is decreased dietary intake. Alcoholics often present with folate deficiency. Drugs such as phenytoin, TMP/SMX, and sulfasalazine may also impair the absorption of folate.

Causes of normocytic anemia are many and include acute blood loss as well as the hemolytic anemias, which may be inherited or acquired. A full review of the many causes of normocytic anemia is beyond the scope of this book.

DIAGNOSTIC EVALUATION

The classification of an anemia as microcytic, macrocytic, or normocytic helps direct the workup. In addition, the reticulocyte count is an important test because it helps to differentiate between hemolytic anemias, blood loss, and bone marrow disorders. The reticulocyte count must be corrected for the level of anemia. **(Corrected reticulocyte count = reticulocyte count × patient Hct/expected Hct.)** A corrected reticulocyte count of 2% or less suggests decreased RBC production and a hypoproliferative bone marrow. Follow-up tests should screen for renal, hepatic, and endocrine etiologies and may also include examination of the bone marrow. A hypoproliferative state may also be seen in hematinic deficiencies such as low iron or B_{12}.

If the reticulocyte count is greater than 3%, blood loss or **hemolytic anemia** should be suspected. A low haptoglobin, elevated lactate dehydrogenase, and an increase in unconjugated bilirubin can confirm hemolysis. A Coombs test helps distinguish between immune and nonimmune hemolysis.

The serum iron level should be checked in cases of microcytic anemia. A decreased serum iron level suggests either iron deficiency or anemia of chronic disease. In iron deficiency, the total iron-binding capacity (TIBC) is elevated and the percent saturation is low, while in anemia of chronic disease, the TIBC is low and the percent saturation is normal or increased. The ferritin level is also decreased in iron deficiency, but it is elevated or normal in anemia of chronic disease. Typically in anemia of chronic disease, the hemoglobin does not fall below 8 g/dL, the MCV is usually only mildly decreased, and the reticulocyte count is low and does not respond to iron therapy. Although rarely needed, bone marrow aspiration and staining for iron stores is the definitive test for iron deficiency. If the serum iron is increased, a **sideroblastic anemia** should be suspected. If the serum iron level is normal, hemoglobin electrophoresis should be performed to evaluate the possibility of hemoglobinopathy, such as thalassemia, as the cause of anemia.

B_{12} and folate levels should be measured if there is a macrocytic anemia. RBC folate levels are more accurate than serum folate levels. Another useful test to differentiate between B_{12} and folate deficiency is to measure the serum methylmalonic acid and homocysteine (HC) levels. Both methylmalonic acid and HC are elevated in B_{12} deficiency, whereas only HC is elevated in folate deficiency.

It is important to examine the peripheral blood smear. If sickled cells are found, a hemoglobin electrophoresis is required to rule out sickle cell anemia. Spherocytes suggest a hemolytic process causing the anemia. Basophilic stippling with microcytic anemia is seen in lead poisoning and thalassemia. In thalassemia, liver disease, and hemolysis, target cells are also found in the peripheral smear. Teardrop cells seen in myelofibrosis and abnormal types of circulating cells such as blast cells suggest a malignancy. Howell–Jolly bodies are common in postsplenectomy patients and sickle cell anemia. Hypersegmented neutrophils may indicate the presence of a megaloblastic anemia.

TREATMENT

Management of anemia depends on an accurate diagnosis. Oral ferrous sulfate ($FeSO_4$) is preferred for iron therapy, since it is soluble, inexpensive, and easily administered. The required amount of elemental iron is 150 to 200 mg/day, which can be achieved by taking 325 mg of $FeSO_4$ two to three times daily. Although food, such as milk or other foods that raise the gastric pH, can impair iron absorption, side effects such as nausea, constipation, and heartburn may require giving $FeSO_4$ with meals. Absorption can be increased especially if given with foods that lower the gastric pH, such as vitamin C rich foods. Other iron preparations such as ferrous gluconate and ferrous fumarate may be better tolerated than ferrous sulfate but are more expensive. Indications for parenteral iron therapy are an inability to tolerate oral therapy, malabsorption or inflammatory bowel disease, severe iron deficiency, and ongoing blood loss. Iron deficiency anemia responds to treatment within 7 to 10 days, evidenced by an elevated reticulocyte count. Hemoglobin levels should return to normal within 1 to 2 months unless there is continued blood loss, and iron supplements should be continued for 6 months or until ferritin is greater than or equal to 50 ng/L. Definitive therapy of iron deficiency anemia involves identifying and treating the underlying cause. Most men and women above 35 to 40 years of age or without a history of significant menstrual bleeding require an evaluation for GI bleeding.

Patients with renal failure or AIDS, or who are undergoing chemotherapy may benefit from recombinant erythropoietin. In thalassemia major, only symptomatic therapy is available, and patients may need multiple transfusions. Since this can lead to iron overdose, chelation therapy with deferoxamine may be required. Other therapies include splenectomy and bone marrow transplant.

For patients with B_{12} deficiency from IF deficiency, parenteral replacement of B_{12} is indicated. If folate deficiency is suspected, 1 mg/day of folate should be given, along with B_{12}. If both B_{12} and folate deficiencies are present, it is important to replace both, since folate replacement alone may improve the anemia while masking the B_{12} deficiency and allowing the neurologic symptoms of B_{12} deficiency to worsen. In normocytic anemias, the underlying process causing the anemia should be treated.

KEY POINTS

- Anemia can result from blood loss, increased destruction of RBCs, or inadequate RBC production.
- Anemia can result in an inadequate supply of oxygen to the tissues, causing symptoms in vulnerable organ systems. Most individuals do not experience symptoms unless their hemoglobin is below 8 g/dL or there is an acute drop in hemoglobin.
- The classification of anemia as microcytic, macrocytic, or normocytic helps direct the workup.
- The three major causes of microcytic anemia are iron deficiency, thalassemia, and anemia of chronic disease, whereas the most common causes of macrocytic anemia are B_{12} and folate deficiency.
- In a normocytic anemia, the reticulocyte count is the most important test because it helps to differentiate between hemolytic anemias, blood loss, and bone marrow disorders.
- Oral ferrous sulfate ($FeSO_4$) is preferred for iron therapy, since it is soluble, inexpensive, and easily administered.

37 Anxiety

Anxiety is the experience of dread, foreboding, or panic, accompanied by a variety of physical symptoms. The distress can be both physical and psychological. It is a very common complaint and accounts for approximately 11% of all visits to a family physician. Box 37-1 lists brief definitions for the different types of anxiety disorders. Anxiety may also be a symptom of other psychological diseases, intoxication or withdrawal, or a medical illness.

■ BOX 37-1 Glossary of Terms

Generalized Anxiety

Excessive or unrealistic worry over at least two issues for more than 6 months.

Panic Disorder

Episodic periods of intense fear or apprehension accompanied by at least four somatic complaints: for example, diaphoresis, dyspnea, dizziness, or flushing, accompanied by behavior changes because of unrealistic and persistent worry.

Phobia

Persistent or irrational fear of a specific object, activity, or situation.

Obsessive–Compulsive Disorder

Intrusive, unwanted thoughts (obsession), and repetitive behaviors performed in a ritualistic manner (compulsion).

Post-traumatic Syndrome

Anxiety symptoms lasting at least 1 month, which develop after an individual experiences a distressing event outside the normal human response (e.g., combat, natural catastrophe). There may be delayed onset and the patient may experience flashbacks.

Adjustment Disorder with Anxious Mood

Anxiety develops as a maladaptive response to an identifiable stressor.

PATHOGENESIS

Anxiety is a normal response to many situations. Pathologic anxiety results when the anxiety occurs in the absence of appropriate stimulus or is of excessive duration and intensity. Both behavioral and biological theories exist for anxiety disorders. Biological theories implicate the involvement of several different monoamine and neuropeptide neurotransmitters. The locus ceruleus, which is the main CNS nucleus responsible for distributing norepinephrine throughout the brain, exhibits increased activity and is implicated in the pathology of some anxiety disorders. The inhibitory neurotransmitter gamma-aminobutyric acid may serve an anxiolytic function in the nervous system.

CLINICAL MANIFESTATIONS

HISTORY

The history is an essential element of the evaluation. Inquiring about stresses, fears, substance use, and precipitating factors is important. Psychological complaints include apprehension, agitation, poor concentration, feeling "on edge," difficulty sleeping, and heightened arousal. Physical symptoms are usually related to increased autonomic activity. Typically, symptoms involve the cardiopulmonary system, GI system, urinary system, and neurologic system. Dyspnea, dizziness, palpitations, sweating, nausea, abdominal pain, diarrhea, frequent urination, sweaty palms, and difficulty swallowing are common symptoms. Anxiety may also cause heightened motor tension, with trembling, twitching, muscle spasms, and easy fatigability.

PHYSICAL EXAMINATION

A physical examination is helpful in detecting medical illness that may present as anxiety. For example, an enlarged thyroid, abnormal lung examination, or irregular heart rhythm may suggest an underlying organic etiology.

DIFFERENTIAL DIAGNOSIS

In addition to anxiety disorders, similar symptoms can be seen in a wide variety of psychological and medical illnesses. Medications such as sympathomimetics (pseudoephedrine), antihistamines, bromocriptine, and bronchodilators as well as excessive caffeine may all cause anxiety-like symptoms. Neuroleptics (e.g., phenothiazines) may cause akathisia and anxiety, while some antidepressants [e.g., selective serotonin reuptake inhibitors (SSRIs)] may cause anxiety-like reactions. Drug or alcohol withdrawal is an important differential consideration. Stimulant abuse (e.g., cocaine, amphetamines) can cause agitation, irritability, and anxiety. Other psychiatric disorders that may have anxiety as a prominent component include depression, manic-depressive disease, alcoholism, psychosis, and grief reaction. Medical illnesses may present with signs and symptoms of anxiety. Box 37-2 lists some of the conditions that may present as anxiety.

BOX 37-2 Medical Conditions That May Mimic Anxiety

Cardiopulmonary
Arrhythmias
Hypoxia
Ischemic heart disease
Mitral valve prolapse
Pulmonary edema
Pulmonary embolus
Asthma
Congestive heart failure
Neurologic Diseases
Encephalopathies
Temporal lobe epilepsy
Primary sleep disorders
Postconcussion syndrome
Endocrine
Hyperthyroidism
Pheochromocytoma
Hypoglycemia
Hypocalcemia
Hypercalcemia
Cushing disease
Carcinoid syndrome
Stimulant Toxicity
Withdrawal syndrome
Hematologic Disorders
Anemia

DIAGNOSTIC EVALUATION

The diagnostic goal is to assess the anxious patient for medical causes and psychiatric illnesses. The initial focus should be on any clinical conditions the patient may currently have and to review all his or her medications. Attention should be given to disorders such as hyperthyroidism, arrhythmia, and drug withdrawal that are more common and often have anxiety as a prominent feature. Laboratory testing may not be necessary and should be focused by clinical findings. For example, pulmonary function testing may be indicated in patients with wheezing or a CBC in patients with pallor and dizziness. Recently, new validated screening tools have been introduced in primary care offices to detect generalized anxiety disorder, in addition to panic, social anxiety, and post-traumatic stress disorders. These screening tools are assisting in improved detection and treatment of anxiety disorders once thought to be uncommon in the primary care setting.

TREATMENT

Treatment strategies for anxiety include psychotherapeutic and pharmacologic interventions. The family physician can provide supportive counseling consisting of empathetic listening, meaningful reassurance, education, guidance, and encouragement. Understanding that a patient may be unable to identify the cause of his or her anxiety coupled with an empathetic willingness to listen may help to alleviate symptoms. Education begins with informing the patient of the diagnosis and discussing the underlying problems and potential treatment. Discussing the patient's fears of serious illness and of "going crazy" may have a cathartic effect.

An important element of treatment is assessing the degree of anxiety. Severely affected patients merit referral to a psychiatrist or psychologist. Nonpharmacologic treatment that has been found beneficial includes psychotherapy, behavioral therapy, relaxation techniques, reconditioning, and cognitive-behavioral therapy. These therapies are often augmented and enhanced by the use of anxiolytic agents. The goal of medication is to help the patient resume function and alleviate anxiety symptoms that interfere with the patient's life. Medications should generally be of limited duration and administered using a scheduled dose, rather than on an "as-needed" basis. Fixed goals should be set; for example, improved sleep or reduction in intrusive symptoms.

Benzodiazepines (BZDs) are the most frequently used medications and are regarded as the anxiolytic medications of choice. Side effects include physical dependency, tolerance, sedation, and impaired memory. To avoid dependence, physicians should prescribe a fixed amount and remain aware of signs of misuse, such as "lost" prescriptions. The patient should be seen regularly, and if symptoms are under control, chronic therapy should be discontinued by tapering doses over several weeks. Abrupt cessation can result in withdrawal symptoms or even seizures. Antidepressants, beta blockers, buspirone, neuroleptics, and gabapentin are also used.

SSRIs are also first-line therapeutic agents. They can benefit patients with panic disorder, general anxiety disorder, post-traumatic stress disorder, and Obsessive compulsive disorder (OCD). SSRIs may take a few weeks to become effective, so a BZD may be prescribed concomitantly for immediate relief and then tapered as the SSRI takes effect. Tricyclic antidepressants and monoamine oxidase inhibitors (MAOIs) are also effective. Buspirone and gabapentin are non-BZD medications that have mild anxiolytic effects. They are nonaddictive and have no withdrawal effects, thus making them good choices for patients at risk of abuse.

Beta blockers blunt adrenergic symptoms such as palpitations, tremors, and tachycardia. They can help patients, who suffer from cardiovascular symptoms, with panic attacks and are useful for treating stage fright on an as-needed basis.

KEY POINTS

- Anxiety is the experience of dread, foreboding, or panic accompanied by a variety of body symptoms.

- Pathologic anxiety results when the anxiety occurs in the absence of an appropriate stimulus or is of excessive duration and intensity.

- Medications such as sympathomimetics (pseudoephedrine), antihistamines, bromocriptine, and bronchodilators as well as excessive caffeine may cause anxiety-like symptoms.

- Treatment strategies for anxiety include psychotherapeutic and pharmacologic interventions.

- BZDs are the most frequently used medications and are regarded as the anxiolytic medications of choice. Side effects include physical dependency, tolerance, sedation, and impaired memory.

38 Asthma

Asthma is a chronic inflammatory disease of the airways triggered by exposure to airborne allergens, irritants, cold air, or exercise.

EPIDEMIOLOGY

Asthma affects 5% to 7% of the U.S. population. Approximately 5 million children have asthma, which makes it the most common chronic disease of childhood, with the greatest prevalence and mortality among inner-city residents. Death rates for asthma are highest among African-American youth between the ages of 15 and 24 years. Risk factors for mortality include a previous history of intubation, admission to an intensive care unit, two or more hospitalizations, or more than two emergency room visits in a single year. Other risk factors include the use of two canisters of short-acting beta$_2$-agonists in a single month, inability to perceive airway obstruction, and the use of systemic steroids.

Recognition of the importance of the underlying inflammatory process of asthma has made anti-inflammatory therapeutic agents the cornerstone of asthma management. Effective outpatient treatment of asthma can prevent exacerbations and reduce emergency room visits and hospitalizations.

PATHOGENESIS

The initial inflammatory event involves the degranulation of presensitized mast cells as a result of re-exposure to the triggering agents and release of inflammatory mediators (histamine, cytokines, leukotrienes, platelet activating factor, etc.), resulting in increased bronchiolar vascular permeability and edema, increased glandular and mucous secretions, and induction of bronchospasm. All this narrows the airway diameter and increases airway resistance, making it difficult to "breathe in" air and even more difficult to "breathe out" air. These events result in the early-phase asthmatic response, producing classic symptoms of wheezing, cough, and dyspnea. Degranulation of mast cells also stimulates alveolar macrophages, T-helper lymphocytes (Th2 cells), and bronchial epithelial cells to release chemotactic factors for the recruitment and activation of additional mediator-releasing leukocytes (eosinophils and neutrophils). The migration and activation of eosinophils and neutrophils occur 6 to 12 hours after the mast cell degranulation phase (acute-phase reaction) and constitute the late-phase asthmatic response, which can last up to 48 hours if left untreated. During this phase, the release of mediators from eosinophils causes epithelial damage, hypersecretion of mucus, and hyper-responsiveness of bronchial smooth muscles, as well as further airway edema, bronchiolar constriction, and mast cell degranulation. Therefore, the recruited eosinophils amplify and sustain the initial inflammatory response without additional exposure to the triggering agent.

Over time, chronic inflammation can change the morphology of the bronchioles, resulting in an increase in the number of mucus-producing goblet cells at the epithelial surface, hypertrophy of submucosal mucous glands (more mucus production), thickening of the basement membrane (thus decreasing airway compliance), edema and inflammatory infiltrates in the bronchial walls with prominence of eosinophils, and hypertrophy of bronchial wall muscle. These changes in bronchiole morphology are referred to as airway remodeling and are signs of chronic, long-standing airway inflammation.

CLINICAL MANIFESTATIONS

HISTORY

Patients with asthma present with symptoms of wheezing, dyspnea, cough, and sputum production. In the classification of a patient's asthma, the asthma is described as being either intermittent or persistent. As outlined in Table 38-1, persistent asthma is further classified as mild, moderate, or severe. These classifications are important in determining the recommendations for therapy.

The frequency of symptoms and presence of nocturnal symptoms are important elements of the history. In addition, identification of the triggers of the patient's asthma, his or her current symptoms, and previous attempts at treatment should be determined. The past medical history should cover the onset of the disease, prescribed and OTC medications, use of alternative medical therapies, history of allergies, past hospitalizations, and the use of steroids. A history of intubation for the treatment of asthma is a significant predictor of its severity and the need for

TABLE 38-1 Asthma Classifications

Classification	Symptoms	Nighttime Symptoms	Lung Function
Intermittent	Symptoms ≤2 times per week	≤2 times per month	FEV_1 or PEF ≥80% predicted
	Brief exacerbations		PEF variability <20%
	Asymptomatic between attacks		
Persistent–mild	Symptoms >2 times per week	>3–4 times per month	FEV_1 or PEF ≥80% predicted
	But <1 time a day		
	Attacks may affect activity		PEF variability 20%–30%
Persistent–moderate	Daily symptoms	>1 time a week but not nightly	FEV_1 or PEF 60%–80%
	Daily use of beta$_2$-agonists		Predicted
	Attacks affect activity		PEF variability >30%
	Exacerbations may last for days		
Persistent–severe	Continual symptoms with use of beta$_2$-agonist multiple times in 1 day	Frequent; at times almost each night	FEV_1 or PEF ≤60% predicted
	Limited physical activity		
	Frequent attacks		PEF variability >30%

FEV_1: forced expiratory volume in 1 second.

aggressive therapy. The family history may be significant for atopy or asthma. Assessment of the home environment—including exposure to smoke, pets, and other irritants or potential triggers—is important in determining the proper treatment.

PHYSICAL EXAMINATION

Vital signs may reveal tachypnea and tachycardia during acute episodes. Fever suggests an underlying viral or bacterial illness as a trigger. The physical examination focuses on the lung examination and listening for the wheezing, rhonchi, and prolonged expiration characteristic of asthma. With severe exacerbations and limited air movement, the lung fields may be deceptively quiet. In some cases, one can appreciate the difficulty with airway movement with physical exam findings such as nasal flaring, tracheal tugging, intercostal retractions and use of accessory muscles, and abdominal breathing.

DIFFERENTIAL DIAGNOSIS

In children, conditions that can also present with wheezing, cough, and increased sputum production include bronchiolitis, cystic fibrosis, croup, epiglottitis,

bronchitis, and foreign-body aspiration. Bronchiolitis has many similarities to asthma but presents as an acute illness and is not a chronic disease. Cystic fibrosis is a chronic disease that initially may be confused with asthma, but patients also develop GI symptoms, growth disturbances, recurrent sinus infections, and pneumonia. Croup, epiglottitis, bronchitis, and foreign-body aspiration are discrete episodes and not chronic diseases. In adults, the primary diseases confused with asthma are COPD and CHF. Both of these diseases usually have their onset in adulthood. A chest x-ray, ECG, spirometry, and other testing can help to distinguish between CHF and pulmonary disease.

DIAGNOSTIC EVALUATION

The history and physical examination suggest the diagnosis. Peak flow testing can provide additional evidence of airway obstruction and support the clinical impression. Airway obstruction exists when the peak flow is less than 80% of the predicted value based on the patient's age, height, and gender. In cases where the diagnosis is still uncertain, complete pulmonary function testing can also be obtained. A chest x-ray is recommended during the initial evaluation of the wheezing patient to detect pneumonia, a foreign body, CHF, or other nonasthmatic causes of wheezing. The chest x-ray in the asthmatic patient may be normal or show hyperinflation due to air trapping. In patients with suspected allergic triggers, allergy testing may be helpful. For patients with suspected cystic fibrosis, sweat testing can be a useful screen.

TREATMENT

For appropriate management, asthma can be divided into four categories (see Table 38-1). The goals of asthma therapy are to prevent symptoms, maintain normal pulmonary function and activity level, prevent emergency room visits and hospitalizations, and minimize the adverse effects of medications.

Effective asthma treatment has four components:

1. Objectively assessing and monitoring lung function using a peak expiratory flow (PEF) meter. PEF monitoring is advocated for patients with moderate and severe persistent asthma. Patients first establish their personal best and are then asked to respond to PEF measurement on the basis of a "color zone" system. The green zone, defined as more than 80% of personal best PEF,

indicates good control. The yellow zone, between 50% and 80% of personal best, indicates the need for prompt inhaled short-acting beta$_2$-agonists and contact with a physician about adjustments in current medication. The red zone, 50% or less of personal best, indicates immediate use of inhaled beta$_2$-agonists and emergency assessment by a physician.

2. Environmental control of asthma triggers to limit exacerbations. It is imperative that patients be made aware not only of the basic facts of their disease but also of the things that trigger their asthma (e.g., "respiratory infections," pollen, change of weather, tobacco smoke, animal dander, mold, dust), so that they can take appropriate environmental control measures to limit their exposures.

3. Treatment for long-term management (Table 38-2).

4. Thorough and detailed patient education. This includes basic facts about the disease and the role of medication, proper use of inhalers, establishing a plan of action for episodes of exacerbation, and recognizing signs of airway obstruction.

Asthma medications are classified into **long-term control medications** (anti-inflammatories) **to prevent** exacerbations and symptoms and **quick-relief med-**

■ **TABLE 38-2** Stepwise Approach to Asthma Management		
	Long-Term Control	**Quick Relief Medication**
Step 1		Short-acting inhaled beta$_2$ agonist
Step 2	**Preferred:** low-dose inhaled corticosteroid **Alternative:** Cromolyn or Nedocromil, leukotriene modifiers or theophylline	Short-acting inhaled beta$_2$ agonist
Step 3	**Preferred:** low-dose inhaled corticosteroid plus long-acting beta$_2$-agonist OR medium dose inhaled corticosteroid **Alternative:** low-dose inhaled corticosteroid, plus leukotriene receptor agonist, theophylline, or zileuton	Short-acting inhaled beta$_2$ agonist
Step 4	**Preferred:** medium-dose inhaled corticosteroid, plus, long-acting inhaled beta$_2$ agonist **Alternative:** medium-dose inhaled corticosteroid, plus leukotriene receptor agonist, theophylline, or zileuton	Short-acting inhaled beta$_2$ agonist
Step 5	**Preferred:** high-dose inhaled corticosteroid, plus long-acting beta$_2$ agonist AND consider omalizumab for patients with allergies	Short-acting inhaled beta$_2$ agonist
Step 6	**Preferred:** high-dose inhaled corticosteroid, plus long-acting beta$_2$ agonist, plus oral corticosteroid, AND consider omalizumab for patients with allergies	Short-acting inhaled beta$_2$ agonist

ications (bronchodilators) **to treat** symptoms and exacerbations. All patients with persistent asthma need both types of medication.

Inhaled short-acting bronchodilators are useful for treating acute symptoms and are the only therapy needed by those with intermittent disease. Albuterol is the most commonly used beta$_2$ agonist and is generally administered as two puffs every 4 to 6 hours, as needed to control acute symptoms. Side effects may include flushing, tremors, and tachycardia.

Inhaled corticosteroids are the most potent and effective anti-inflammatory agents used for the long-term treatment of persistent asthma. They prevent irreversible airway injury, improve lung function, and reduce asthma deaths. Most patients can be adequately maintained on twice-daily doses. Patients should be advised to gargle and rinse their mouths with water after using inhaled steroids in order to prevent oral candidiasis. As the severity of asthma increases, so must the strength of the inhaled corticosteroid. High-dose inhaled steroids used for severe asthma may interfere with the normal vertical growth of children. For this reason, oral leukotriene inhibitors, which have an additive effect when given in conjunction with inhaled steroids, can be added to low- or moderate-dose inhaled corticosteroids in order to reduce the need for high-dose steroids.

Cromolyn sodium and nedocromil are mast cell stabilizers; they prevent mast cell degranulation in addition to inhibiting bronchoconstriction. They have mild to moderate anti-inflammatory effects and are relatively safe to use in children and pregnant women with persistent-mild asthma. They are also effective agents against exercise-induced asthma in a single inhaled dose taken 15 to 30 minutes before exercise.

Salmeterol, a long-acting beta$_2$-agonist, is useful in the management of nocturnal symptoms and exercise-induced asthma. It is more effective than nedocromil in the treatment of exercise-induced asthma, since its duration of action is only 9 hours, as opposed to 2 to 3 hours for nedocromil. It is also useful as additive therapy to low-dose inhaled corticosteroids to avoid high-dose steroids. Studies have shown that salmeterol combined with low-dose steroids is more efficacious in improving symptoms and reducing the use of rescue medication than simply doubling the dose of inhaled steroids.

Oral (systemic) corticosteroids are recommended and effective as "burst" therapy for gaining initial control of asthma when therapy is being initiated or during an acute exacerbation. One method of administering burst therapy is to give prednisone (adults, 40–60 mg/day, children 1–2 mg/kg/day) for 3 to 10 days or until the

PEF improves to 80% of personal best. Long-term use of oral steroids should be considered only for patients who are refractory to all other therapies because of their potential for causing side effects and growth retardation.

Anticholinergics for asthma include inhaled ipratropium (Atrovent), which inhibits vagally mediated bronchoconstriction and mucus production. It is effective when used in conjunction with a short-acting beta$_2$-agonist for the treatment of severe asthma exacerbations.

Nonadherence and poor asthma control are usually related to inadequate understanding of the disease and its treatment, improper use of inhaled medication, lack of environmental control of asthma triggers (e.g., outdoor allergens, tobacco smoke, animal dander, dust, cockroaches, molds), or poor continuity of care. Patient education remains the cornerstone of a successful asthma management strategy: increasing patient involvement, and fostering a strong partnership between patients, their families, and the physician. This relationship is imperative to help ensure not only the patient's adherence to the treatment regimen but also the continuous follow-up with his or her family physician.

KEY POINTS

- Asthma is a chronic inflammatory respiratory condition (type I hypersensitivity reaction).
- The symptoms of asthma include cough, wheezing, and dyspnea.
- The pathophysiology of asthma includes airway edema, increased mucus production, and bronchospasm.
- Asthma can be classified into intermittent, mild-persistent, moderate-persistent, and severe-persistent types.
- Short-term control includes short-acting inhaled bronchodilators (beta$_2$-agonists); long-term control includes inhaled corticosteroids.
- Intermittent asthma does not require daily medication; persistent asthma is controlled by inhaled corticosteroids as well as short-acting inhaled bronchodilators.
- Table 38-2 outlines a stepwise approach to the management of asthma.

39 Atopic Dermatitis

"Atopic dermatitis" (AD) is a clinical term describing one of the most common skin diseases and the most common form of eczematous dermatitis. The term "atopy" describes a genetic condition involving a personal or family history of hay fever, asthma, dry skin (xerosis), or eczema. AD is itchy, recurrent, symmetric, and commonly involves the skin in the flexural creases (e.g., popliteal and antecubital regions). It begins early in life, followed by periods of remission and exacerbation, and usually resolves by age 30. The highest incidence is among children, with 65% of cases presenting within the first 12 months of life.

PATHOGENESIS

The precise pathogenesis of AD is unclear. Genetic factors, altered immune function, and abnormalities within the epidermis are thought to play a role in the development of AD. Individuals with AD appear to inherit cellular changes that lead to mast cell and basophil hyperactivity in association with IgE-mediated cross-linking and activation of these cells. With activation, histamine, leukotrienes, and other factors are released, leading to vascular leakage, which is manifest as erythema, edema, and pruritus. During the late phase response and with chronic disease, inflammatory cells are present in the skin. These abnormalities in mast cell and basophil reactivity are not specific to the skin, and patients with AD frequently have other manifestations of atopic disease, such as asthma or allergic rhinitis.

CLINICAL MANIFESTATIONS

HISTORY

AD may present in slightly different patterns at different ages. The age of the patient and any past history of skin disease are helpful in narrowing the differential diagnosis. In addition, it is important to ask about family history of atopic disease and to get detailed information about potential triggers for the patient's AD. Infants may present around 3 months of age with inflammation occurring initially on the cheeks and later involving the forehead and extensor surfaces of arms and legs while sparing the diaper area. AD will resolve in approximately 50% of infants by 18 months of age and the rest will progress into childhood with this condition.

During childhood, there may be lichenification and inflammation of flexural areas, including the antecubital and popliteal fossae, neck, wrists, and ankles. Exudative lesions, which are more typical of the infant phase, are less common. Other areas—such as the hands, eyelids, and anogenital regions—are more commonly involved in adolescents and adults.

AD tends to be cyclic, with remissions and exacerbations. Factors that cause dryness of the skin or increase the desire to scratch will worsen and often trigger AD. These include excessive washing (especially with hot water), decreased humidity, occlusive clothing, sweating, contact with irritating substances (wool, cosmetics, some soaps, fabric softeners, household chemicals, etc.), contact allergy, and aeroallergens (dust mites, pollen, animal dander, molds, etc.). Stress and foods such as eggs, milk, seafood, nuts, wheat, or soy can also provoke exacerbations of AD.

PHYSICAL EXAMINATION

The location and nature of any skin lesion should be noted. During an acute eruption of AD, the skin may have papules and vesicles, with eventual crusting of the vesicles. Chronic skin lesions suggesting possible AD include scaling plaques and lichenification of the skin, particularly in the flexural creases. Dry skin and keratosis pilaris are other commonly associated skin findings. Signs of secondary bacterial infection should be noted, as the skin of patients with AD is more susceptible to infections with staphylococcal or streptococcal bacteria. The examination should also include a search for other manifestations of atopic disease, such as asthma, allergic rhinitis, and allergic conjunctivitis.

DIFFERENTIAL DIAGNOSIS

Eczema can also include diseases other than AD, such as dyshidrotic eczema and lichen simplex chronicus. In addition to these, the differential diagnosis for eczema includes other skin and systemic diseases, as outlined in Box 39-1.

BOX 39-1 Differential Diagnosis of Atopic Dermatitis

Hand dermatitis
Dyshidrotic eczema
Lichen simplex chronicus
Stasis dermatitis
Seborrheic dermatitis
Contact dermatitis
Psoriasis
Scabies
Fungal infections
Immunodeficiency diseases

DIAGNOSTIC EVALUATION

The diagnosis of AD can be made clinically by the presence of three essential criteria: personal or family history (first-degree relative) of atopy, pruritus, and the specific patterns of eruption.

AD is an itch that, when scratched, will erupt, leading to the phrase "**the itch that rashes**." The skin lesions generally do not appear before rubbing or scratching traumatizes the skin. Patients with AD often have abnormally dry skin and a lowered threshold for itching. The finding of papules, vesicles, and plaques located in the flexural creases is supportive of the diagnosis of eczema. In addition, lichenification and dry, scaly skin should raise suspicion for eczema even in the absence of active lesions. Allergy testing should be considered in order to identify triggers of the patient's eczema, particularly in those who are refractory to therapy and with no triggers identified by history.

TREATMENT

The goal of the therapy is to decrease inflammation, promptly treat secondary infections, and preserve and restore the stratum corneum barrier. In general, steroids are used to suppress the inflammation of acute flare-ups. Antibiotics are used to treat any secondary infection of the atopic lesions. The most common pathogen is *Staphylococcus aureus*. Trigger avoidance, emollients, and antihistamines are used in efforts to maintain the integrity of the skin.

During an acute exacerbation, weeping and vesiculated lesions may be dried with aluminum subacetate (Domeboro) compresses, and baths with an oatmeal-based emollient like Aveeno may help to relieve itching. **Antihistamines** are useful in helping to control the pruritus. Sedating antihistamines are best used at night for those patients who have sleep disturbances secondary to the pruritus.

Both types of skin lesions are then treated most commonly using **topical steroid ointments or creams**. Emollients are most effective when used after a shower or bath when the skin can absorb the most moisture. Many physicians prefer to use ointments rather than creams in patients with AD because of the ointment's added moisturizing effects. Topical steroid treatment has been shown to be effective and safe for use in acute flare-ups for up to 4 weeks, although in many cases the AD flare-up can be adequately treated in a shorter time period. Important side effects of long-term daily use of topical steroids include skin atrophy, striae, telangiectasia, and worsening of acne conditions and all patients must be educated on these adverse reactions prior to implementing topical steroid treatment.

Chronically, trigger avoidance and keeping the skin moist are important aspects of treatment. Chemical irritants should be avoided. The hands should be protected from prolonged water exposure. Cotton clothing should be worn and mild soaps, such as Dove or Basis, are recommended. Bathing should be in warm but not hot water and daily moisturizing creams, oils, or petroleum jelly applied. Scratching should be kept to a minimum through use of antihistamines and topical steroids. Other medications that have been used for treating AD include tars, oral steroids, and ultraviolet (UV) light. Patients do not usually tolerate topical tar medications because of their inconvenience and the staining associated with their use. Patients not controlled with topical steroids, antihistamines, use of emollients, and trigger avoidance merit referral to a dermatologist or allergist. The treatment of eczema is summarized in Table 39-1.

Nonsteroidal immunomodulators like tacrolimus (Protopic) and pimecrolimus (Elidel) are second-line treatment options for moderate-to-severe and mild-to-moderate eczema, respectively, refractory to standard treatment. Tacrolimus is available in 0.1% and 0.03% ointments for adults and 0.03% ointments for children 2 years of age and above; pimecrolimus is available in 0.1% ointment for adults and children 2 years of age and above. Side effects include temporary stinging and burning on initial application, which eventually abate as the skin heals, and adverse effects in the sun with UV exposure. Of note, there has been controversy whether or not these agents induce local or distant malignancy. Recently, new label revisions that include second-line treatment indications, patient education, and enhanced warnings of adverse effects were approved by the FDA. These ointments are used for short treatment periods and are contraindicated in children less than 2 years of age and in breast-feeding women and those who plan to become pregnant.

People with AD, regardless of severity, should not receive a smallpox vaccination or be exposed to those

TABLE 39-1 Treatment of Atopic Dermatitis	
Topical	Topical steroids
	Topical immunomodulators as second-line treatment
	Tar
	Moisturizers should be applied after showers and handwashing
	Lipid-free lotion cleansers
Antibiotics	Erythromycin (250 mg qid)
(suppress *S. aureus*)	Dicloxacillin (250 mg qid)
	Cephalexin (250 mg qid) or
	Cefadroxil (500 mg bid)
Antihistamines	Hydroxyzine
(sedation and controlling pruritus)	Doxepin
Severe Cases	Oral prednisone
	Intramuscular triamcinolone
	Psoralen plus Type A ultraviolet light
	Tar plus Type B ultraviolet light
	High potency topical steroids

who have newly received the smallpox vaccination as the live virus can cause severe and even life-threatening reactions in those with eczema. Exposure includes touching the inoculation site before it has healed and transmission of the live virus through towels, clothing, or bandages worn by the person vaccinated. The transmission period may last from 3 weeks to 1 month.

KEY POINTS

- The highest incidence of AD is among children, with 60% of cases presenting within the first 12 months of life.
- Lichenification and inflammation of flexural areas (antecubital/popliteal fossae, neck, wrists, and ankles) are common findings in atopic dermatitis.
- The mainstays of therapy are steroids, trigger avoidance, emollients, and antihistamines.

Chronic Obstructive Pulmonary Disease

The obstructive lung diseases include asthma, cystic fibrosis, bronchiectasis, and COPD. "COPD" is a collective term used to describe emphysema, chronic bronchitis, or both and is characterized by an airflow limitation that is not fully reversible. Chronic bronchitis is defined as a productive cough that occurs for at least 3 months a year for more than 2 consecutive years. Emphysema is defined as an abnormal dilatation of the terminal airspaces with destruction of alveolar septa. Thus, chronic bronchitis is defined clinically while emphysema is defined pathologically. It is estimated that 16 million Americans are diagnosed with COPD and an equal number have the disease but are as yet undiagnosed. COPD is the fourth leading cause of death in the United States for individuals 65 to 85 years of age. Cigarette smoking is the most common cause of COPD, accounting for up to 90% of these cases.

PATHOGENESIS

The pathogenesis of COPD is not completely understood, but it is thought to result from chronic inflammation. Smoking and other inhaled irritants may promote an inflammatory response in the airways, resulting in the mucosal edema, increased mucus production, and reactive airways characteristic of chronic bronchitis. Bronchospasm may result in airway narrowing, which—along with impaired ciliary function—results in difficulty clearing secretions, air trapping, and alterations in gas exchange. Host susceptibility also plays a role and explains why only 15% of smokers develop COPD.

Similar changes may occur in patients with emphysema; however, the inflammatory response may predominantly affect the smaller airways, leading to tissue destruction and loss of the normal elastic recoil of the lung. This results in increased dead space and air trapping, in essence creating functionless lung tissue where there is minimal to no air exchange.

There is great overlap between these two categories of COPD and many patients will have features of both chronic bronchitis and emphysema. In addition to cough and increased mucus production, changes that occur as a result of COPD include decreased concentration of oxygen in the blood and decreased clearance of carbon dioxide from the blood. This results in lower oxygen delivery to the various organs and can lead to compromised organ function. For example, decreased oxygen delivery to the lung tissue will result in elevation of pulmonary artery blood pressure, which can cause right-sided heart failure or cor pulmonale.

CLINICAL MANIFESTATIONS

HISTORY

Early in the course of the disease, COPD patients will have minimal or no symptoms. Often a productive chronic cough is the first symptom, followed by shortness of breath with exertion as the disease progresses. Ultimately, the cough may become disabling and patients may develop dyspnea in the recumbent position, requiring them to sleep in the upright position.

Other important historical factors include smoking history, defined in pack-years (packs per day times number of years smoking), personal or family history of respiratory disorders, and exposure to secondhand smoke or environmental irritants. An assessment of the patient's limitations in activities may help to assess the severity of his or her disease prior to pulmonary function testing.

PHYSICAL EXAMINATION

The patient with COPD may appear overweight and cyanotic, as typified by the "**blue bloater**" associated with chronic bronchitis. Alternatively, he or she may appear thin and barrel-chested, typical of the "**pink puffer**" associated with emphysema. Use of accessory muscles of respiration should be noted. On percussion, hyper-resonance associated with the air trapping may be present and auscultation may reveal diminished peripheral breath sounds due to the limited air movement. Many patients with chronic bronchitis or those with an acute exacerbation of chronic bronchitis have rhonchi or wheezing. Skin examination can reveal the presence of cyanosis as well as clubbing of the digits. Heart sounds may be more distant due to the altered chest configuration and increased air between the chest wall and the heart. In addition, the presence of rhonchi and wheezing may obscure the heart sounds. With cor pulmonale and right-sided heart failure, other symptoms and signs such as peripheral edema, jugular venous distention, and hepatojugular reflux may be present.

DIFFERENTIAL DIAGNOSIS

Respiratory symptoms and cough may have several different etiologies. In addition to COPD, other diseases such as upper respiratory infections, bronchitis, or pneumonia may cause shortness of breath and cough. Allergies, asthma, and cystic fibrosis are chronic conditions that typically present in childhood and may include increased cough, mucus production, shortness of breath, and wheezing. Patients with decompensated CHF commonly have shortness of breath and on examination may have wheezing, rales, and peripheral edema.

Alpha$_1$ antitrypsin deficiency should be considered in patients below 45 years of age with a family history of respiratory disease who present with features of COPD, particularly in the absence of smoking. Up to 10% of these patients will also have serious liver disease and may have findings consistent with hepatitis or cirrhosis.

DIAGNOSTIC EVALUATION

Evaluation of the patient suspected of having COPD should include a detailed history and physical examination, which will provide the diagnosis in most cases. Other tests that may be performed to confirm the diagnosis and exclude other diseases include a chest x-ray and pulmonary function testing. In patients with a diagnosis of COPD, arterial blood gases, pulse oximetry, and an ECG may be obtained to assess disease severity and detect cor pulmonale.

Chest radiographs are not diagnostic of COPD, and findings in patients with COPD may vary depending on the predominant component (bronchitis or emphysema). The classic findings in patients with chronic bronchitis are increased lung markings, termed a "**dirty-chest**" appearance. In patients with predominantly emphysema, there are decreased lung markings, hyperlucency of the lung fields, and flattening of the diaphragms, all consistent with the hyperinflation of the lungs found in emphysema. In advanced COPD, the ECG may show evidence of right atrial enlargement, right ventricular hypertrophy, and right axis deviation.

Pulmonary function testing measures air exchange and lung volumes. With COPD, there is difficulty and delay in the movement of air out of the lungs, resulting in prolonged expiration on both physical examination and pulmonary function testing. In addition, because of the air trapping that occurs from incom-

plete emptying of the lungs, residual volumes are increased. The forced expiratory volume in 1 second (FEV_1) is a measure of the maximum air that can be expired from the lung in 1 second after a full inspiration. The FEV_1 is the most accurate and reproducible measure of outflow obstruction. It is significantly decreased in patients with COPD and is the primary measure used to assess disease severity. The FEV_1 also correlates with patient symptoms and disease severity and is the best predictor of survival. Patients with stage-1 disease will have minimal limitations in activities and an FEV_1 50% or more of their predicted FEV_1 (based on age, gender, height, and weight). Stage-2 disease occurs when patients are limited in their activities because of the COPD; they have FEV_1 measures of 35% to 49% of their predicted FEV_1. Patients with stage-3 disease are severely limited in activity; their FEV_1 is less than 35% of their predicted level. In patients with stage-2 or -3 disease, arterial blood gases, pulse oximetry, or ECGs may help in management of the disease and are important in identifying patients who might benefit from supplemental oxygen.

TREATMENT

Preventing the progression of disease through early identification and aggressive smoking cessation programs should be the primary goal in approaching patients with COPD. Pulmonary function testing to detect a decrease in lung function and the accelerated decline in lung function associated with smoking is helpful in motivating patients to stop smoking. With smoking cessation, lung function will show a modest improvement initially and then follows the normal age-related decline, as with nonsmokers.

For patients with established COPD, goals of therapy are improvement in lung function, avoiding or reducing hospitalizations, early treatment or prevention of acute exacerbations, and minimizing disability to improve quality of life. Smoking cessation and oxygen therapy for hypoxic individuals are the only therapies that can improve survival. Other long-term benefits of oxygen supplementation include decrease in polycythemia, pulmonary artery pressure, dyspnea, hypoxemia during sleep, and decreased nocturnal arrhythmia events. To get the effect of long-term oxygen therapy, patients should use oxygen for at least 15 h/day with maximum effect seen at 20 hours of use. Pulmonary rehabilitation does not actually improve pulmonary function testing but may enhance physical endurance and thus overall function. Preventive medicine is extremely important and patients should receive a pneumococcal vaccine and annual influenza vaccinations.

Other mainstay treatments include bronchodilators, steroids, antibiotics, and oxygen. Box 40-1 outlines steps used in the treatment. Bronchodilators, in

■ **BOX 40-1** Treatment Guidelines for COPD
1. For mild, variable symptoms
Selective beta$_2$-agonist metered-dose inhaler (MDI) aerosol, 1–2 puffs every 2–6 hours as needed, not to exceed 8–12 puffs per 24 hours
2. For mild-to-moderate continuing symptoms
Ipratropium bromide (Atrovent) MDI aerosol, 2–6 puffs every 6–8 hours
PLUS:
Selective beta$_2$-agonist MDI aerosol, 1–4 puffs as required four times daily for rapid relief as needed or as regular supplement
3. If response to step 2 is unsatisfactory or there is a mild to moderate increase in symptoms
Add sustained-release theophylline, 200–400 mg three times a day or 400–800 mg at bedtime for nocturnal bronchospasm
AND/OR:
Consider use of a mucokinetic agent
4. If control of symptoms is suboptimal
Consider a course of oral corticosteroids for 10–14 days
If improvement occurs, wean to low daily or alternate-day dose
If no improvement occurs, stop abruptly
If corticosteroid appears to help, consider possible use of aerosol MDI, particularly if patient has evidence of bronchial hyper-reactivity
5. For severe exacerbation
Increase beta$_2$-agonist dosage, such as MDI with spacer, 6–8 puffs every 30 minutes to 2 hours, or inhalant solution, unit dose every 30 minutes to 2 hours, or subcutaneous administration of epinephrine or terbutaline sulfate (Brethine), 0.1–0.5 mL
AND/OR:
Increase ipratropium dosage, such as MDI with spacer, 6–8 puffs every 3–4 hours, or inhalant solution of ipratropium, 0.5 mg every 4–8 hours
AND:
Provide theophylline dosage intravenously with calculated amount to bring serum level to 10–12 mg/mL
AND:
Provide methylprednisolone acetate (Depoject, depMedalone 40, Depo-Medrol, etc.) dosage intravenously, giving 50–100 mg immediately, then every 5–8 hours; taper as soon as possible
AND ADD:
An antibiotic if indicated
A mucokinetic agent if sputum is very viscous
Adapted from American Thoracic Society. Standards for the diagnosis and care of patients with chronic obstructive pulmonary disease. *Am J Respir Crit Care Med.* 1995;152(5 Pt 2):S77–S121.

the form of anticholinergics (e.g., ipratropium), which cause bronchodilation through inhibition of vagal stimulation, or beta$_2$-agonists (e.g., albuterol) are used to treat acute exacerbations of COPD and can be used in patients who have daily symptoms. When used together, anticholinergics and beta$_2$-ago-nists have a synergistic effect. For patients with daily symptoms, a long-acting beta$_2$-agonist, such as salme-terol, is available for twice-daily use. Short-acting bronchodilators can then be used for breakthrough symptoms. Theophylline also has a bronchodilating effect and may improve diaphragmatic function.

Serum levels must be monitored, since nausea, palpitations, and seizures can result from toxic levels.

Oral steroids are used to treat acute exacerbations of COPD in a 2-week tapering dose. Long-term use of oral steroids has the potential for significant side effects, and their use is not well defined. Inhaled corticosteroids may be helpful in limiting inflammation, improving airway reactivity, and reducing the frequency of COPD exacerbations. However, like oral steroids, they have not been shown to affect survival and their role in COPD is not clearly defined. Still, inhaled corticosteroids are an option of treatment but should be used in conjunction with long-acting $beta_2$-agonist.

Antibiotics are useful for treating acute exacerbations of COPD, particularly in those patients with an increase in dyspnea, cough, and mucus production. Antibiotics commonly used include tetracyclines, sulfonamides, penicillins (e.g., amoxicillin with or without clavulanic acid), fluoroquinolones, macrolides, and cephalosporins. Antibiotics should include coverage for the most common organisms associated with COPD exacerbations, namely *Streptococcus pneumoniae, Haemophilus influenzae*, and *Moraxella catarrhalis*. For those requiring frequent antibiotics or with severe underlying disease, many experts recommend using fluoroquinolones for an acute exacerbation.

Patients with severe disease will often need supplemental oxygen. Candidates for oxygen supplementation are those with a PO_2 of less than 55, pulse oximetry less than 88%, and cor pulmonale. The use of continuous positive airway pressure (CPAP), either daily or at night, can improve functional status, oxygenation, and arterial blood gases. Use of CPAP is generally reserved for those patients with COPD who are hypercapneic. For patients with cor pulmonale and right-sided heart failure, treatment of the heart failure and the use of diuretics may be beneficial. Pneumococcal and influenza vaccines are indicated for patients with COPD.

KEY POINTS

- COPD is smoking-related in over 90% of cases.
- Pulmonary function testing (FEV_1) can help in assessing disease severity.
- Smoking cessation is an important aspect of therapy for COPD.
- Bronchodilators, steroids, antibiotics, and oxygen are the mainstays of therapy.

Congestive Heart Failure

CHF affects an estimated 4.9 million Americans and is the most frequent cause of hospitalization in the elderly. One percent of adults aged 50 to 60 and 10% of those in their eighties are affected by it. The overall 5-year mortality is 60% for men and 45% for women. The three major risk factors for heart failure are hypertension, CAD, and valvular heart disease.

PATHOGENESIS

Heart failure occurs if the heart is unable to perfuse body tissues adequately. Cardiac output depends on three factors: preload, contractility, and afterload. **Preload** (also referred to as the left ventricular end-diastolic pressure) is the pressure required to distend the ventricle at a given volume. The relationship of pressure and volume defines compliance. **Contractility** describes the functional state of the myocardial muscle. Normally, as preload increases, the cardiac output and the amount of blood pumped by the heart muscle increase. **Afterload** is the resistance against which the heart contracts and is clinically reflected by the systolic blood pressure.

Heart failure begins with symptoms that occur only during periods of stress, as during illness or exercise; but as the disease progresses, symptoms may occur with rest. Heart failure may be due to either systolic or diastolic dysfunction. Systolic dysfunction is characterized by decreased contractility of the left ventricle, resulting in a reduced ejection fraction. A decreased ejection fraction leads to a compensatory increase in preload to maintain cardiac output. Eventually, there is a limit to which increases in preload can compensate, and pulmonary congestion occurs, resulting in signs and symptoms such as orthopnea, paroxysmal nocturnal dyspnea (PND), rales, jugular venous distention (JVD), and edema.

Decreases in cardiac output trigger a host of compensatory mechanisms, including activation of the renin–angiotensin–aldosterone system, increased levels of catecholamines, and the secretion of atrial natriuretic hormone. These compensatory mechanisms result in systemic vasoconstriction, fluid retention, and increased afterload, which further inhibits cardiac output, thus creating a vicious feedback cycle. Late changes effected by these compensatory mechanisms include myocardial and vascular remodeling and fibrosis.

About 40% of patients have diastolic dysfunction. Diastolic dysfunction results from an inability of the ventricle to relax properly, which leads to a higher filling pressure, pulmonary congestion, and decreased cardiac return. Changes that occur with aging predispose elderly individuals to developing diastolic dysfunction. Other causes include ischemia, hypertension, ventricular hypertrophy, volume overload, and pericardial disease. It is also common for patients with systolic dysfunction to have some element of diastolic dysfunction.

CLINICAL MANIFESTATIONS

HISTORY

Symptoms of CHF include dyspnea, orthopnea, PND, nocturia, edema, weight gain, fatigue, chest pain, abdominal pain, anorexia, and mental status changes (Box 41-1). In taking the patient's history, it is useful to determine what activities make the patient short of breath, since classification of severity of disease is based on whether the patient is asymptomatic, has dyspnea with exertion, or has dyspnea at rest. The need to sleep

---

■ BOX 41-1 Initial Assessment Questions to Determine Severity of CHF

Dyspnea, orthopnea, PND
Recent weight increase, edema, ascites
Chest pain or palpitations
Causes of anemia (blood loss, etc.)
Recent signs and/or symptoms of recent illness
Exercise tolerance
Claudication
Fatigue
Dietary changes (increased salt intake, eating a balanced diet)
Social history: smoking history, alcohol and/or illicit drug abuse

on more than one pillow suggests orthopnea. Chest pain, palpitations, and excessive salt intake are additional important historical factors associated with heart failure. Previous and current medical conditions and risk factors for CAD should be thoroughly reviewed.

PHYSICAL EXAMINATION

Checking general appearance and vital signs is important in order to determine whether the patient has an arrhythmia, is hypertensive, or is in respiratory distress (Box 41-2). Examination of the neck may reveal JVD, a sign of elevated filling pressures. The point of maximal impulse (PMI) of the left ventricle is often displaced laterally and downward in individuals with cardiomegaly. Auscultation of the lungs may reveal bibasilar rales. When rales are present, measurement of the lung field level at which they are heard is a useful way of following treatment. Cardiac auscultation may reveal third and fourth heart sounds, which are often present in patients who are fluid-overloaded and/or who have a stiff ventricle. Murmurs may indicate valvular pathology as the cause of heart failure. Abdominal examination often reveals hepatomegaly, which is a sign of right-sided heart failure and indicates moderate-to-severe venous congestion. Lower extremity edema is a common finding; if this is of long standing, it is often accompanied by stasis dermatitis. Quantifying the degree of edema is useful for following the treatment.

DIFFERENTIAL DIAGNOSIS

The differential diagnosis depends on the presenting symptom. For patients complaining of dyspnea, the major differential is pulmonary diseases such as COPD, interstitial lung disease, pulmonary infections, and PE. Dyspnea may also be a sign of anemia.

For patients with fluid retention and edema, the differential diagnosis includes hypoalbuminemic states, cirrhosis, nephrotic syndrome, and chronic venous stasis. In the elderly, some common signs of heart failure may be misleading. For example, many patients have edema from chronic venous insufficiency and may not have heart failure. In these patients, the examination and constellation of symptoms combined with diagnostic testing are needed to establish the presence or absence of heart failure.

DIAGNOSTIC EVALUATION

The goals of the diagnostic evaluation are to determine the underlying reason for heart failure and search for causes of acute decompensation. Box 41-3 lists some causes of heart failure.

The chest x-ray remains an excellent, readily available test for identifying heart failure. Characteristic findings include cardiomegaly, redistribution of vascular markings, prominent interstitial markings, Kerley B lines, and perihilar haziness. In more advanced cases, pleural effusions may be identified. The chest x-ray may also identify pulmonary disease, which may be causing or contributing to symptoms. An ECG is useful for detecting an arrhythmia or for

---

■ BOX 41-2 Physical Exam Findings

Vital signs: increase of weight from documented baseline
General: diaphoresis
Skin: skin changes (pallor, cyanosis, jaundice)
Neck: elevated jugular venous pressure, hepato-jugular reflex
Cardiovascular: tachycardia, bradycardia, arrhythmias, S3, S4 heart sounds, murmur, lateral displacement of PMI, diminished peripheral pulses
Respiratory: labored breathing with use of assessory muscles, rales above the lower 25% of the lung that do not clear after cough
Abdomen: hepatomegaly, tender liver, or ascites
Extremities: edema in lower extremities without evidence of venous insufficiency

---

■ BOX 41-3 Causes of Heart Failure

Myocardial Damage
Ischemia
Infarction
Hypertensive cardiomyopathy
Infiltrative heart disease (e.g., amyloid, sarcoid)
Dilated cardiomyopathy
Toxins (e.g., alcohol, Adriamycin, cocaine, radiation)
Diastolic Dysfunction
Valvular heart disease
Infections: bacterial, viral, and parasites
Congenital heart disease, including metabolic disorders (Pompe disease and McArdle disease)
Constrictive pericarditis
Extracardiac
Anemia
Renal failure
Thyroid disease
Connective tissue disease

providing evidence of ischemic disease, left ventricular hypertrophy (LVH), or left atrial enlargement.

Virtually all patients with heart failure should have an echocardiogram. The echocardiogram can determine whether the mechanism of heart failure is primarily systolic or diastolic dysfunction. In patients with systolic dysfunction, the ejection fraction is reduced (<45%), whereas in diastolic dysfunction the ejection fraction is preserved or even high. Doppler US techniques help confirm diastolic dysfunction by identifying abnormal flow across the mitral valve. Echocardiograms can also detect LVH, valvular disease, pericardial disease, and wall motion abnormalities suggestive of ischemia.

Blood work should include a CBC, UA, electrolytes including liver function tests (LFTs), BUN, creatinine, albumin, PT/INR, and TSH. In patients with acute symptoms, cardiac markers are useful for detecting acute myocardial damage. BNP can assist in distinguishing between pulmonary disease and heart failure as the cause for dyspnea. The BNP is elevated in CHF and can be used along with clinical assessment to monitor disease status. Depending on the patient's initial clinical evaluation, other tests may be useful. For example, an exercise or pharmacologic ECG stress test is helpful for detecting ischemic heart disease.

Common causes of cardiac decompensation are listed in Box 41-4 and should be considered in patients with previously stable heart failure. CAD, atrial fibrillation, valvular disease, alcohol abuse, thyroid disease, and hypertension are examples of potentially treatable causes of heart failure.

TREATMENT

The goals of management are to reduce symptoms, prevent complications, slow or reverse deterioration in myocardial function, and improve survival. All patients should follow a no-added-sodium diet (<2 to 3 g of sodium daily), stop smoking, limit alcohol, monitor their daily weight, and stay as active as possible.

■ BOX 41-4 Causes of Cardiac Decompensation

Myocardial ischemia	Myocardial infarction
Arrhythmia	Anemia
Acute valvular disease	Superimposed medical illness
Pneumonia	Pulmonary embolus
Uncontrolled hypertension	Dietary indiscretion
Fever	Emotional stress
Excess exertion	

■ BOX 41-5 Treatment Principles of Heart Failure

Identify and correct reversible causes
Identify and correct causes for decompensation
Determine if heart failure is primarily systolic or diastolic
Use vasodilators in patients with systolic dysfunction
Initiate low sodium diet to control fluid retention
Cautious use of beta blockers in systolic dysfunction to minimize the risk of cardiac decompensation
Control heart rate in diastolic dysfunction
Digoxin in patients with systolic dysfunction who remain symptomatic despite vasodilators/diuretics

Box 41-5 outlines the goals of heart failure therapy. **Diuretics** are a mainstay of therapy for systolic dysfunction and acute pulmonary congestion in patients with diastolic dysfunction. Loop diuretics are introduced first for fluid control in patients in overt CHF with the goal to reduce symptoms such as dyspnea and edema. Single larger doses of loop diuretics are more effective than smaller divided doses. Symptom improvement can be seen in hours to days, whereas other agents may show benefits weeks to months after initiation. Hypokalemia is a common side effect and requires treatment if the potassium level is below 4.0 meq/L. Close monitoring of BUN and Cr as well as daily weights is important, as an increase in either may indicate the need to adjust diuretic therapy.

ACE inhibitors slow the progression of heart failure, decrease the number of hospitalizations, and decrease mortality in patients with left ventricular systolic dysfunction (LVSD). ACE inhibitors are generally started prior to beta blockers because they provide rapid hemodynamic benefit. Patients should start on a low dose of an ACE inhibitor (e.g., 6.25 mg of captopril twice daily, 2.5 to 5 mg of lisinopril daily) to reduce the risk of hypotension and azotemia while reducing concurrent diuretic therapy. Common side effects include hypotension, hyperkalemia, dehydration, and cough. Patients with pre-existing renal artery stenosis may experience renal impairment with an ACE inhibitor. Deterioration of renal function (>25%) should result in either a dose reduction or discontinuation of the medication. If a patient cannot tolerate an ACE inhibitor, an angiotensin receptor blocker (ARB) and the combination of hydralazine and nitrates are alternative therapies.

Randomized trials demonstrate a decrease in mortality and sudden death in patients with heart failure who are treated with **beta blockers.** These should be added after ACE inhibitors and diuretics in patients with stable heart failure since they have delayed hemodynamic benefits. Beta blockers are also helpful in heart failure secondary to ischemia, diastolic dysfunction, and atrial arrhythmia. In adding beta blockers to heart failure therapy, start with a low dose (e.g., 3.25 mg/day of carvedilol or 12.5 to 25 mg/day of metoprolol) and titrate slowly upward to achieve a resting heart rate of 50 to 60 beats per minute, as some patients are more sensitive to the effects of beta blockers. Long-term benefits of left ventricular ejection fraction (LVEF) improvements and survival are dose dependent in patients who tolerate the heart rate goal achieved at a target therapeutic dose. Patients should be monitored closely for fluid retention and clinical deterioration. Relative contraindications to beta blocker use are listed in Box 41-6. Diuretic doses may have to be adjusted upward if fluid retention occurs.

Spironolactone, which blocks the effects of aldosterone, also lowers the risk of hospitalization and sudden cardiac death from heart failure. Spironolactone is indicated for patients with symptoms at rest who are already being treated with ACE inhibitors, beta blockers, and loop diuretics. Important side effects include renal and electrolyte abnormalities, especially hyperkalemia. The risk of hyperkalemia is especially high in patients on an ACE inhibitor and spironolactone; however, spironolactone and other aldosterone antagonists may be used to assist in managing diuretic-induced hypokalemia in those patients classified as having mild-to-moderate CHF.

Digoxin is useful in individuals with systolic dysfunction and moderate-to-severe heart failure whose symptoms, such as fatigue, dyspnea, and exercise intolerance, are uncontrolled with an ACE inhibitor and diuretics. Digoxin therapy reduces hospitalizations but not mortality from CHF. Digoxin is not useful in patients with diastolic dysfunction or those with acutely decompensated heart failure.

Recently, exercise training has been added as an ancillary approach to improve symptoms and clinical status in patients with reduced LVEF and CHF. Exercise training, also known as cardiac rehabilitation, has been shown to improve symptoms, increase exercise capacity, reduce hospitalizations, and improve quality of life along with survival in those with CHF. Exercise training should be used in conjunction with medications and should be used in those patients with mild-to-moderate CHF, as there is no reported data to recommend this adjuvant of treatment in those with advanced heart failure.

Treatment goals for diastolic dysfunction are prevention of LVH and control of symptoms by reducing end-diastolic pressure without reducing cardiac output. Rate control and the maintenance of sinus rhythm are essential. Slowing of the heart rate allows more time for ventricular filling during diastole. Diuretics are indicated for volume overload and for correcting precipitating factors such as hypertension. If calcium channel blockers are used for diastolic failure, they should be in the nondihydropyridine class, such as verapamil and diltiazem. The dihydropyridine class causes a reflex tachycardia that decreases filling time.

KEY POINTS

- One percent of adults aged 50 to 60 and 10% of those in their eighties are affected by CHF.
- Systolic dysfunction is characterized by decreased contractility of the left ventricle, resulting in a reduced ejection fraction.
- About 40% of patients with CHF have diastolic dysfunction. Diastolic dysfunction results from the ventricle's inability to relax properly, which leads to a higher filling pressure, pulmonary congestion, and decreased cardiac return.
- Characteristic chest x-ray findings in CHF include cardiomegaly, redistribution of vascular markings, prominent interstitial markings, Kerley B lines, and perihilar haziness.
- The goals of management are reduction of symptoms, prevention of complications, and improvement of survival.
- ACE inhibitors slow the progression of heart failure, decrease the number of hospitalizations, and decrease mortality in patients with LVSD; they are recommended in patients with LVSD.
- Randomized trials demonstrate a decrease in mortality and sudden death in patients with heart failure who are treated with beta blockers.

■ **BOX 41-6** Relative Contraindications for Beta Blocker Use in CHF
Heart rate <60 bpm
Symptomatic hypotension
Signs of peripheral hypoperfusion
PR interval >0.24 seconds
Second- or third-degree AV block
History of asthma or lung disease
Peripheral artery disease with resting limb ischemia

42 Depression

Feeling blue or sad is an appropriate response to a difficult situation. Clinical depression occurs if the reaction is more severe or prolonged than expected. Major depression is a mood disorder characterized by at least 2 weeks of depressed mood, a loss of interest or pleasure in usual activities, and a feeling of hopelessness associated with other findings such as sleep disturbances or loss of energy. Major depression is a chronic debilitating disease with a lifetime prevalence of 7% to 12% in men and 20% to 25% in women. It often accompanies chronic medical illnesses and substance abuse.

A less severe form of depression is dysthymia. It lasts at least 2 years and is described by some as a depressive type of personality. Although symptoms are not as severe as seen in major depression, they persist too long to be considered an adjustment reaction. Most patients with depression seek help from a family physician rather than a psychiatrist, making it important that the family physician feels comfortable managing this illness. Despite the prevalence of depression, the diagnosis is missed in up to 50% of family practice patients; even when diagnosed, it is often undertreated. Table 42-1 lists the indications for screening for depression in adults, children, and adolescents.

PATHOGENESIS

Most theories explaining depression emphasize a biologic model. Depression is thought to be related to dysregulation of the brain's neurotransmitters. Although an imbalance in neurotransmitters provides an explanation for symptoms, it is still unclear why the imbalance develops. Research suggests that genetic factors play a role and that some individuals appear to be predisposed to developing depression

▪ TABLE 42-1 Depression: Indications for Screening	
Adults	**Children and Adolescents**
First-degree biologic relative with history of depression	Antisocial behavior
Two or more chronic diseases	Diminished school performance
Obesity	Withdrawal from friends or social activities
Chronic pain (e.g., backache, headache)	Excessive weight gain or loss
Impoverished home environment	Substance abuse, such as alcohol or street drugs
Financial strain	Aggression
Experiencing major life changes	Agitation or irritability
Pregnant or postpartum	
Socially isolated	
Multiple vague symptoms (e.g., gastrointestinal, cardiovascular, neurologic)	
Fatigue or sleep disturbance	
Substance abuse, such as alcohol or street drugs	
Loss of interest in sexual activity	
Elderly age	

Table from: Sharp LK, Lipsky MS. Screening for depression across the lifespan: a review of measures for use in primary care settings. Am Fam Physician. 2002;66:1001–8,1045–6,1048,1051–2.

in response to stressors. Potential stressors include medical illness, stressful life events, unresolved losses, poor support systems, and life changes affecting lifestyle, such as divorce or financial loss. The process by which environmental factors interact with biologic factors to cause depression is still poorly understood.

CLINICAL MANIFESTATIONS

HISTORY

Depression can cause a wide range of psychological and somatic complaints. Box 42-1 lists a summary of the criteria used for diagnosing depression. The average age of onset of depression is from 20 to 40 years of age, although it can first present at any age. Identifiable stressors often play a role in the first episode of depression but may play a limited role or have no role in subsequent episodes. A concern expressed by a family member or friend about crying spells or depressed mood should prompt the physician to ask questions about depression. The patient's past medical history should be reviewed, since illnesses such as stroke, epilepsy, cardiovascular disease, chronic fatigue syndrome, dementia, diabetes, cancer, rheumatoid arthritis, and HIV are frequently associated with depression. A family history of depression significantly increases the risk for depression. A careful review of medications is indicated, since some medications can precipitate depression. Box 42-2 lists medications associated with depressive symptoms as a side effect.

Many patients with depression first seek treatment for physical symptoms, and depression should be considered in patients with somatic complaints such as headache, backache, fatigue, chronic abdomi-

■ **BOX 42-2** Common Medications Causing Depression
Alpha-methyldopa
Amphetamine withdrawal
Beta blockers
Digitalis
Cimetidine
Clonidine
Indomethacin
Isotretinoin
Levodopa
Oral contraceptives
Phenothiazines
Reserpine
Steroids

nal or pelvic pain, sleep disorders, sexual dysfunction, and a generalized positive review of systems. An old adage states that if there are more than four complaints, consider depression.

Eliciting the patient's social history, particularly regarding alcohol and other substance use, is important. Some individuals presenting with depression have manic-depressive illness, so it is important to ask about episodes of mania. The severity of depression may be assessed by asking about suicidal thoughts and psychotic symptoms. Risk factors for suicide include social isolation (e.g., divorced, widowed, living alone), substance use, elderly male, persons with terminal or chronic illnesses, and those who have developed a specific plan. Although women attempt suicide more often, men succeed more often.

PHYSICAL EXAMINATION

A physical examination helps screen for medical disorders. Assessing mental status and appearance, mood, affect, speech, thought content, perceptual disturbances, and cognition is important. Psychomotor retardation, poor eye contact, tearfulness, poor grooming, somber affect, and impaired memory are characteristics of depression.

DIFFERENTIAL DIAGNOSIS

Several conditions besides depression can cause a depressed mood. An adjustment disorder with a depressed mood occurs when an identifiable stressor

■ **BOX 42-1** Diagnostic Criteria of Major Depression
The diagnosis requires 2 weeks of a depressed mood and/or disinterest with an impairment of function accompanied by four of the following:
Weight changes
Sleep disturbance
Loss of energy
Feelings of worthlessness or guilt
Poor concentration
Psychomotor retardation or agitation
Thoughts of death
Recurrent suicidal ideations

causes more symptoms than expected but does not last more than 6 months. Grief reactions may also present with symptoms mimicking depression; however, symptoms begin to improve after a few months. An anxiety disorder can mimic depression but is not usually accompanied by depressive symptoms such as loss of appetite and fatigue. Anxiety disorder is dominated by feelings of apprehension, whereas depression is dominated by sadness and hopelessness. A bipolar disorder or substance abuse may also present with symptoms similar to those of depression. In addition to psychological diseases, certain medications (see Box 42-2) and medical illnesses such as chronic infections (e.g., HIV, TB), endocrine disorders (e.g., hypothyroidism, hyperthyroidism, Cushing disease, and Addison disease), connective tissue diseases, neurologic disorders, and cancers are associated with depression.

DIAGNOSTIC EVALUATION

The clinical interview is the most effective means of diagnosing depression. Laboratory testing such as a CBC, basic chemistries, UA, Venereal Disease Research Laboratories (VDRL) testing, HIV testing, and a vitamin B_{12} level may be helpful in ruling out a medical disorder. A baseline ECG should be performed in patients with a history of cardiac disease or those who are over age 40 if tricyclic antidepressants are going to be prescribed. Neuroimaging and an electroencephalogram (EEG) should be considered for patients with new onset psychotic depression.

TREATMENT

Common treatments include **supportive counseling** and **pharmacotherapy**. Examples of supportive counseling include providing education, empathizing with the patient, challenging a patient's exaggerated negative or self-critical thoughts, and encouraging him or her to be more active and schedule enjoyable activities. Sometimes encouraging patients to break their problems down into smaller components is helpful. Often a willingness to explore issues is therapeutic, although the physician should not be expected to address and solve all problems. Patients with family or marital issues may benefit from therapy. Patients with persistent symptoms or major depression should be treated pharmacologically.

The different classes of antidepressant medications are equally effective. The choice of medication depends on the patient's symptoms, current medications, and side-effect profile. If the patient has insomnia, a more sedating medication such as a tricyclic antidepressant, trazodone, or mirtazapine is a good choice. If somnolence is a problem, a more energizing antidepressant such as a SSRI or bupropion might be chosen.

Although SSRIs are typically energizing, about 15% of patients experience sedation as a side effect. If anxiety or agitation is a complaint, SSRIs should be avoided as a first choice. Sedative antidepressants should be given in this situation. Although tricyclic antidepressants (TCAs) have been available for years, they have many unpleasant side effects. Their anticholinergic properties can precipitate an attack of acute angle glaucoma or bladder outlet obstruction. They can also cause constipation, dry mouth, orthostatic hypotension, tachycardia, cardiac arrhythmias, tremor, and weight gain. SSRIs appear to be safe in patients with cardiac disease and cause less orthostatic hypotension in elderly patients. Common side effects include GI disturbances, headache, agitation, insomnia, sexual dysfunction, tremor, and somnolence. Trazodone has minimal anticholinergic side effects but is very sedating and on rare occasion causes priapism in males. Venlafaxine combines SSRI properties with noradrenergic effects. It is often used for refractory depression, but its side effects limit its use as a first-line agent. MAOIs are effective but less commonly used because of their potential for drug and food interactions.

About 60% of patients will respond to a given antidepressant and 80% will respond to a second alternative or added antidepressant medication. Patients should be assessed for therapeutic response and adverse effects of their medication within the first 2 weeks; however, therapy should be continued for 6 to 8 weeks before evaluating for effectiveness or changing the medication. The greatest risk of increased suicidal thoughts and behaviors is in the first to second month of treatment and close follow-up is recommended to identify these events early. For severe cases of major depression, some patients may require multiple medications to achieve a therapeutic response to treatment.

For a first episode of depression, antidepressants should be continued for 4 to 9 months after symptoms improve. Following a major depressive episode, about 50% of the patients relapse; the highest risk for recurrence is within the first few months of tapering an antidepressant. Patients suffering relapses should promptly be restarted on medications. The risk of relapse increases with each progressive episode, and patients who relapse should be considered for long-term therapy. Patients who fail to respond to therapy, abuse substances, are suicidal, have accompanying psychosis, or show symptoms of mania should be referred to a psychiatrist.

KEY POINTS

- Major depression is a mood disorder character-ized by at least 2 weeks of depressed mood, a loss of interest or pleasure in usual activities, and a feeling of hopelessness associated with other findings such as sleep disturbances or loss of energy.

- Major depression is a chronic debilitating dis-ease with a lifetime prevalence of 7% to 12% in men and 20% to 25% in women.

- Despite the prevalence of depression, the diag-nosis is missed in up to 50% of family practice patients; even when diagnosed, it is often un-dertreated.

- Conditions such as stroke, myocardial infarction, pregnancy, chronic fatigue syndrome, dementia, diabetes, cancer, rheumatoid arthritis, and HIV are frequently associated with depression.

- The different classes of antidepressant medica-tions are equally effective. The choice of medica-tion depends on the patient's symptoms, current medications, and side-effect profile.

Chapter 43

Diabetes Mellitus Type 2

Diabetes mellitus is the most common endocrine problem encountered in family medicine. Diabetes is a group of heterogeneous metabolic disorders characterized by the abnormal metabolism of glucose with defects in insulin secretion, insulin action, or both. Diabetes is generally divided into type 1 diabetes, which is characterized by little or no insulin production, and type 2 diabetes, in which the initial defect appears to be a resistance to the action of insulin.

EPIDEMIOLOGY

Diabetes mellitus affects about 6% of the population. Type 2 diabetes accounts for approximately 90% to 95% of individuals with diabetes. Of the 18.2 million patients with type 2 diabetes, many have few symptoms and about 5.2 million remain undiagnosed. Worldwide in 2000 there were an estimated 171 million cases of type 2 diabetes and in 2030 an estimated 366 million cases are projected. This was previously a disease of the middle aged and elderly; however, there has been an increase in incidence in young adults and children as a result of the obesity epidemic seen in the United States.

PATHOGENESIS

Type 1 diabetes is believed to be an autoimmune disorder, with the production of autoimmune antibodies against pancreatic islet cells. The disease typically develops during childhood, possibly triggered by a viral infection. Type 1 patients are vulnerable to ketoacidosis and always require exogenous insulin. In type 2 diabetes, insulin is produced but cells are resistant to its action. However, since insulin is produced, individuals with type 2 diabetes generally do not develop ketoacidosis.

Early in type 2 diabetes, elevated levels of insulin may be present as the pancreas attempts to compensate for insulin resistance. Eventually the beta-cell can no longer compensate for the insulin resistance and hyperglycemia occurs. In addition to hyperglycemia, lipid metabolism is also affected. Patients with type 2 diabetes frequently have low levels of high-density lipoprotein (HDL), moderately elevated cholesterol levels, and high triglycerides. Type 2 diabetes

develops more commonly in African-Americans, Hispanics, and American-Indians. Other risk factors include having a first-degree relative with diabetes mellitus, obesity—especially central obesity—and a sedentary lifestyle.

Gestational diabetes mellitus (GDM) affects 1% to 2% of pregnancies, usually during the third trimester. Blood sugars usually return to normal after delivery, but up to 30% of women with GDM develop diabetes mellitus later in life. Acute complications of diabetes include ketoacidosis, hyperosmolar nonketotic diabetic coma (HNKDC), and hypoglycemic reactions from treatment. HNKDC is a syndrome characterized by severe fluid deficits induced by hyperglycemic diuresis. It generally develops in debilitated patients, such as nursing home residents, who are unable to take in adequate fluids.

Most of the morbidity and mortality associated with diabetes mellitus results from long-term complications. These can be divided into microvascular and macrovascular types. Microvascular complications include retinopathy, neuropathy, and nephropathy. Macrovascular complications are related to the premature atherosclerosis, which affects the cardiovascular, cerebrovascular, and peripheral vascular systems. MI is the primary cause of the excess morbidity seen in diabetic individuals. Foot problems including ulcers, deformities, and infections can also manifest from neurologic and microvascular complications.

CLINICAL MANIFESTATIONS

HISTORY

Patients with type 1 diabetes usually present abruptly, often with ketoacidosis caused by an acute stress, such as an infection. Other common initial symptoms are nausea, abdominal pain, polyuria, polydipsia, polyphagia, and weight loss.

Patients with type 2 diabetes present more gradually. Classic symptoms include polyuria, polydipsia, and polyphagia. Patients may initially complain of fatigue, blurred vision, or recurrent infections. Many patients are asymptomatic and are first diagnosed by blood tests that reveal an elevated glucose. Others may present with symptoms related to complications such as a burning sensation in the feet due to a painful neuropathy. The history should also seek to identify risk factors for cardiovascular disease and ask about symptoms such as chest pain or claudication, which may indicate macrovascular disease.

PHYSICAL EXAMINATION

The physical examination should focus on weight, body habitus, and—for younger individuals—growth. Most findings are not diagnostic but result from complications of the disease. An eye examination may show evidence of retinopathy, such as exudates, hemorrhages, and microaneurysms. A cardiovascular examination—including blood pressure, listening for carotid bruits, and assessing peripheral pulses—is important. A skin and foot examination looking for ulceration, deformities, and skin infection should be performed. Neurologic examination can detect signs of neuropathy such as sensory loss.

DIFFERENTIAL DIAGNOSIS

Transient hyperglycemia may result from stresses such as an infection or a heart attack that subsequently resolves when the inciting event is under control. Elevated blood sugars may also be related to pancreatic disease from pancreatitis, pancreatic cancer, pancreatic resection, and hemochromatosis, which is often referred to as "bronze diabetes." Endocrinopathies such as Cushing disease, pheochromocytoma, and acromegaly and medications such as high-dose steroids, beta blockers, oral contraceptives, phenytoin, and hydrochlorothiazide may also cause hyperglycemia.

DIAGNOSTIC EVALUATION

The American Diabetes Association (ADA) recommends that high-risk individuals be screened for diabetes with a fasting blood sugar. The ADA also recommends that all patients over age 45 should be screened with a fasting blood sugar every 3 years; those with risk factors should be screened earlier (see Box 43-1 for risk factors). The diagnosis of diabetes mellitus can be established by one of three criteria: (1) fasting blood glucose greater than 126 mg/dL on two or more separate occasions; (2) random blood glucose greater than 200 mg/dL with polyuria, polydipsia, and polyphagia; and (3) a 2-hour postprandial glucose greater than 200 mg/dL. If any of these criteria are met, confirmation of the diagnosis with random or fasting blood glucose level should be made on another day within 1 week of the initial blood work. Although an HbA$_{1C}$, or glycosylated hemoglobin level, is not one of the diagnostic criteria, it is a crucial test to assess the degree of blood sugar control.

■ **BOX 43-1** Risk Factors for Diabetes Mellitus Type 2
Family history of DM2
Age
BMI >25 kg/m²
Low HDL cholesterol (<35 mg/dL) and/or high triglycerides (>250 mg/dL)
Blood pressure >140/90 mmHg
History of gestational diabetes or birth of macrosomic baby (birth weight >9 lb)
Previous impaired fasting glucose with fasting plasma glucose 110–125 mg/dL
Previous impaired glucose tolerance with oral glucose tolerance test 2 hour glucose value 140–199 mg/dL
Clinical condition associated with insulin resistance such as polycystic ovarian syndrome (PCOS) or acanthosis nigricans
Habit of physical inactivity
Vascular disease
Ethnic groups at increased risk of DM2: African-Americans, Native Americans, Hispanic Americans, Asian-Americans, and Pacific Islanders

Normally about 4% to 6% of hemoglobin is glycosylated. The percent of glycosylated hemoglobin rises with the average level of blood glucose. Since the average lifespan of a red blood cell is 120 days, the HbA$_{1C}$ reflects the average glucose levels over the past 2 to 3 months.

A new category termed **"Prediabetes"** has been developed to identify those at risk for subsequent diabetes. When fasting, blood glucose values fall between 100 and 125 mg/dL, a person is considered a prediabetic.

In addition to establishing the diagnosis of diabetes, the initial evaluation should be aimed at evaluating risk factors and detecting diabetic complications. Routine laboratory testing should include a fasting lipid profile, glycosylated hemoglobin, UA, electrolytes, BUN, creatinine, and an ECG in patients over 40. For patients over 30 years of age or those with diabetes mellitus of more than 5 years' duration, screening for microalbuminuria should be performed annually.

TREATMENT

This section focuses mainly on type 2 diabetes, which is more common in the family practice setting. The goals of treatment are to alleviate symptoms, minimize development of long-term complications, improve quality of life, and reduce motility. Diet and exercise are the cornerstones of treatment. Eighty to 90% of individuals with type 2 diabetes are overweight. Even a modest weight loss of 10 to 20 lb may be sufficient to improve glycemic control. Reducing fat intake is also important, since diabetic patients are at risk for developing hyperlipidemia and vascular disease. Exercise is important for controlling weight and may also improve insulin resistance. Lifestyle modifications are also warranted for patients considered to be prediabetic in order to delay progression of glucose intolerance and the diagnosis of diabetes.

If lifestyle modifications fail to control the blood sugar, then pharmacologic therapy is the next step. In addition to insulin, there are five classes of oral agents: sulfonylureas, biguanides, thiazolidinediones, meglitinides, and alpha-glucosidase inhibitors. All of these agents need the presence of endogenous insulin to be effective.

Sulfonylureas stimulate insulin release from pancreatic beta-cells. Contraindications include allergy, pregnancy, and significant renal dysfunction. The most common serious side effects of these medications are hypoglycemia and weight gain. About 50% to 70% of patients can initially be controlled solely with a sulfonylurea. As beta-cell function worsens, 5% to 10% of patients per year previously controlled with a sulfonylurea will lose glycemic control. Sulfonylureas generally improve fasting blood sugars by 30 to 60 mg/dL and HbA$_{1C}$ by 1.5% to 2.0%. The **meglitinides** (Prandin, Starlix) are used to stimulate insulin release and used preprandial. They stimulate insulin release in the presence of glucose by increasing calcium and decreasing potassium in pancreatic beta-cells. The two FDA approved medications include repaglinide and nateglinide; both are taken 1 to 30 minutes before meals to maximize the release of insulin. Both medications have been shown to improve HbA$_{1C}$. Adverse effects associated with meglitinides include weight gain up to 3 kg and nonsevere hypoglycemia.

Metformin is the only biguanide available in the United States. It works by inhibiting hepatic gluconeogenesis and increasing glucose uptake in the peripheral tissues. When used alone, metformin does not cause hypoglycemia, but it can potentiate hypoglycemia when used in conjunction with insulin or sulfonylureas. The most common side effects are nausea, diarrhea, and dyspepsia. A rare but often fatal complication is lactic acidosis. The risk of lactic acidosis can be reduced by avoiding the use of metformin in patients with renal dysfunction (creatinine greater than or equal to 1.5 mg/dL in men and 1.4 mg/dL in women), CHF, acute or chronic acidosis, or hepatic dysfunction. Metformin is similar in effectiveness to the sulfonylureas.

Thiazolidinediones work by decreasing insulin resistance in skeletal muscle and the liver. They can be used with insulin or other medications. They can cause hepatotoxicity and require monitoring of liver enzymes. Recently, there have been new FDA warnings regarding thiazolidinediones use and the increased risk of CHF and MI in patients with cardiac conditions. Therefore, although these medications are still used to achieve adequate glucose control, they are used with caution in patients with cardiac conditions. **Alpha-glucosidase inhibitors** inhibit an enzyme found in the intestinal brush border that hydrolyzes disaccharides, thus limiting the rate of carbohydrate absorption and reducing postprandial elevation of glucose. The major side effects are flatulence, diarrhea, and abdominal pain. Recently, the FDA approved exenatide as a synthetic peptide that enhances glucose-dependent insulin secretion from beta-cells, regulates gastric emptying, promotes satiety, and decreases postprandial glucagon secretion, which in turn reduces hepatic glucose output. It is recommended as adjunctive therapy for patients with type 2 diabetes who have inadequate glycemic control with metformin and/or sulfonylurea, and/or thiazolidinedione. The addition of this incretin/glucagon-like peptide-1 mimetic helps improve glycemic control and may reduce body weight since it slows gastric emptying. Side effects include hypoglycemia when added to a sulfonylurea, nausea, vomiting, diarrhea, and a very rare complication of pancreatitis. This medication is only indicated in those patients who do not use insulin. Another recently released oral agent, sitagliptin, acts as an inhibitor of the breakdown of incretin by inhibiting the enzyme dipeptidyl peptidase-4 and can improve glycemic control without weight gain or risk of hypoglycemia.

Eventually, as beta-cell function worsens over time, about 50% of type 2 patients will end up taking insulin. Given in sufficient doses, insulin can usually control even the most refractory hyperglycemia. Characteristics of insulin preparations vary in terms of onset and duration of action. Patients on insulin usually require self-monitoring at home using a glucometer.

Type 2 diabetes is a progressive disease, and a single agent may be ineffective at the outset or lose effectiveness over time. Combination therapy with two or more agents that work by different mechanisms may reduce the blood sugar to an acceptable level. A biguanide with a sulfonylurea is the most widely studied combination. The effect of the two medications is additive; switching from one to another does not improve control.

All individuals with diabetes who receive medication to lower blood sugar must be warned about the possibility of a hypoglycemic reaction manifest by confusion, loss of consciousness, tachycardia, shakiness, headache, or sweatiness. Persons at risk for hypoglycemia should be instructed about the symptoms of a reaction and should carry either a hard candy or glucose gel to take if hypoglycemic symptoms develop.

Monitoring, preventing, and treating complications are important elements in managing patients with diabetes mellitus (Box 43-2). Hypertension and hyperlipidemia should be aggressively treated. Many experts recommend a target blood pressure of 130/80 mmHg and initiating treatment for a low-density-lipoprotein (LDL) cholesterol over 70 mg/dL. The ADA also recommends prophylactic aspirin use in patients of age 50 years or above.

The ADA recommends monitoring the HbA_{1C} every 3 to 6 months, with a target goal of below 7% to prevent microvascular complications. Levels above 8% usually suggest the need to re-examine treatment, either by re-emphasizing adherence to current therapy or by changing management. With the elderly population, glucose control may be complicated by hypoglycemic episodes, and adjustments of target blood sugar to higher levels may be reflected in the HbA_{1C}. For the elderly population, target HbA_{1C} is generally below 8% in order to avoid complications of hypoglycemic episodes.

Currently the ADA recommends annual dilated eye examinations and screening for microalbuminuria in patients with diabetes. Patients with retinopathy need monitoring by an ophthalmologist. Microalbuminuria is defined as the excretion of 30 to 300 mg of urinary protein over 24 hours. The presence of microalbuminuria should prompt a careful retinal evaluation, since retinopathy usually precedes nephropathy. Reducing blood pressure to 130/80 mmHg and using an ACE inhibitor are strategies that may slow the progression of nephropathy. For patients who cannot tolerate an ACE inhibitor, an angiotensin receptor blocking agent is an alternative. Neuropathy is one of the most common diabetic complications. In addition to sensory loss, diabetic neuropathy can cause bladder and bowel problems, impotence, and orthostatic hypotension. Patients with sensory neuropathies frequently also have peripheral vascular disease and are especially prone to develop foot problems. Painful neuropathies may respond to tricyclic antidepressants, carbamazepine, or gabapentin.

Another important intervention to reduce complications in diabetic patients includes tobacco cessation with support groups and counseling. Annual influenza vaccines and a one-time pneumococcal vaccination are also recommended to prevent severe infection. Dental exams every 6 months are also recommended to maintain proper oral hygiene, again to deter serious infections that can be complicated with type 2 diabetes.

■ **BOX 43-2** Targets of Optimal Diabetes Type 2 Management
Blood Glucose Monitoring:
Monitor glucose two to four times each day
Premeal: 70–140 mg/dL
Postmeal: <160 mg/dL (2 hours after start of meal)
Bedtime: 100–160 mg/dL
More than 50% of glucose readings within target range with no severe hypoglycemic episodes
HbA_{1C}:
<7%
Test every 3 months and use to verify home glucose monitoring readings
Blood Pressure:
Goal <130/80
Lipids:
LDL <100 mg/dL (some advocate for <70 mg/dL)
HDL >40 mg/dL
Triglycerides <150 mg/dL

KEY POINTS

- There are two main types of diabetes mellitus: type 1, characterized by little or no insulin production, and type 2, in which the initial defect is insulin resistance.

- Many individuals with type 2 diabetes are asymptomatic and are identified by blood testing.

- Glycemic control reduces the risk of developing complications and slows the progression of diabetes in those who already have established complications.

- The cornerstones of treatment in type 2 diabetes are diet and exercise, with pharmacologic treatment reserved for those who do not reach treatment goals with diet and exercise alone.

Diverticulitis

Diverticuli are herniations in the colonic mucosa; they are present in 20% of individuals over the age of 40 and up to 70% of people over age 70. Most patients with diverticuli are asymptomatic; however, up to 15% will develop complications such as diverticulitis, GI obstruction, or bleeding. Diverticulitis is an inflammation of the diverticuli that most commonly affects the sigmoid colon. Risk factors for the development of diverticulitis include older age, a low-fiber diet, a previous history of diverticulitis, constipating conditions, hereditary diseases such as polycystic kidney disease, Marfan syndrome, Ehlers–Danlos syndrome, and the presence of a large number of diverticuli in the colon.

PATHOGENESIS

Diverticuli are outpouchings, or herniations, of the colonic mucosa through the muscularis layer. These occur in areas of mucosal weakness where an artery penetrates the muscularis to reach the submucosa and the mucosa. The sigmoid colon is more commonly involved because the luminal size is smaller and the pressures generated are greater than in other areas of the colon. Normally, diverticuli are asymptomatic; however, they may become obstructed with fecal material, which can cause inflammation and microabscess formation within and around the diverticulum. This inflammatory process is called diverticulitis. The inflammation may progress to involve a larger segment of colon and cause a narrowing or stricture. Larger abscesses may form and encroach on neighboring structures, leading to development of fistulas. Diverticular bleeding is usually not associated with pain and occurs when fecal matter traumatizes one of the perforating arteries at the site of a diverticulum.

CLINICAL MANIFESTATIONS

HISTORY

The clinical manifestations of diverticular disease vary from asymptomatic disease to abdominal pain or bleeding. Only 10% to 25% of diverticulosis sufferers will develop symptoms. Patients with diverticulitis usually present with complaints of colicky left-lower-quadrant abdominal pain that may be aggravated by

eating and relieved by a bowel movement. On occasion, the abdominal pain may occur in other locations, such as the right lower quadrant. These patients also experience fever, chills, nausea, vomiting, and decreased appetite; they are often constipated. Patients may present with massive GI bleeding but without other symptoms or pain. Colon cancer should be suspected in elderly patients with weight loss, abdominal pain, and changes in bowel habits.

PHYSICAL EXAMINATION

General symptoms such as fever may or may not be present. The physical examination may reveal peritoneal signs such as rigidity, rebound tenderness, and guarding. The abdomen may be distended and tympanic. Often a mass or fullness is palpated in the left lower quadrant. Bowel sounds are either decreased or normal early in presentation; however, they may be increased with obstruction. The physical examination should include a rectal examination to exclude the presence of a mass or bleeding. In cases of severe bleeding, patients may have signs of hypovolemia and anemia.

DIFFERENTIAL DIAGNOSIS

Box 44-1 lists some causes of lower abdominal pain. The differential diagnosis for rectal bleeding includes polyps, colon cancer, angiodysplasia, and diverticular disease. Patients with left-lower-quadrant abdominal pain may have infectious, inflammatory, or ischemic colitis, IBS, or colon cancer. In right-sided abdominal pain, appendicitis should be considered. Nephrolithiasis may cause abdominal pain but is usually not associated with tenderness or fever. In women, gynecologic complaints such as an ovarian mass, ruptured ovarian cyst, torsion, and endometriosis are part of the differential diagnosis.

DIAGNOSTIC EVALUATION

Diverticulitis is initially a clinical diagnosis, supported by laboratory and diagnostic testing. An elevated WBC count along with a left shift suggests an inflammatory process. Hemoglobin testing is useful for evaluating GI bleeding and UA is useful in evaluating

BOX 44-1 Causes for Lower Abdominal Pain

Inflammatory bowel disease (Crohn disease, ulcerative colitis)
Irritable bowel syndrome
Large bowel obstruction or ileus
Carcinoma of the colon
Ischemic colitis
Nephrolithiasis
Appendicitis
Mesenteric ischemia
Colon spasm
Incarcerated hernia
Urinary tract infections
Gynecologic disorders (ovarian pathology, ectopic pregnancy, endometriosis)

urinary tract disorders such as stones or infection. Plain abdominal films do not point to any specific findings with diverticulitis but may show an ileus pattern. CT of the abdomen is the imaging test of choice for patients with suspected diverticulitis and provides diagnostic evidence of diverticulitis in more than 90% of cases (sensitivity 90% to 100% and specificity 95% to 100%). CT findings may include pericolic fat infiltration (considered diagnostic finding), thickened fascia, muscular hypertrophy, and "arrowhead sign" that shows localized colonic wall thickening with arrowhead-shaped lumen pointing to inflamed diverticuli. A CT scan can also be helpful in detecting other causes for a patient's abdominal pain. Barium enema can reveal diverticulitis but is often not advisable during an acute episode for fear of causing perforation and spillage of barium into the abdomen. In patients with diverticulitis and no recent colonoscopy, follow-up testing should include a colonoscopy 6 to 8 weeks after resolution of symptoms in order to detect an underlying malignancy. Avoidance of immediate colonoscopy is important to avoid colonic perforation.

TREATMENT

Patients with diverticulosis should be encouraged to eat high-fiber diets and to engage in daily exercise. Traditionally, these patients were counseled to avoid foods with small seeds and nuts, but recent research findings have shown no correlation between diverticulitis and these foods; still, some providers may counsel patients to avoid these foods if the patient reports abdominal upset with their ingestion. Fiber supplements such as psyllium are helpful. In addition to dietary maneuvers, anticholinergic or antispasmodic drugs may be helpful for the relief of crampy abdominal pain. Stool softeners may be helpful in those with firm stools or constipation. 5-Aminosalicylic acids, such as mesalazine 800 mg twice daily and/or rifaximin 400 mg twice daily each for 7 to 10 days every month, may reduce symptoms in uncomplicated diverticular disease.

Patients with diverticulitis may be treated as outpatients or inpatients depending on the severity of illness and their reliability in adhering to therapy and follow-up. Patients with mild symptoms and stable vital signs who are not vomiting may be placed on a clear liquid diet and oral antibiotics with follow-up in 2 to 3 days. If the patient is improving, the diet may be advanced and the antibiotic continued for 7 to 10 days. The patient should undergo colonoscopy in 6 to 8 weeks to evaluate the possibility of colon carcinoma. Patients with more severe pain, vomiting, or unstable vital signs will require hospitalization. The patient initially takes nothing by mouth and is provided with intravenous fluids and antibiotics. Adequate pain relief is provided with opiates, with meperidine being the optimal choice as it provides decreased intraluminal pressure. As the pain subsides, a diet is introduced and the patient is placed on oral antibiotics. Again, follow-up colonoscopy is recommended. Both inpatients and outpatients with diverticulitis are monitored for complications that may require surgical intervention. These include abscess formation, stricture formation with obstruction, fistulas, and peritonitis. Recurrent episodes may prompt surgical intervention.

Antibiotic selection for patients with diverticulitis should provide coverage for gram-negative and anaerobic bacteria. Common oral outpatient choices are amoxicillin/clavulanate, trimethoprim/sulfamethoxazole, or ciprofloxacin plus metronidazole with duration of treatment being 7 to 10 days. Common inpatient treatment includes metronidazole or clindamycin, plus aminoglycoside, aztreonam, or third-generation cephalosporin (ceftriaxone, ceftazadime, cefotaxime). Ampicillin/sulbactam or piperacillin/tazobactam may also be used. Improvement should be expected within 48 to 72 hours of initiation of treatment.

Diverticular bleeding is managed with supportive care and evaluation of the source of the bleeding. The bleeding will generally stop without intervention but may recur in up to 25% of cases.

KEY POINTS

- Diverticular disease is common in the elderly.
- Risk factors for diverticulitis include age over 40 years, low-fiber diet, history of diverticulitis, and the number of diverticuli in the colon.
- The clinical manifestations of diverticular disease vary from totally asymptomatic disease to severe pain, bleeding, or diverticulitis.

- Patients with diverticulitis will often have left-lower-quadrant pain along with fever and chills.
- Elderly patients with weight loss, abdominal pain, and changes in bowel habits should be suspected of having colon cancer.
- In acute cases of diverticulitis, CT scan is the test of choice.

Human Immunodeficiency Virus

A 1997 study found that approximately 1% of family practice patients were HIV-positive. Because HIV infection is often a disease of families, involving spouse and children, the family physician has an important role in the diagnosis, treatment, and prevention of AIDS.

PATHOGENESIS

HIV-1 is a retrovirus that infects lymphocytes bearing the CD4 marker. CD4 lymphocytes are T cells involved in cell-mediated immunity. The depletion of CD4 lymphocytes also impairs B-cell activation against foreign antigens and limits antibody production. Together, these effects contribute to the immunocompromised state termed AIDS.

HIV is transmitted from person to person through blood and body fluids. HIV transmission is linked to sexual contact (80%), intravenous drug use (24%), and transfusions (4%) pre-1980. HIV may also be transmitted to health care workers from needle-stick injuries or from mother to infant in utero, during labor, or through breast-feeding. With sexual activity the transmission rate from a male to a female is 0.5 to 1.5 per 1000 episodes, whereas the transmission rate from female to male is 0.3 to 0.9 per 1000 episodes. Viral load is the most powerful predictor of risk of heterosexual transmission. There is a 1.5 times greater risk of transmission during menstruation. Health care workers suffering from an infected needle stick have a risk of seroconversion of approximately 3.2 per 1000 with hollow-bore needles and a lower rate with a suture needle. Blood splashed on intact skin poses a very low risk of transmission.

CLINICAL MANIFESTATIONS

HISTORY

Manifestations of acute HIV infection are fever, fatigue, rash, headache, lymphadenopathy, pharyngitis, myalgia, GI upset (i.e., diarrhea, vomiting), night sweats, aseptic meningitis, and oral or genital ulcers. Symptoms of acute HIV infection usually develop within days to weeks after exposure and usually last less than 14 days. During the acute infection, HIV disseminates widely and spreads into lymphoid tissue. Seroconversion, or the development of antibodies to the virus, takes 3 to 4 weeks. A prolonged asymptomatic period of clinical latency (up to 12 years) may ensue, with measurable HIV-1 ribonucleic acid (RNA) and antibody levels as the only evidence of infection. Ultimately AIDS develops, characterized by immune deficiency, high-level viremia, opportunistic infections, and death.

A complete history should include risks for transmission, pre-existing comorbid conditions, social history, and previous antiretroviral treatments. The patient's spouse or partner(s) and children should be evaluated for HIV infection. Patients should be questioned about symptoms associated with opportunistic infections, such as dyspnea, dysphagia, and skin lesions. Past and current history of genital symptoms or lesions should be obtained. Even though HIV patients live longer because of new combinations of antiretroviral regimens, many still view HIV infection as untreatable and may become depressed or even suicidal. Learning about patients' previous psychiatric illnesses and family support can help them to cope with the disease and adhere to treatments. Inquiring about prior medications used by the patient, duration of use, response, intolerance, and toxicities helps clinicians choose appropriate medications and antiviral therapy.

PHYSICAL EXAMINATION

The physical examination should focus on weight change, the presence of fever, skin lesions, signs of opportunistic infections, presence of STDs, neurologic function, and emotional state. A weight loss of more than 10% requires aggressive evaluation and treatment. *Pneumocystis carinii* pneumonia is the most common cause of fever, and patients may have a normal lung examination despite active infection. Sinusitis is also common in early-stage disease, and the presence of sinus tenderness should be noted. Other opportunistic infections that may be apparent on physical examination include oral thrush (candidiasis), CMV retinitis (with a ketchup-and-cottage-cheese fundus), toxoplasmosis (an intracranial lesion manifested as deficits in extraocular movements), and cryptococcal meningitis (headache, fever, mental status change). Common skin lesions are Kaposi sarcoma, an exacerbation of psoriasis, seborrheic dermatitis, drug-related eruptions, dry skin, molluscum contagiosum, and herpes zoster. HIV infection increases the risk of pelvic inflammatory disease and cervical carcinoma in women, making a gynecologic exam including Pap smear and STD evaluation (including syphilis) necessary. Mild confusion and memory loss may occur early in HIV disease and suggest AIDS dementia complex. Myopathies, sensory and motor neuropathies, and central lesions (CNS lymphoma) may also be found in HIV disease.

DIFFERENTIAL DIAGNOSIS

Box 45-1 lists the differential diagnosis. Early HIV infection can be confused with acute viral infections or other immunocompromised states. Family physicians should be alert to the possibility of HIV in patients presenting with fever, fatigue, and STDs.

DIAGNOSTIC EVALUATION

HIV is defined as the presence of HIV antibodies confirmed by a positive enzyme-linked immunosorbent assay (ELISA) and a positive Western blot test. A positive ELISA test should always be followed by a Western blot test. A positive Western blot test reacts with two out of three (p24, gp41, and gp120/180) different antigens. A false-negative ELISA or indeterminate Western blot tests may occur in the first 3 to 4 weeks after HIV exposure (acute seroconversion state). Rapid HIV tests have >99% sensitivity for detecting HIV antibodies; however, positive results require confirmatory testing. Plasma viral load (PVL) can detect HIV infection as early as 11 days. Laboratory evaluation is performed to determine the

■ **BOX 45-1** Differential Diagnosis for Acute HIV Infection
Infectious Diseases
Infectious mononucleosis, influenza, primary cytomegalovirus infection, streptococcal pharyngitis, viral hepatitis, secondary syphilis, primary herpes simplex virus infection, toxoplasmosis, malaria
Immunocompromised State
Primary immunodeficiency disease in both B/T cells (i.e., immunoglobulin A deficiency, most commonly found in adults >21 years old), lymphoma
Others
Drug reactions

■ **BOX 45-2** Initial Laboratory Evaluation of an HIV-Positive Patient
(1) CD4 cell counts, PVL[a], CBC for HIV-related anemia or thrombocytopenia
(2) Pap smear, GC/chlamydial infection, syphilis (VDRL test)
(3) Hepatitis C, hepatitis B panel, tuberculin skin test, toxoplasma titer, cytomegalovirus titer
(4) Basic metabolic profile: BUN, creatinine, electrolytes, liver function tests, total protein, serum albumin

aPVL can be done via branched DNA (bDNA) assay, polymerase chain reaction (PCR), or the nucleic acid sequence-based amplification (NASBA). Sensitivity of all three assays is between 200 and 500 HIV RNA copies/mL. The new ultrasensitive assay can detect as low as 20–50 copies/mL.

stage of HIV disease, preferably using the CD4 count and PVL. Other suggested screenings for related cancers, STDs, and HIV-related infections are listed in Box 45-2.

TREATMENT

The primary goals of initiating treatment with antiretroviral therapy include improving quality of life, reducing HIV-related mortality and prolonging survival, restoring and preserving immunologic functions, maximizing and maintaining suppression of viral load, and preventing vertical transmission of HIV. Before initiating treatment, the patient should be counseled and educated about the potential risks and benefits; this includes long-term and short-term adverse drug effects and the need for long-term commitment and adherence to the antiretroviral therapy. The U.S. Department of Health and Human Services (USDHHS) updated guidelines for antiretroviral therapy in adults and adolescents with HIV infection in 2008. The current recommendation is to offer antiretroviral therapy to those patients who have a history of an AIDS-defining illness or with a CD4 T-cell count <350 cells/mm[3]. Antiretroviral therapy should also be started in patients who are pregnant, patients with HIV-associated nephropathy, and patients coinfected with hepatitis B (HBV) when treatment for HBV infection is indicated, regardless of CD4 T-cell count. Antiretroviral treatment may be considered in some patients with CD4 T-cell count >350 cells/mm[3].

Treatment should be instituted aggressively in advanced HIV disease, and antiretroviral therapy may have to be adjusted to overcome resistance. The effectiveness of treatments is measured against baseline CD4 and PVL, with follow-up laboratory tests

■ **TABLE 45-1** Primary Prophylaxis against Opportunistic Infections			
Infection	**Indications**	**Primary Treatment**	**Secondary Treatment**
PCP[a]	CD4 cells <200/mm³	Bactrim	Dapsone
Toxoplasmosis	CD4 cells <100/mm³	Bactrim	Dapsone
MAC[b]	CD4 cells <50/mm³	Azithromycin or Clarithromycin	Rifabutin
TB	PPD >5 mm	INH w/pyridoxine	Rifampin
VZV[b]	exposure	VZIG	Acyclovir

[a]In neonates, PCP prophylaxis treatment (Bactrim or dapsone) begins when zidovudine therapy is stopped or the child reaches age 6 weeks, and is continued until the child is found to be HIV-free or for at least 1 year.
[b]MAC, *Mycobacterium avium* complex; VZV, varicella zoster virus; PCP, pneumocystic carinii pneumonia; TB, tuberculosis; VZV, varicella zoster virus; VZIG, varicella-zoster immunoglobulin; INH, Isoniazid

done 4 to 6 weeks after the start of therapy. Desired results would be a 1- to 2-log reduction in PVL (i.e., 50,000 to 500 copies) and a rise in CD4 count of 50 to 150 cells/mm³ per year with an accelerated response expected within the first year of treatment. The viral load should become undetectable after 16 to 24 weeks of therapy. CD4 counts and PVL should be measured every 3 to 4 months to determine when to initiate therapy in patients who are untreated, assess immunologic response to treatment, and assess the need to start or discontinue prophylactic therapy for opportunistic infections.

The treatment regimens for HIV infection should include a combination of antiretroviral medications and be continued indefinitely. Three different categories of antiviral agents are available, the nucleoside reverse transcriptase inhibitors (NRTIs), protease inhibitors (PIs), and non-nucleoside reverse transcriptase inhibitors (NNRTIs). Two NRTIs (e.g., zidovudine plus didanosine or zidovudine plus lamivudine) plus a PI (e.g., ritonavir-boosted darunavir or indinavir) or an NNRTI (e.g., efavirenz) are recommended for initial therapy in treatment-naïve patients. Resistance to antiretroviral therapy can develop, and a change of medications as well as resistance testing may be necessary in cases of therapeutic failure. Guidelines for providing prophylaxis against opportunistic infections are presented in Table 45-1. Dosages for adolescents and children must be adjusted on the basis of weight and Tanner stages. A full discussion of medication dosing and side effects is beyond the scope of this chapter.

Studies in obstetric HIV patients have shown that elective cesarean section appears to decrease the vertical transmission rate by 50% and, with concurrent zidovudine therapy, by 87%. Since maternal immunoglobulins against HIV cross the placenta, all neonates born to an HIV-positive mother will have a positive ELISA test/Western blot test for HIV in the first 6 months. Current recommendations for children born to HIV-positive mothers state that infants should receive zidovudine for at least the first 4 to 6 weeks of life. Repeat testing at 1 month, 2 to 3 months, and 4 months of age is indicated until two tests are concordant. The mother should be counseled about avoiding breast-feeding.

The U.S. Public Health Service (USPHS) has recommended prophylactic antiviral treatment for occupational exposure to HIV infection. Since there are 3 to 4 weeks before seroconversion occurs, early chemoprophylaxis may destroy the virus and prevent long-term infection. The optimal window to initiate prophylaxis is 24 to 72 hours after exposure and duration of treatment is at least 4 weeks.

PROGNOSIS

Median survival rate has increased from 30 to 35 years during 2000 to 2005 period. The rates of AIDS and death among HIV infections decreased with introduction of highly active antiretroviral therapy (HAART).

KEY POINTS

- Symptoms of acute HIV infection usually develop within days to weeks after exposure and usually last less than 14 days. The development of antibodies (seroconversion) takes place at 3 to 4 weeks after the exposure.

- HIV is officially defined as presence of HIV antibodies confirmed by a positive ELISA and a positive Western blot test.

- Treatment regimens for HIV infection should include a combination of antiretroviral medications continued indefinitely.

EPIDEMIOLOGY

Hypertension (HTN) is defined as a systolic blood pressure (BP) greater than or equal to 140 or diastolic pressure greater than or equal to 90.

EPIDEMIOLOGY

HTN affects about 50 million Americans (25% of the adult population) and remains a major risk factor for the development of cardiovascular and cerebrovascular disease. Prevalence increases with age, such that by the age of 60, HTN is present in approximately 71% of African-Americans, 61% of Mexican-Americans, and 60% of non-Hispanic whites. Primary HTN accounts for 90% to 95% of all cases of HTN; secondary HTN causes about 5% to 10% of all adult HTN.

PATHOGENESIS

HTN can be either **primary (essential) or secondary**. Primary HTN is a complex process that results from a variety of physiological and environmental factors. Secondary HTN includes exogenous substances (e.g., stimulants, alcohol, NSAIDs), renal failure, sleep apnea, renovascular disease, primary aldosteronism, pheochromocytoma, and Cushing syndrome.

Insulin resistance is also associated with increased arterial BP. Hyperinsulinemia can increase vascular tone by any of the following four mechanisms: (1) promoting Na^+ retention; (2) promoting hypertrophy or hyperplasia of vascular smooth muscles through its mitogenic properties; (3) modifying ion transport, leading to an increase in intracellular calcium; and (4) sympathetic activation.

Poorly controlled HTN leads to complications or damage in several target organs. The risk of cardiovascular complications correlates with the degree of BP elevation.

CLINICAL MANIFESTATIONS

HISTORY

HTN is referred to as the "**silent killer**" because it is generally asymptomatic until there is end-organ damage. HTN is usually diagnosed during a routine office visit screening. Clinical manifestations include ischemic heart disease, stroke, peripheral vascular disease, renal insufficiency, retinopathy characterized by exudates or hemorrhages, and, in severe HTN, papilledema.

The history for hypertensive individuals should focus on symptoms of end-organ damage, additional risk factors for cardiovascular disease, and secondary causes of HTN. It is essential to ask about cardiovascular symptoms, such as chest pain, shortness of breath, prior TIAs or strokes, and renal disease. It is important to inquire about a family history of heart disease, HTN, hyperlipidemia, diabetes, and renal disease. Additional behavioral risk factors such as tobacco and alcohol use, exercise, and dietary habits should be assessed. Inquiring about medications is important, since drugs such as NSAIDs, decongestants, estrogen, progesterone, appetite suppressants, and MAOIs may elevate BP. Features of the history that suggest a secondary cause include the following:

1. Early or late onset of HTN (younger than 20 and older than 50 years of age).
2. An associated history of tachycardia, sweating, and headache.
3. A personal or family history of renal disease.
4. Resistant HTN in a compliant patient.
5. Symptoms consistent with sleep apnea.
6. History of amphetamine, cocaine, or alcohol abuse.
7. Use of oral contraceptives, estrogens, corticosteroids, NSAIDs.
8. History of hirsutism or easy bruising.

PHYSICAL EXAMINATION

The diagnosis of HTN requires an elevated BP (SBP ≥ 140 or DBP ≥ 90 mmHg) on at least two consecutive visits 2 weeks apart. The exception is one SBP greater than or equal to 210, one DBP greater than or equal to 120, or the presence of significant end-organ damage at the time of the first reading. Because several factors—such as pain, fear, anxiety, physical activity, and exogenous substances or medication—can influence BP readings, a standard approach must be followed to ensure accurate BP readings and avoid incorrectly labeling a patient as hypertensive (Box 46-1).

BOX 46-1 Essentials of Blood Pressure Measurement

1. Seated at rest for 5 minutes
2. No caffeine or cigarettes in preceding 30 minutes
3. Bladder of blood pressure cuff encircles 80% of arm
4. Arm supported at heart level
5. Inflate cuff and determine systolic range by palpably checking for obliteration of radial pulse
6. Auscultate over brachial artery after inflating cuff 10–20 mmHg above palpable systolic pressure
7. Systolic pressure=onset of Korotkoff sounds
8. Diastolic=muffling or cessation of Korotkoff sounds

Additional elements of the physical examination include the skin examination, looking for signs of Cushing syndrome or neurofibromatosis; funduscopic examination, looking for target-organ damage such as retinal hemorrhages, increased vascular tortuosity, and "arteriovenous (AV) nicking"; checking the thyroid for enlargement or nodularity; auscultating the carotids for bruits; listening to the lungs for signs of heart failure; palpating the chest for displacement of the PMI (suggestive of cardiomegaly); listening to the heart for murmurs and S_3 or S_4 heart sounds; examining the abdomen for bruits or masses; conducting a neurologic examination for focal deficits; and checking the extremities for pulses and the presence of edema.

DIFFERENTIAL DIAGNOSIS

The differential diagnosis generally involves distinguishing between primary and secondary HTN. Additional considerations in evaluating elevated BP readings are transient factors, such as stress or an acute illness causing the elevated reading, as well as "white coat" HTN and "pseudohypertension."

Primary HTN tends to run in families; the physical examination and laboratory screening do not identify a specific etiology for the elevated BP. Although secondary HTN accounts for only 5% of hypertensive individuals, it is important to identify these cases because they are potentially curable.

White coat HTN and pseudoHTN are conditions where the patient does not truly have HTN, but the BP is elevated under the conditions or time it is being measured. For example, with white coat HTN, the patient's BP is elevated in the physician's office but not at other times. In pseudoHTN, the patient is generally elderly; has calcified, rigid blood vessels; and the intra-arterial BP is actually lower than what can be measured with the BP cuff.

DIAGNOSTIC EVALUATION

Once the diagnosis of HTN has been made, four main questions must be addressed:

1. Is this HTN primary (essential) or secondary?
2. How many risk factors are present?
3. Is there evidence of target-organ damage?
4. Are there any comorbid conditions that would affect the choice of therapy?

Laboratory and diagnostic studies are indicated to assess end-organ damage, identify additional cardiovascular risk factors, exclude secondary causes, and assist in the choice of medications. A CBC is recommended as a baseline for future evaluation in the event of medication-induced neutropenia or agranulocytosis. A fasting serum glucose, K+, serum creatinine, UA, and lipid profile are recommended for newly diagnosed hypertensive patients. A high fasting serum glucose can indicate diabetes mellitus, unprovoked hypokalemia (<3.5 meq/L) suggests hyperaldosteronism, an elevated creatinine may indicate renal insufficiency, and proteinuria or microalbuminuria may indicate renal end-organ damage. Two other recommended tests are serum calcium (with albumin) and uric acid, since hypercalcemia or hyperuricemia may preclude the use of thiazide diuretics and hypercalcemia can identify hyperparathyroidism.

An ECG is helpful in assessing for prior MI, heart block, or left ventricular hypertrophy. A plain chest x-ray can detect cardiomegaly and CHF and help assess for coarctation of the aorta. In patients with suspected white coat HTN, ambulatory BP monitoring may help determine whether HTN is an appropriate diagnosis. A serum TSH can help diagnose thyroid disease, which can elevate BP.

TREATMENT

Once the diagnosis of HTN has been established, treatment should be initiated. The seventh report of the Joint National Committee (JNC) on Detection, Evaluation and Treatment of High Blood Pressure in 2003 classified HTN into three stages (Table 46-1).

Diabetic patients and those with evidence of renal disease warrant aggressive therapy to achieve a BP of <130/80 (Box 46-2). The first step in treatment for patients with normal renal function and nondiabetic patients with preHTN is lifestyle modification. About 60% of hypertensive patients are salt-sensitive and may benefit from sodium restriction (<2.4 g/day) by avoiding added salt and salty or processed food.

TABLE 46-1 Stages of Hypertension

Stage	Systolic Pressure	Diastolic Pressure
	Range	Range
Optimal	<120	<80
Prehypertension	120–139	80–89
Stage 1	140–159	90–99
Stage 2	>160	>100

Other lifestyle changes include weight reduction, regular aerobic exercise (30- to 60-minute sessions three to four times a week), and limiting alcohol intake (<24 oz beer per day, <8 oz of wine per day, <2 oz of whisky per day). Lifestyle modification alone effectively controls about 10% of patients.

If patients remain hypertensive after 3 to 6 months of lifestyle modification, it is appropriate to start antihypertensive medication. Patients with stage 2 HTN and diabetic patients with SBP over 130 or DBP over 80 warrant earlier initiation of pharmacologic therapy in addition to lifestyle recommendations. The therapeutic goal for all patients is a BP of 120/80 mmHg or less. Isolated systolic HTN (SBP ≥140 mmHg) is a common form of HTN in the elderly. The Systolic HTN in the Elderly Program (SHEP) demonstrated that the treatment of patients over age

BOX 46-2 JNC 7 Treatment Overview

Treat to BP <140/90 or <130/80 in patients with diabetes or chronic renal disease

Most patients require two medications for optimal control

Encourage lifestyle modifications:

- Weight loss
- DASH diet
- Sodium restriction
- Aerobic physical activity for at least 30–40 minutes per day
- Moderate alcohol consumption
- Smoking cessation

Initial drug treatment:

- Stage 1 hypertension (140–159/90–99 mmHg): thiazide-type diuretics; may consider ACEI, ARB, BB, CCB, or combination
- Stage 2 hypertension (>160/100 mmHg): 2-drug combination using thiazide-type diuretic plus ACEI, ARB, BB, or CCB

60 with isolated systolic HTN by using low-dose diuretics and beta blockers (BBs) significantly reduces the incidence of strokes and MIs.

The four classes of medications that are most commonly used as **first-line agents** are **diuretics, BBs, calcium channel blockers,** and **ACE inhibitors.** Most patients will require two or more antihypertensive medications to achieve adequate control. For patients with BP more than 20/10 mmHg above goal BP, consideration should be given to initiating therapy with two agents.

DIURETICS

Thiazides were the first major drugs introduced for the treatment of HTN and are still the most widely used. They inhibit Na^+ reabsorption from the renal tubules and thus reduce total blood volume. In addition, they blunt the effect of endogenous vasoconstrictors on the vascular smooth muscles, causing a decrease in peripheral vascular resistance. Thiazides are useful in patients without renal impairment (GFR > 25 or creatinine levels <2 and <1.5 in the elderly). Although thiazides may cause adverse metabolic side effects—such as hypokalemia, hyperuricemia, carbohydrate intolerance, and hyperlipidemia; these effects can be held to a minimum if the dose is kept below the equivalent of 25 mg/day of hydrochlorothiazide (HCTZ). Most patients can be successfully treated with 12.5 to 25 mg of HCTZ. Side effects include sexual dysfunction, dyslipidemia, hyperglycemia, and elevations in uric acid levels.

For patients with renal impairment (Cr >2 to 2.5), loop diuretics (i.e., furosemide) are more effective. They tend to produce more diuresis and hypokalemia than thiazides. Concomitant use of NSAIDs interferes with the delivery of loop diuretics to their site of action. Loop diuretics tend to lower serum calcium, whereas thiazides tend to cause hypercalcemia.

Before diuretics are administered, the serum K^+ level should be checked and then monitored periodically after diuretic therapy is initiated.

BETA BLOCKERS (BBs)

Beta-adrenergic receptor blockers work by decreasing heart rate and cardiac contractility. In addition, they modulate the output of the central and peripheral sympathetic nervous systems and decrease release of renin from the juxtaglomerular apparatus. Their renin-mediated mechanism of action may account for the decreased responsiveness in "low-renin" patients (elderly, African-Americans).

Within the BB class of medications, there are nonselective and selective beta-receptor blockers. Nonselective agents block both beta$_1$ and beta$_2$ receptors, whereas selective agents block only beta$_1$ receptors. Use of a selective agent is indicated in patients with a history of reactive airway disease, where the selectivity may lessen the likelihood of medication-induced bronchospasm. In addition to selective and nonselective subcategories, there are BBs with intrinsic sympathomimetic activity (ISA). BBs with ISA are thought to be less likely to elevate triglycerides or lower HDL cholesterol, and they cause less of a decrease in heart rate.

Side effects of BBs include bradycardia, fatigue, depression, insomnia, sexual dysfunction, and adverse effects on the lipid profile. BBs should be avoided or used cautiously in patients with asthma, COPD, second- or third-degree heart block, peripheral vascular disease, and insulin-dependent diabetes mellitus. Sudden withdrawal of these medications should be avoided, as it can cause tachyarrhythmias and rebound HTN due to the upregulation of beta receptors associated with chronic therapy.

ACE INHIBITORS (ACEIs)

ACEIs act through the renin–angiotensin system by inhibiting the enzyme that converts angiotensin I to angiotensin II. ACEIs are particularly beneficial in patients with CHF and provide renal protection for those with diabetes. Patients epidemiologically associated with "low-renin" states, such as the elderly and African-American populations, may be less likely to respond to the antihypertensive effects of these medications. ACEIs are generally well tolerated; the most common side effect is cough. Other less common but serious reactions include angioedema and neutropenia. In those with renal artery stenosis, ACEIs may cause an acute reversible renal failure. ARBs act by blocking the receptor site. They appear to be equipotent for lowering BP but may not be as effective as ACEIs in treating CHF and diabetic nephropathy. Unlike ACEIs, they do not cause a cough and only rarely cause skin rashes, making these agents useful for patients who cannot tolerate ACEIs because of these side effects.

CALCIUM CHANNEL BLOCKERS (CCBS)

CCBs include diltiazem, verapamil, and dihydropyridines. CCBs lower BP through a peripheral vasodilatory action. Diltiazem and verapamil depress the AV node and myocardial contractility. The dihydropyridines have a purer vasodilatory action and can cause a reflex tachycardia, but they have less effect on cardiac contractility. The use of short-acting dihydropyridines to lower BP may precipitate ischemic events in individuals with coronary artery disease because of reflex tachycardia. No such association has been found with use of long-acting dihydropyridines. Other side effects of CCBs include dizziness, edema, constipation, headache, and flushing. Diltiazem and verapamil should be avoided or used cautiously in patients with second- or third-degree heart block, CHF, and those already taking BBs.

OTHER HYPERTENSIVE MEDICATIONS

Less commonly used but still important classes of antihypertensives include the centrally acting agents and alpha-adrenergic blockers. The centrally acting sympatholytic inhibitors include agents such as clonidine, methyldopa, guanfacine, and reserpine, one of the first available antihypertensives. They lower BP by stimulating alpha-adrenergic receptors in the CNS, which in turn reduces peripheral sympathetic outflow. These agents are usually second-line medications because of the high frequency of side effects, including sedation, fatigue, dry mouth, sexual dysfunction, and postural hypotension. Rebound HTN has been reported with their abrupt withdrawal. Alpha blockers block the alpha-adrenergic receptors, thereby relaxing smooth muscle and decreasing peripheral resistance. These agents include prazosin, terazosin, and doxazosin. Tachyphylaxis, headache, and postural hypotension are relatively common. The hypotension includes a marked first-dose phenomenon. Therefore, the first dose should be small and given at bedtime. The alpha blockers also relax smooth muscle in the prostate and are good choices for men with HTN and BPH.

KEY POINTS

- HTN affects 50 million Americans and is a major risk factor for the development of cardiovascular disease and cerebrovascular disease.

- Primary HTN accounts for 90% to 95% of all cases of HTN.

- The history, physical examination, and laboratory evaluation of hypertensive individuals involve assessment for end-organ damage, additional risk factors for cardiovascular disease, and secondary causes of HTN.

- The first step in therapy generally involves lifestyle modifications; if patients still remain hypertensive after 3 to 6 months, antihypertensive medications should be started.

47 Hyperthyroidism

Thyroid diseases are second only to diabetes as the most common endocrine problems encountered in medicine. Thyroid hormone affects virtually every cell in the human body. Family physicians must be aware of the many and varied clinical manifestations of thyroid disease as well as their different causes and treatment options.

PATHOGENESIS

The thyroid gland is derived from pharyngeal epithelium and, during development, it descends in the neck to its final location just anterior to the larynx, with the thyroglossal duct indicating its path of descent. TSH is released by the pituitary gland via stimulation from hypothalamic thyrotropin-releasing hormones (TRHs). TSH causes increased trapping of iodine by the thyroid, elevated production and release of triiodothyronine (T3) and thyroxine (T4), and growth of the gland itself. Thus elevated levels of TSH may lead to diffuse or nodular enlargement of the thyroid gland (i.e., goiter). Heightening levels of thyroid hormone cause the pituitary gland to be less sensitive to TRH and thus create an effective feedback loop that normally maintains a euthyroid state.

T4 and T3 are the active thyroid hormones and are 99% protein bound by thyroxine-binding globulin (TBG) and other serum proteins. In the peripheral tissues, T4 is converted into free T3, which has a 40 times greater affinity for the cellular receptors than T4. Thus, at the cellular level, T3 is the metabolically active thyroid hormone and is principally responsible for the metabolic effects of the thyroid hormone. However, due to extremely low concentrations of serum T3, free T4 is more easily measured.

Many states alter the amount of TBG and thus may affect measured thyroid hormone levels. Circumstances that increase TBG include pregnancy, acute liver disease, the newborn state, and medications such as oral contraceptive pills (OCPs) and tamoxifen. Elevated levels of androgens, chronic liver disease, glucocorticoid excess, severe illness, and nephrotic syndrome all diminish TBG levels.

Graves disease, in which circulating antibodies mimic the activity of TSH, causes enlargement of the thyroid gland and abnormally elevated levels of circulating thyroid hormone. Thyroid nodules occasionally release T3 and T4 independent of TSH. These autonomously functioning nodules often produce excessive levels of thyroid hormone, resulting in systemic abnormalities and atrophy of the remaining normal thyroid tissue. Postpartum and autoimmune thyroiditis (Hashimoto) are inflammatory conditions of the thyroid that can result in hyperthyroidism early in the process as a result of excess release of preformed thyroid hormone associated with thyroid cellular injury.

CLINICAL MANIFESTATIONS

HISTORY

Patients with symptomatic hyperthyroidism (also known as thyrotoxicosis) often complain of weight loss despite normal or high caloric intake, nervousness, heat intolerance, fatigue, increased perspiration, more frequent bowel movements, and inability to sleep. Older patients may complain of angina, palpitations, and shortness of breath. Women who are premenopausal often experience irregular vaginal bleeding. Those with Graves disease may describe a doughy, swollen appearance of their pretibial area (i.e., myxedema); they may have visual changes secondary to exophthalmos and are more likely to suffer from other endocrine disorders. In patients with a thyroid nodule, it is important to obtain a history of head and neck radiation because these patients have a higher rate of thyroid carcinoma.

PHYSICAL EXAMINATION

Individuals suffering from hyperthyroidism often appear restless and fidgety. Their skin may be moist and velvety and palmar erythema is often detectable. Patients often have a fine resting tremor and a "frightened" facial appearance secondary to ocular abnormalities that include widened palpebral fissures, infrequent blinking, and lid lag. The cardiovascular examination may reveal atrial fibrillation, sinus tachycardia, widened pulse pressure, and heart failure. Examination of the neck may demonstrate the presence of a goiter or nodule. Patients with thyroiditis may have thyroid tenderness in addition to enlargement of the gland. If a goiter is present, auscultation may reveal a bruit or venous hum. Deep tendon reflexes are typically brisk and symmetric.

DIFFERENTIAL DIAGNOSIS

The most common causes of hyperthyroidism are Graves disease, toxic multinodular goiter, and thyroiditis. Other potential causes are thyroid adenomas (a variant of toxic multinodular goiter) and, rarely, factitious thyrotoxicosis or pituitary disorders. A nonendocrine etiology that may cause hyperthyroidism related to pregnancy or presence of a hydatidiform mole is hypersecretion of hCG, which may bind to the TSH receptor and act as a thyrotropic substance. In areas of the world where there is insufficient iodine, ingestion of iodine or amiodarone may stimulate the thyroid and lead to hyperthyroidism.

DIAGNOSTIC EVALUATION

The diagnosis of hyperthyroidism is established by a raised serum total or free T4 or T3 hormone levels, reduced TSH level, and high radioiodine uptake in the thyroid gland with features of hyperthyroidism. The TSH is often the initial test ordered in evaluating for thyroid disease. TSH is very sensitive for detecting both hyper- and hypothyroidism. Follow-up testing of abnormal TSH results formerly involved measurement of total serum T4, T3, resin uptake, and free T4 index. These tests may still be used, but free T4 and T3 have largely supplanted their use, since the free levels of these hormones define disease activity in hyperthyroidism. TSH is decreased in patients with Graves disease, toxic multinodular goiter, toxic nodule, and occasionally with thyroiditis. Patients with these conditions have primary hyperthyroidism and will have elevated levels of thyroid hormone (free T4 and T3). A thyroid radioactive iodine uptake scan is useful in the setting of hyperthyroidism to differentiate between a diffuse process (e.g., Graves disease or thyroiditis) and a nodular disorder. The thyroid scan will show diffusely increased uptake in Graves disease, nodular hyperfunctioning in toxic multinodular goiter, and decreased uptake in thyroiditis. In patients with a palpable nodule, the thyroid scan also helps to differentiate between hot (hyperfunctioning) and cold (hypofunctioning) nodules. Thyroid scanning, US, and fine-needle aspiration are often used to monitor thyroid nodules. US can determine whether the nodule is solid or cystic. Thyroid antibodies are commonly found in patients with thyroiditis (Hashimoto) and Graves disease. In hyperthyroid patients with abnormally high levels of TSH, MRI is useful in evaluating for pituitary pathology.

TREATMENT

Initial therapy for hyperthyroidism is targeted toward controlling thyroid hormone production with medications. Definitive treatment will depend on the underlying disease process, patient's age, comorbidities, and patient's preferences. There are three distinct treatments for hyperthyroidism: antithyroid medications, thyroidectomy, and radioiodine.

Antithyroid medications as definitive therapy are most commonly used in patients below 40 years of age; they include propylthiouracil (PTU) and methimazole (Tapazole). These medications are relatively safe and inhibit iodine processing during the production of thyroid hormone; they also inhibit the peripheral conversion of T4 to T3. Agranulocytosis is a rare but serious side effect of these medications, so CBCs should be monitored during treatment. Other side effects include nausea, arthropathy, skin rashes, allergic reactions, and elevations of liver enzymes. Both medications are typically introduced in a loading dose for about 4 to 6 weeks and then as the patient's condition improves the dose can usually be reduced. Treatment typically lasts 1 year, followed by a gradual taper. Roughly 50% of those with Graves disease will have no further episodes. For those in whom hyperthyroidism returns, options include retreatment, radioactive iodine, and surgery. Radioactive iodine (iodine 131 or ^{131}I) is very commonly used in the treatment of thyrotoxicosis but is contraindicated in young children and pregnant women. The main disadvantage is resultant hypothyroidism, for which lifelong treatment with thyroid replacement is necessary. Maximum treatment effects are noted after 3 to 4 months and treatment may be repeated after 6 months if hyperthyroidism returns. Pretreatment with antithyroid medications is often initiated to avoid excess release of thyroid hormone resulting from radiation-induced damage to the thyroid tissue.

Symptomatic treatment of thyrotoxicosis is another important consideration. Beta blockers like propranolol are given and increased in dose until the symptoms of anxiety, restlessness, and tachycardia are adequately controlled. For patients with thyroiditis, this may be the only therapy required, as these patients typically progress to become euthyroid and ultimately hypothyroid and require thyroid replacement therapy. Definitive treatment of other forms of hyperthyroidism is typically achieved by radioactive iodine treatment, antithyroid medications, or surgery.

Surgery is a useful treatment and offers a quick and definitive cure. It is most often performed in younger patients and those with a hyperfunctioning nodule. Postsurgical hypothyroidism occurs but is less common than in those undergoing radioactive iodine treatments. The main risks include those associated with neck surgery, such as recurrent laryngeal nerve damage, damage to the parathyroid gland, infection, bleeding, and hypothyroidism.

Thyroid storm is a rare, life-threatening syndrome of severe thyrotoxicosis. Symptoms include nausea, fever, heart failure, tachycardia, and diaphoresis and usually occur in an individual with unknown or inadequately treated hyperthyroidism. Treatment is similar to that used to treat hyperthyroidism but more aggressive; it includes high-dose antithyroid medications, intravenous iodine, intravenous beta blockers, and high-dose steroids.

Patients with Graves disease and exophthalmos are at risk for corneal ulcers and permanent visual deficits secondary to optic nerve compression and extraocular muscle involvement. To prevent corneal ulcers, eye patches, protective glasses, and artificial tears are often employed. Steroids tapered over several weeks are also commonly used in preventing permanent ocular damage. In severe cases, radiation of the extraocular muscles or orbital decompression is indicated. Treatment of the pretibial myxedema usually consists of a topical steroid.

Patients with thyroid nodules must be evaluated over time to detect malignancies. Those with hyperfunctioning solitary nodules may be treated surgically or with thyroid suppression, using exogenous thyroid hormone. Because roughly 1 out of 20 nodules (functioning and nonfunctioning) are malignant, all thyroid nodules must be evaluated using US and biopsy.

KEY POINTS

- Patients with symptomatic hyperthyroidism (also known as thyrotoxicosis) often complain of weight loss despite normal or high caloric intake, nervousness, heat intolerance, fatigue, increased perspiration, more frequent bowel movements, and inability to sleep.

- The most common causes of hyperthyroidism are Graves disease, toxic multinodular goiter, and thyroiditis.

- The TSH is often the initial test ordered in evaluating for thyroid disease. If abnormal, it is followed by serum-free T4 and T3 to define disease activity in hyperthyroidism.

- A thyroid radioactive iodine uptake scan is useful in hyperthyroidism to differentiate between a diffuse process (e.g., Graves disease or thyroiditis) and a nodular disorder.

- Definitive treatment of hyperthyroidism is typically achieved by radioactive iodine treatment, antithyroid medications, or surgery.

Chapter

48 Hypothyroidism

Hypothyroidism occurs in about 1% to 3% of the population and affects people of all ages, including newborns and the elderly. The incidence is higher in women than in men (10:1 ratio) and also higher in elderly individuals. The range of symptoms experienced by those with hypothyroidism extends from mild fatigue to myxedema coma. Family physicians must have a high index of suspicion for the diagnosis of hypothyroidism because of its many symptoms.

PATHOGENESIS

Thyroid hormone regulates cellular metabolism and affects virtually every cell in the human body. Hypothyroidism may be due to agenesis of the thyroid, failure of the pituitary gland to produce TSH, or inadequate production of thyroid hormone by the thyroid gland. Because iodine is a core constituent of thyroid hormone, geographic areas that lack sufficient iodine have an increased rate of endemic hypothyroidism, cretinism, and goiter. To avoid this, most developed nations currently provide iodine as a dietary supplement. Because thyroid hormone is necessary for normal neurologic and physical development, all newborns in the United States are screened for congenital hypothyroidism.

Autoimmune destruction of the thyroid gland is the most common cause of noniatrogenic hypothyroidism. Hashimoto thyroiditis is the most common autoimmune disease affecting the thyroid and is characterized by elevated levels of antibodies to thyroid peroxidase and thyroglobulin. These antibodies cause inflammation of the thyroid gland, which can result in a goiter and lead to diminished production of thyroid hormone. Hashimoto thyroiditis is much more common in women, has a genetic predisposition, and is often associated with other autoimmune disorders.

Therapies for hyperthyroidism such as radioactive iodine and surgery are common causes of iatrogenic hypothyroidism. Medications such as lithium, iodine, and interferon may also cause hypothyroidism. Any disorder causing dysfunction of the hypothalamus or pituitary glands, such as pituitary adenoma or postpartum pituitary necrosis, may lead to lower levels of TRH and TSH. This then results in diminished production of thyroid hormone.

Myxedema from severe hypothyroidism causes systemic problems secondary to abnormal cellular metabolism and increased deposition of mucopolysaccharides in subcutaneous tissues. This results in a variety of abnormalities, including fluid accumulation in the pericardial sac, firm and tense swelling of the skin, connective tissue abnormalities, and neurologic dysfunction.

Rarely, individuals with long-standing hypothyroidism may experience myxedema coma. This life-threatening condition most often occurs after significant cold exposure or infection and results in hypothermia, mental status changes, and respiratory depression.

CLINICAL MANIFESTATIONS

HISTORY

Symptoms of hypothyroidism include weakness, fatigue, cold intolerance, constipation, dry skin, headache, and thinning hair. Although very mild weight gain can occur secondary to a slowing metabolism, excessive weight gain is uncommon. Women may complain of altered menstruation and infertility. Patients with long-standing hypothyroidism often experience a delay in thought, hoarse voice, muscle cramps, and diminished acuity of taste, smell, and hearing.

Congenital hypothyroidism has a subtle presentation that may include feeding problems, a hoarse cry, jaundice, and constipation. Later findings include developmental delay, short stature, and delayed dentition.

PHYSICAL EXAMINATION

Physical examination findings often vary according to the degree of hypothyroidism. The general appearance often reveals coarse, dry hair; pallor; thin, brittle nails; large tongue; thinning of the outer halves of eyebrows; and facial puffiness. Vital signs may show hypothermia, bradycardia, and normal-to-low BP. The neck should be evaluated for the presence of goiter, which may or may not be tender. Cardiovascular examination may reveal evidence of a pericardial effusion or cardiac enlargement. The skin is typically hard and doughy, while deep tendon reflexes are usually prolonged, with a slow return phase. Children who have had hypothyroidism since infancy have a cretinous appearance, which includes a large head, short limbs, wide-set eyes, and a broad, flat nose.

DIFFERENTIAL DIAGNOSIS

Box 48-1 lists the differential diagnosis of hypothyroidism. The two most common causes are thyroid gland failure due to Hashimoto thyroiditis and hypothyroidism secondary to surgery or radiation therapy. Endemic goiter due to iodine deficiency is rare in the United States because of the iodine supplementation of salt, but it is fairly common in other parts of the world.

DIAGNOSTIC EVALUATION

TSH, which is synthesized and secreted by the pituitary gland, is the most sensitive indicator of hypothyroidism due to thyroid dysfunction. It is elevated in patients with hypothyroidism except in the rare cases of central hypothyroidism, where the pituitary fails to secrete TSH. TSH and free T4 are both low in cases of hypothalamic or pituitary dysfunction. In subclinical hypothyroidism, TSH is elevated while the free T4 normal. High titers of thyroid antibodies are seen most commonly in those with Hashimoto thyroiditis, but they may be present in other conditions as well, such as subacute lymphocytic thyroiditis. A radioactive iodine uptake (RAIU) scan is often low or low normal in Hashimoto disease and shows a variable pattern with goitrous hypothyroidism. Pituitary failure can be confirmed by the failure of TSH to respond to TRH stimulation.

Hypothyroid patients may have elevations of cholesterol due to depressed degradation of lipids, crea-

tine phosphokinase (CPK), and liver enzymes. A CBC may show a mild normocytic, normochromic anemia due to diminished oxygen requirements and decreased production of erythropoietin or, less commonly, may demonstrate a macrocytic anemia secondary to decreased absorption of vitamin B_{12}. Serum electrolytes occasionally show hyponatremia. The ECG and chest x-ray may reveal findings consistent with a pericardial effusion. Patients with low TSH and low free T4 should have a MRI to evaluate for abnormalities of the pituitary or hypothalamus.

TREATMENT

Hypothyroidism is a most gratifying disease to treat because of the ease and completeness with which it responds to treatment. Levothyroxine is nearly always the treatment of choice. Widely available and inexpensive, it is converted to T3 in the peripheral tissues at a rate similar to that seen in euthyroid individuals. Most patients require a daily dose between 75 and 150 μg. Thyroid levels in the hypothyroid newborn must be corrected quickly and maintained in order to avoid irreversible damage. Young adults with mild hypothyroidism are typically given a starting dose of 50 μg, with increase in increments of 25 to 50 μg every 3 to 4 weeks. Older patients and those with cardiovascular disease are often very sensitive to thyroid replacement. In order to avoid precipitating an anginal attack or palpitations, these patients should be started on lower doses of levothyroxine, such as 25 μg, with gradual incremental increases to therapeutic levels over 4 to 6 months. After therapy is started, serum TSH should normalize and then be assessed every 6 to 12 months.

Patients with subclinical hypothyroidism have an elevated TSH and normal free T4 levels. These patients are at much higher risk for subsequently developing hypothyroidism and should be retested every 6 to 12 months. Therapy is initiated if the patient becomes symptomatic, if the TSH levels rise above 10 mU/L, or if free T4 levels fall below normal. Treating patient with TSH levels between 5 and 10 mIU/L remains controversial. Treatment should be individualized based on patient preference, symptoms, age, and associated medical conditions. Factors favoring treatment included younger age, symptoms consistent with hypothyroidism, abnormal lipids, a persistent and gradual increase of TSH, presence of antithyroid antibodies, and an enlarged thyroid.

Myxedema coma is the ultimate stage of long-standing untreated hypothyroidism and is associated with a high rate of mortality. This state almost invariably affects the elderly. Intravenous levothyroxine and steroids, warming blankets, and mechanical ventilation in an intensive care unit are the mainstays of treatment.

■ BOX 48-1 Differential Diagnosis of Hypothyroidism
Iatrogenic hypothyroidism (postablative hypothyroidism)
Surgery
Radioactive iodine
Hashimoto thyroiditis (chronic lymphocytic)
Subacute lymphocytic thyroiditis
Subclinical hypothyroidism
Hypothalamic or pituitary dysfunction
Iodine deficiency (endemic goiter)
Congenital hypothyroidism (agenesis)
Tracheotomy
Medications

KEY POINTS

- Hypothyroidism occurs in about 1% to 3% of the population and affects people of all ages, including newborns and the elderly.

- Symptoms of hypothyroidism include weakness, fatigue, cold intolerance, constipation, dry skin, headache, and thinning hair.

- Physical examination findings often reveal coarse, dry hair; pallor; thin, brittle nails; large tongue; thinning of the outer halves of eyebrows; and facial puffiness.

- The two most common causes are thyroid gland failure due to Hashimoto thyroiditis and hypothyroidism secondary to surgery or radiation therapy.

- TSH, which is synthesized and secreted by the pituitary gland, is the most sensitive indicator of hypothyroidism due to thyroid dysfunction.

49 Obesity

Obesity is the presence of an abnormally large amount of adipose tissue. The preferred method to assess obesity is to use a measure known as the BMI. BMI is calculated by dividing the weight in kilograms by the height in meters squared. The BMI has the advantage of being independent of gender and frame size and serves as a surrogate measure of body fat. Using BMI, **overweight** is defined as **BMI of 25 to 29.9 kg/m²** and **obesity** as a **BMI greater than 30 kg/m²**. Morbid obesity is defined as a BMI greater than 40.0 kg/m². In the United States, approximately 20% of men and 25% of women meet the criteria for obesity. Unfortunately, the percentage of obese Americans is increasing, particularly among children and adolescents. Minority populations are disproportionately affected. About one-third of Mexican-American and African-American women are obese.

Several studies suggest that central obesity may be associated with more adverse health conditions than lower body obesity. Central obesity can be determined by calculating a waist-to-hip ratio. Central obesity is present if the waist-to-hip ratio is greater than 0.85 in women and 1.0 in men.

PATHOGENESIS

People gain weight when the caloric intake exceeds the body's energy expenditure. The reason why an individual's caloric intake exceeds demand is complex and represents a heterogeneous disorder reflecting genetic, socioeconomic, and environmental influences. Clinically, physicians should view obesity as a chronic metabolic disease with health consequences rather than solely as a cosmetic or behavioral problem.

The current American social environment has contributed to the increased incidence of obesity. Many individuals have sedentary jobs and lifestyles that reduce or eliminate calorie-burning activities. More people can afford to eat at restaurants, where large portions of high-calorie foods contribute to added weight. In addition to environmental and social influences, some individuals overeat in response to emotional stress or have become conditioned to eat not for sustenance but for the pleasure associated with various activities (e.g., watching television and movies and attending parties).

Studies of identical twins indicate that energy expenditure and fat distribution appear to be influenced by heredity. Recent studies have also explored the role of leptin, an appetite-controlling hormone. This hormone is secreted by fat cells and may signal the hypothalamus with a measure of the level of stored fat. There have been case reports of obese individuals having mutations of the leptin gene. In a few cases, genetic syndromes such as Prader–Willi cause obesity. These syndromes are usually identified in childhood.

There is some evidence that the body regulates its weight around a certain weight or set point. The body defends the set point by adjusting the metabolic rate, and one theory proposes that obese patients regulate their weight around a higher set point. Some experts believe that physical activity and the amount of dietary fat may help modify this set point. Despite advances in understanding the pathophysiology of obesity, it is unlikely that these advances will lead to significant improvements in treatment in the near future.

CLINICAL MANIFESTATIONS

HISTORY

Obese patients generally have symptoms related to decreased exercise tolerance or to illnesses associated with obesity. Box 49-1 lists some health conditions associated with obesity. In addition, obese individuals may suffer from psychological impairments, such as a poor self-image or social isolation.

The history should also include information about current diet, previous diets attempted and their outcome, motivation to lose weight, and knowledge about health and diet. A complete review of medical problems associated with obesity is listed in Box 49-1.

PHYSICAL EXAMINATION

The physical examination should include the patient's BP, height, weight, and BMI. Although anthropomorphic measures are important, visual assessment of the patient is generally accurate—that *is*, if the patient *looks* overweight, then he or she *is* overweight. In addition, signs of obesity-influenced conditions

BOX 49-1 Conditions Associated With Obesity

Cancer of the uterus, breast, prostate, and colon	Coronary disease
Degenerative arthritis	Diabetes
Fatty liver	Gallbladder disease
Gout	Hyperlipidemia
Hypertension	Increased operative risk
Low back pain	Reflux esophagitis
Sleep apnea	Low self-esteem
Thromboembolic disease	Intertrigo

should be sought and an assessment made of the patient's mobility.

DIFFERENTIAL DIAGNOSIS

Obesity can be either primary or secondary. Secondary causes of obesity account for less than 1% of cases. Medicines associated with weight gain include tricyclic antidepressants, beta blockers, phenothiazines, glucocorticoids, oral contraceptives, sulfonylureas, and insulin.

Neuroendocrine problems such as hypothyroidism, Cushing syndrome, and hypothalamic disease can also cause obesity. Genetic disorders causing obesity are extremely rare and are usually clinically evident in childhood.

DIAGNOSTIC EVALUATION

Few tests are routinely indicated in the obese patient. Laboratory evaluation will depend on the individual and his or her age, but should usually include a fasting blood glucose and lipid profile. A TSH is helpful in cases of suspected hypothyroidism.

TREATMENT

Obesity is a chronic problem that can be frustrating for both the patient and the physician. Individuals must be motivated to lose weight and to make lifestyle changes in diet and exercise. Poorly motivated patients are unlikely to adhere to a weight-loss program.

Treatment options include diet, exercise, drugs, and surgery. The degree of obesity and the presence of associated illness should influence management strategies. Conservative therapy relying on diet and exercise forms the basis of most weight-loss programs. High-cost programs or hazardous procedures such as surgery should be reserved for morbidly obese patients and those at greatest risk from obesity who have failed more conservative treatment.

Most obese people would like to achieve an "ideal body weight." Unfortunately, short of surgery, most diet, exercise, or drug programs result in about a 10% weight loss. For many individuals, the goal might be to achieve a healthful weight rather than an ideal weight. Even modest weight reduction (5% to 10%) can be clinically significant, especially in obese individuals with diabetes or hypertension. Emphasizing realistic goals and then reinforcing them can help to prevent failure, which would only contribute further to poor self-esteem. Sometimes prevention of further weight gain may be the most appropriate goal for an individual who is unwilling or unable to lose weight.

Ideally, the patient and the physician should work together to create a nutritionally sound diet that incorporates the patient's food preferences. A dietitian can also be helpful in planning a diet.

Avoiding behaviors associated with obesity such as the consumption of restaurant and fast food, large portion sizes and sugar-added beverages are standard advice. Conversely, behaviors associated with weight loss such as recommending an increase intake of fruits, vegetables, and eating a healthy breakfast should be recommended. Weight is a product of energy balance and the loss of 1 lb of fat requires a 3500-calorie deficit. Therefore, a calorie deficit of 500 to 1000 calories per day will result in a weight loss of 1 to 2 lb/week, which is appropriate for most patients. Gradual dietary changes tend to produce better, longer-lasting results. Simple suggestions include eating three meals a day, eating only at mealtimes, and limiting portions to one serving. Reducing dietary fat to 20% to 30% of total calories also enhances weight loss and is consistent with recommendations to reduce the risk of cardiac disease. Low-carbohydrate diets are more acceptable to many patients because of the increased satiety associated with them. The low-carbohydrate diets have achieved better short-term weight loss, but long-term results are comparable to those with traditional low-fat calorie-restricted diets. Very low calorie, medically supervised diets have a limited role in management and are usually reserved for the morbidly obese or individuals at very high risk, such as those with sleep apnea. A minimum of 800 calories per day is recommended. Risks for very low calorie diets include cardiac arrhythmias and gallstones. Exercise alone, without calorie restriction, is not an efficient weight loss strategy. However, exercise enhances overall health, improves waist-to-hip ratio, and helps to keep an individual's metabolic rate from resetting during periods of caloric restriction. Studies show that people who exercise regularly with an expenditure of 2000 kcal/week are more likely to maintain weight loss.

Exercise is most likely to be sustained if the exercise is something that the patient enjoys and can fit into his or her lifestyle. Opportunities should be explored to integrate exercise into daily activities whenever possible, such as climbing stairs instead of taking the elevator. Even if exercise produces only minimal weight loss, it still improves cardiovascular risk factors and obese patients with good fitness levels have been shown to have a reduced mortality risk from cardiovascular disease compared to lean but unfit individuals.

Drug therapy should be considered for morbidly obese individuals or those with significant comorbidities. Medications include appetite suppressants such as phentermine. Side effects include insomnia, hypertension, tachycardia, nausea, diarrhea, and anxiety. Amphetamines and amphetamine-like products are rarely used because of their side effects and addictive potential.

Sibutramine is a serotonin-norepinephrine reuptake inhibitor that suppresses appetite and is approved for long-term use in obesity management. Side effects include insomnia, dry mouth, headache, constipation, and small increases in pulse and BP in some patients. It is contraindicated in patients with stroke, heart failure, or cardiac arrhythmias and should not be given to patients on MAOIs, SSRIs, dihydroergotamine, meperidine, and fentanyl. Most of the weight loss with sibutramine occurs in the first 6 months and it is approved only for a limited period of time. Until more evidence on its safety and efficacy are available, lifestyle measure should be the mainstay of obesity management over sibutramine.

Orlistat is a GI lipase inhibitor that interferes with fat absorption. Side effects are triggered by dietary indiscretions and primarily affect the GI tract; they include oily stools, diarrhea, and leakage of stool. Symptoms usually improve with time and adherence to a low-fat diet. Surgery for obesity, such as gastric stapling, should be reserved for patients with morbid refractory obesity. Liposuction can remove localized deposits of fat by use of a suction probe. However, serious complications—including fat embolus, hemorrhage, and even death—have been reported.

Childhood obesity is increasing, and children who are overweight by age 6 are at much greater risk for being obese as adults than are other children. Involvement of the parents in managing the diet and activity of younger children is essential. Often, slowing weight gain is the goal, so that the child can grow out of the obesity. In adolescents, the degree of parental involvement should be individualized. Schools may also represent an important opportunity for preventing childhood obesity. Program aimed at decreasing television and video viewing time, increased physical activity, healthy eating, and eliminating sugar-sweetened beverage intake have shown some success in decreasing the prevalence of obesity.

KEY POINTS

- BMI is the weight in kilograms divided by the height in meters squared. BMI is independent of gender and frame size.
- Obesity is defined as a BMI greater than 30.
- Obesity is a heterogeneous disorder reflecting genetic, socioeconomic, behavioral, and environmental influences.
- The loss of 1 lb of fat requires a 3500-calorie deficit.

Chapter

50 Osteoporosis

Osteoporosis is a reduction in bone mass per unit of volume with microarchitectural deterioration of bone tissue that compromises bone strength and increases the susceptibility to fracture. It is seen primarily in elderly individuals.

EPIDEMIOLOGY

As our population has aged, the number of individuals with osteoporosis has grown to over 10 million, with an additional 34 million individuals at high risk for developing this condition. The majority of these are women (80%); one in two women will have an osteoporosis related fracture over their lifetime, and by age 75, one out of three white women will suffer an osteoporotic hip fracture. While the incidence among men is lower, one in four men over age 50 will have an osteoporosis-related fracture over their lifetime. Osteoporosis is responsible for 1.5 million fractures each year, with an annual cost of approximately $17 billion. Approximately 10% to 20% of patients who suffer a hip fracture die of a medical complication within 6 months of the fracture, and those who survive are often unable to live independently.

PATHOGENESIS

The resorption and formation of bone is a continuous process. Under steady state, these processes are equal and linked. At around age 35, bone mass peaks, and both genders begin to lose bone mass after age 40. Estrogen receptors are present on osteoblasts, the cells that form bone, which may explain why estrogen-deficient states result in bone loss. There also appears to be an uncoupling of osteoblasts from the action of osteoclasts, the cells that resorb bone. Several different chemical modulators may mediate this uncoupling, but the precise mechanisms for developing osteoporosis have not yet been determined.

Osteoporosis can either be primary or secondary to an underlying disease, such as hyperparathyroidism. Primary osteoporosis is an age-related bone disorder that results from aging and changes in sex hormones. It is of two types: Type I osteoporosis, or postmenopausal osteoporosis, affects women approximately 20 years after menopause. It primarily affects

trabecular bone and is due to increased osteoclast activity. Trabecular bone is present in the hip, vertebrae, distal radius, and heel. Type II osteoporosis, or senile osteoporosis, involves loss of both cortical and trabecular bones and primarily affects individuals over age 70. Type II changes appear to be related to age-related decreases in calcium absorption and decreases in vitamin D absorption and synthesis. The effects of types I and II osteoporosis are additive and most individuals with osteoporosis have elements of both types. Secondary osteoporosis can be caused by many medical conditions and a variety of medicines, particularly glucocorticoids.

CLINICAL MANIFESTATIONS

HISTORY

Patients with osteoporosis are generally asymptomatic. However, chronic pain and tenderness over the affected area may occur, particularly in association with osteoporotic fractures. The bones most commonly affected by osteoporotic fractures are the spine, hip, and distal radius. It is important to elicit other symptoms that may occur as complications of osteoporosis. For example, a vertebral fracture may result in spinal cord compression and neurologic findings. Osteoporosis of facet joints may also contribute to back pain.

History is useful to identify those patients with risk factors for osteoporosis. These risk factors can be grouped into several different categories: (1) genetic: Caucasian or Asian ethnicity, small stature, and a family history of osteoporosis; (2) lifestyle: tobacco, alcohol, and caffeine consumption, lack of physical activity; (3) nutritional: low calcium and vitamin D intake; and (4) other risk factors such as older age and postmenopausal state.

PHYSICAL EXAMINATION

On physical examination, height reduction greater than 1.5 inches, dorsal kyphosis (dowager or widow hump), exaggerated cervical lordosis, gait deficits, and low body weight are common findings associated with osteoporosis. Dorsal kyphosis is due to wedge-shaped deformity in the middorsal vertebrae. Because of the risk of spinal cord compression, it is important to perform a complete neurologic examination to rule out neurologic involvement from an osteoporotic fracture.

DIFFERENTIAL DIAGNOSIS

While osteoporosis is commonly age-related, other diseases or conditions may secondarily cause osteoporosis. These can be divided into five different categories (Box 50-1). Identification and treatment of these underlying diseases can limit bone loss. Glucocorticoid-induced disease is the most common cause of secondary osteoporosis. When the disease or condition is not modifiable, as in patients requiring chronic corticosteroids, the use of preventive medicines such as a bisphosphonate (e.g., alendronate) may help to prevent bone loss.

■ **BOX 50-1** Secondary Causes of Osteoporosis
Endocrine
Acromegaly
Diabetes mellitus
Cushing disease
Hyperparathyroidism
Hypogonadism
Hyperthyroidism
Nutritional
Malabsorption
Malnutrition
Anorexia nervosa
Liver disease
Vitamin D deficiency
Alcoholism
Collagen Vascular
Rheumatoid arthritis
Ehlers–Danlos syndrome
Marfan syndrome
Osteoporosis imperfecta
Cancer
Multiple myeloma
Bone metastases
Breast cancer
Lymphoma
Leukemia
Medications
Glucosteroid
Phenobarbital
Phenytoin
Heparin
Methotrexate
Excess thyroid hormone replacement

DIAGNOSTIC EVALUATION

Patients at risk for developing osteoporosis are candidates for screening. These include (1) postmenopausal women below 65 years of age with one or more risk factors besides menopause; (2) all postmenopausal women over age 65; (3) postmenopausal women with a history of fractures; (4) those who are on long-term corticosteroid treatment; and more recently (5) men over age 70. In addition, those who are considering treatments or preventive measures for osteoporosis may benefit from information gained through screening. Patients being treated for osteoporosis require repeat testing to assess therapy. Measurement of bone mineral density (BMD) is the standard method for screening and establishing the diagnosis of osteoporosis. Dual energy X-ray absorptiometry (DEXA) is the preferred method for confirming the diagnosis and monitoring therapy because it represents the best combination of sensitivity, technical simplicity, reproducibility, and cost while also minimizing radiation exposure. In using DEXA to determine the effects of therapy, the same machine should be used, if possible, in order to limit variations in measurements between different DEXA scanners. BMD determinations of both the spine and hip provide the best assessments, since the degree of osteoporosis can differ between sites.

The BMD report provides a T score and Z score. The T score compares the patient's BMD with that of a normal adult 25 to 30 years of age and of the same gender. The Z score compares the patient's BMD with that of the same age group and gender. Osteoporosis is defined as a T score of more than 2.5 standard deviations below the mean (–2.5 SD). Osteopenia, or low bone mass, is defined as a T score between –1.0 and –2.5. Z scores of –1.5 suggest a secondary cause of osteoporosis. The risk for an osteoporotic fracture increases two- to fourfold for every standard deviation in reduced BMD.

In addition to a DEXA scan, blood tests are useful for identifying and managing secondary cases of osteoporosis. Initial tests consist of a complete blood count (CBC); erythrocyte sedimentation rate (ESR); 25-hydroxy vitamin D; chemistry panel including serum calcium, phosphorus, and alkaline phosphatase as well as renal function. Calcium and phosphate measurements help detect hyperparathyroidism and vitamin D deficiencies. In patients with anemia and an elevated ESR, multiple myeloma should be considered. Electrolyte abnormalities can identify patients with chronic acidosis or renal tubular acidosis. Serum alkaline phosphatase is a marker of osteoblastic activity and is elevated in malignancy, hyperparathyroidism, and other high-turnover states. More selective tests such as a 24-hour urine calcium tests or parathyroid hormone (PTH) levels should be selectively ordered based on history, physical examination, and preliminary laboratory findings.

TREATMENT

The first line of prevention for osteoporosis is lifestyle changes, while pharmaceutical agents are the first line of treatment for osteoporosis. Smoking cessation, avoiding excess alcohol, weight-bearing exercise, and improved dietary habits are helpful in preserving bone mass. It is recommended that calcium intake should be 1000 mg/day for premenopausal women and 1500 mg/day for postmenopausal women. Vitamin D supplementation increases bone density in patients with an established deficiency. Vitamin D deficiency has also been associated with cardiovascular disease, diabetes, autoimmune disease, and some types of cancer. Stores should be normalized with supplementation over a period of 2 to 3 months with repeat testing to assure adequate levels. As patients age, the risk of falls increases and fall prevention is another priority for reducing the number of osteoporotic fractures. Improving vision, adjusting sedative medications, and incorporating balance exercises are beneficial. Other environmental adjustments such as minimizing clutter, anchoring rugs, adding hand rails, and better lighting in dark hallways are helpful in preventing falls.

Pharmaceutical therapy for osteoporosis should be considered for individuals with a BMD T score below –2.5 without risk factors or T score below –1.5 with multiple risk factors, women above age 70 with multiple risk factors, and patients undergoing long-term corticosteroid treatment. Preventive therapy for osteopenia should be provided to those with T score values below –1.0. Table 50-1 lists some of the medications available for treatment. The bisphosphonates must be taken on an empty stomach with a large glass of water, with the patient remaining upright without eating for at least 30 minutes. More convenient formulations that allow these medicines to be administered in a single weekly dose or in a monthly dose make the therapy easier. More recently annual intravenous therapy has become available. Common side effects include stomach pain, nausea, and musculoskeletal pain. Osteonecrosis of the jaw is a very rare but serious side effect. It occurs primarily in patients with metastatic cancer or multiple myeloma who received high dose therapy.

■ **TABLE 50-1** General Guidelines for Pharmacologic Agents		
Agent	**Benefits**	**Contraindications**
HRT	Inhibits bone reabsorption in estrogen-deficient patients	Breast cancer
		Estrogen-dependent neoplasm
	Control vasomotor symptoms	Undiagnosed vaginal bleeding
		H/O thromboembolic disorder
		H/O migraine
		Low HDL
Bisphosphonates	Inhibits bone resorption	Gastric ulcer
		Abnormal esophageal motility
		Unable to sit upright × 30 min
Calcitonins	Most effective in spine	Allergy to salmon protein
	Analgesic effect in back pain	Unable to tolerate nasal spray
SERM	Pt w/contraindications to HRT use	Vasomotor symptoms not relieved
	Decrease total and low-density-lipoprotein (LDL) cholesterol	
	Not affecting HDL	H/O thromboembolic disorder

HRT, hormone replacement therapy; SERM, selective estrogen receptor modulator.

KEY POINTS

- Osteoporosis is a reduction in bone mass per unit of volume that is seen primarily in older individuals.
- Approximately 20% of patients who suffer a hip fracture die within a year of the fracture.
- Osteoporosis can either be primary or secondary. Secondary causes include medications, cancers, endocrine disorders, collagen vascular disease, or nutritional problems.
- DEXA is the preferred method for detecting osteoporosis and is reported as a T score that compares the patient's BMD with peak bone mass and a Z score that compares the patient's BMD with age- and gender-matched controls.

51 Prostate Disease

Common prostate problems include benign prostatic enlargement, prostatitis, and prostate cancer. BPH is an enlargement of the prostate gland, with or without the cellular changes of true hyperplasia, which affects up to 90% of men by age 80. Prostatitis is an inflammation of the prostate that affects 5% to 9% of men during their lifetimes. Prostatitis occurs secondary to bacterial infection only about 10% of the time and may be acute or chronic. Nonbacterial prostatitis can be subdivided into chronic nonbacterial prostatitis and prostatodynia. "Chronic nonbacterial prostatitis" describes an inflammatory process with no identified bacterial etiology, whereas "prostatodynia" refers to prostate-related symptoms in the absence of inflammation. Prostate cancer is among the most common forms of cancer and is the second leading cause of cancer death in men. However, the clinical incidence of the disease does not match the prevalence noted at autopsy, where small, occult cancers are commonly detected.

PATHOGENESIS

The pathophysiology of prostate disease is not completely understood, but testosterone is thought to stimulate prostatic enlargement and cancer. Bacterial prostatitis may occur through the introduction of bacteria into the prostate in association with sexual activity or as part of a more generalized urinary tract infection (UTI). Chronic nonbacterial prostatitis and prostatodynia (sometimes referred to as chronic pelvic pain syndrome or CPPS) are poorly understood processes. In recent years, some urologists have come to believe that nonbacterial prostatitis may be due to organisms such as *Chlamydia*, *Mycoplasma*, and *Ureaplasma* species, while the pain associated with prostadynia may stem from the neuromuscular structures of the pelvic floor rather than the prostate itself.

Symptoms of prostatic disease may result directly from an inflammatory process causing dysuria, urinary frequency, and urgency, or they may be due to lower urinary tract obstruction. An enlarged prostate from either a benign or a cancerous process can cause obstruction of urinary flow at the neck of the bladder. Early in the process, the detrusor muscle will undergo hypertrophy, but it can still contract effectively, allowing the bladder to empty. However the hypertrophied

detrusor muscle may contract involuntarily, leading to symptoms of urgency, frequency, and nocturia. As the obstructive process progresses, bladder emptying is incomplete and muscle contractility may become less effective, leading to symptoms of incomplete emptying, hesitancy, and a weak urinary stream. More severe obstruction requires abdominal straining in order to establish urinary flow and, ultimately, urinary dribbling and overflow incontinence may occur.

CLINICAL MANIFESTATIONS

HISTORY

Symptoms of prostatic disease include difficulty voiding, a sensation of incomplete bladder emptying, dysuria, urinary frequency, urgency, or nocturia. In addition, patients may complain of vague symptoms such as discomfort in the genital region, perineum, or rectum. Pain with ejaculation may also be present. Signs of prostatic enlargement and the degree of obstruction are indicated by positive responses to the questions about symptoms presented in Box 51-1. Other important historical factors include personal or family history of prostate disease.

PHYSICAL EXAMINATION

Physical examination will focus on the genital and prostate examination. Abdominal examination that can detect bladder distention, indicating at least 200 mL of retained urine, should be performed. Costovertebral angle tenderness may indicate upper UTI. The penis and testicles should be examined for tenderness and signs of inflammation or STDs. Finally, the rectal examination should be performed. The optimal position for examination of the prostate is with the patient standing and bent over the examination table with his elbows resting on the table. The normal prostate is approximately the size of a chestnut, with the consistency of the contracted abductor pollicis muscle in the hand. In the midline, the fissure should be identifiable. Enlargement is indicated by both an increase in size and loss of the midline fissure. Tenderness or a boggy texture on palpation suggests an inflammatory process. Many cancers present with increased firmness of the prostate, indicating induration but no discrete mass. The only time a

■ BOX 51-1 Questions to Elicit Symptoms of Prostate Disease

Do you have the sensation of not emptying your bladder completely after you have finished voiding?
Do you have to urinate again less than 2 hours after you finished urinating before?
Does your urinary stream stop and start again several times during urination?
Do you find it difficult to postpone urination?
Have you noticed a weak urinary stream?
Do you have to push or strain to initiate urination?
Do you awaken to urinate more than one time per night?

prostate examination is not indicated in the evaluation of urinary or prostate-related symptoms is in an ill-appearing febrile patient in whom acute bacterial prostatitis is suspected. In these instances, bacteremia may occur with a prostate examination; therefore, treatment should be initiated without it.

DIFFERENTIAL DIAGNOSIS

Lower urinary tract symptoms of urinary frequency, hesitancy, urgency, dysuria, and nocturia may result from conditions involving the bladder, prostate, urethra, or neurologic systems. Urethral strictures should be suspected in those with a history of urethral catheterization, instrumentation, or urethritis. Bladder lesions such as cancer or cystitis may cause symptoms suggestive of prostatic disease. Neurologic diseases such as MS and spinal cord injury may cause voiding dysfunction, known as vesicosphincter dyssynergia, with symptoms overlapping those seen with prostatic disease. Peripheral neuropathies associated with diabetes mellitus or alcoholism may affect the autonomic fibers to the bladder, leading to obstructive urinary tract symptoms. Pharmacologic agents such as those with anticholinergic or alpha-adrenergic agonist properties may precipitate urinary retention. Finally, psychogenic voiding dysfunction is a cause for failure of relaxation of the striated urethral sphincter and poor bladder emptying.

DIAGNOSTIC EVALUATION

Evaluation begins with a focused history and physical examination. Inquiring about medications, neurologic disease, and prior urologic disease may suggest the underlying cause for the patient's symptoms. Evaluation of the patient begins with a urinalysis (UA) and culture to assess for hematuria, signs of inflammation, and infection. In patients with suspected obstruction, BUN and creatinine values should be obtained, along with

US of the renal system looking for signs of obstruction. Patients found to have hematuria should have either a CT scan of the abdomen or an intravenous pyelogram performed, along with a cystoscopy to assess for renal and bladder carcinoma. Glycosuria should prompt consideration of diabetes with or without neuropathy as a cause of urinary symptoms.

Patients with urinary tract symptoms and fever should have their urine and blood cultured and also treatment with an antibiotic. In those with suspected acute bacterial prostatitis, hospitalization is often warranted. In patients with chronic symptoms, evaluation by UA and culture obtained before and after prostatic massage can help diagnose infectious prostatitis. WBCs present after prostate massage indicate bacterial or nonbacterial prostatitis, with the culture distinguishing between the two. The absence of WBCs in the urine or in prostatic secretions after prostatic massage suggests prostatodynia or CPPS as the underlying cause. Patients with a history of urethral disorders, infections, or instrumentation may be evaluated for stricture by cystoscopy or by performing a urethrogram. In those with suspected ongoing infection, cultures should be obtained.

Cystoscopy is warranted to evaluate patients over age 40 suspected of bladder carcinoma based on either the symptoms or the presence of hematuria—as well as in those without an apparent explanation for symptoms after an initial evaluation. Urine cytology may also be helpful for detecting bladder carcinoma. A PSA determination combined with digital rectal examination (DRE) of the prostate is used to screen for prostate cancer. However, there is some debate over the usefulness of the PSA for universal screening for asymptomatic prostate cancer because of the lack of specificity of testing and the lack of definitive outcomes data supporting prostate cancer screening. Conditions such as benign prostatic enlargement and prostatitis may cause elevated PSA values and thus may lead to invasive procedures such as prostate biopsies. Currently, the U.S. Preventive Services Task Force concludes that data are insufficient to recommend either for or against PSA testing. The American Cancer Society recommendations emphasize the importance of shared decision-making regarding testing, stating that PSA testing and DREs should be offered annually, beginning at age 50 years, to men with a life expectancy of at least 10 years. Information concerning the benefits and limitations of testing should be provided to all patients rather than routinely screening all men. Some physicians limit their screening to those groups that are at a high risk for prostate cancer, such as African-Americans, or those with a family history of prostate cancer. PSA values between 0 and 4 ng/mL are considered normal, although up to 20% of prostate cancers are diagnosed in men with normal PSA levels. Because PSA levels tend to increase with age, some experts advocate the use of age-specific PSA reference ranges as a way of increasing the accuracy of PSA tests. However, others feel that age-specific reference ranges may lead to missing or delaying the detection of prostate cancer in older men. Values between 4 and 10 ng/mL are abnormal but often due to benign conditions. Values greater than 10 ng/mL are suspicious for carcinoma. Additional PSA measures, such as the rate of increase in PSA values and the percent of free PSA or the ratio of free PSA: total PSA can help determine the need for biopsy. Using a cutoff of 25% free PSA in patients with values of 4 to 10 may eliminate many unnecessary biopsies without a significant loss in sensitivity. PSA levels that increase more than 0.75 ng/mL increase the concern of an underlying prostate cancer.

TREATMENT

Acute bacterial prostatitis generally requires 3 to 4 weeks of antibiotic therapy with agents such as TMP/SMX or a fluoroquinolone active against gram-negative bacteria. In those requiring hospitalization, intravenous treatment with a broad-spectrum cephalosporin along with an aminoglycoside is recommended. Patients with chronic prostatitis who have positive cultures should have therapy based upon antibiotic sensitivities. Empiric therapy for those with negative cultures can be provided with TMP/SMX or a fluoroquinolone. Patients may require therapy for 4 to 12 weeks or more. Patients with negative cultures but with WBCs in their prostatic secretions may respond to 2 weeks of therapy with antibiotics such as erythromycin or doxycycline, which are active against atypical organisms. Patients with negative cultures, no signs of inflammation, and a negative urologic workup who do not respond to antibiotics can be difficult to manage. Many different therapies may be tried, including NSAIDs, sitz baths, biofeedback, tricyclic antidepressants, and muscle relaxants. If these patients have urinary urgency as a prominent symptom, an anticholinergic medication such as oxybutynin (Ditropan) may be used. If hesitancy is a predominant symptom, then alpha-adrenergic blocking agents such as tamulosin (Flomax) may be tried. Unfortunately, none of these therapies consistently show benefit for patients with CPPS.

Treatment for benign prostatic enlargement can be directed at attempting to decrease the size of the prostate or to enhancing relaxation of the muscle at the bladder outlet. Finasteride inhibits the conversion of testosterone to dihydrotestosterone, the active metabolite. This blocks the effects of testosterone on the prostate and, over 6 to 12 months, can decrease prostatic size by about 20%; it may provide relief from obstructive symptoms. A baseline PSA should be obtained before starting finasteride because the medication will cause about a 50% decline in PSA values, a factor that must be considered in using PSA for prostate cancer screening for patients on therapy. Alpha-adrenergic blockers such as terazosin, doxazosin, and tamulosin block action at the alpha-adrenergic receptors on the smooth muscle in the bladder neck, allowing for relaxation and enhanced bladder emptying. These agents have an advantage over finasteride in their higher efficacy and prompt onset of action in relieving symptoms. The alpha blockers, doxazosin, terazosin prazosin also lower blood pressure and may be of value in patients with concomitant hypertension. Tamulosin and alfuzosin are more selective agents for treating BPH and have little effect on blood pressure and less associated dizziness. Orthostatic hypotension is increased when these agents are combined with phsophodiesterase inhibitors such as sildenafil (Viagra) used to treat erectile dysfunction and should either be avoided or separated by several hours. Alpha blockers may also be used in combination with finasteride. Patients refractory to medical therapy require referral to an urologist for consideration of surgical procedures such as transurethral resection of the prostate (TURP), transurethral incision, ablation, or resection of the prostate in order to provide symptom relief.

Patients with suspected cancer of the prostate should be referred to a urologist for a transrectal US guided biopsy of the prostate gland. Biopsy is done in the outpatient setting and usually well tolerated, although many patients experience some discomfort and bleeding. If cancer is detected and there are no signs of metastases (negative bone scan, laboratory testing, and chest x-ray), a total prostatectomy, which can be curative, is generally recommended. PSA values should be monitored after surgery and are generally not detectable following curative prostatectomy. Elevation of the PSA level after surgery suggests recurrent or residual disease. For patients who are not candidates for prostatectomy, transurethral procedures may provide symptom relief or radiation therapy may be offered as a nonsurgical treatment. For patients with metastases, hormonal suppression through orchiectomy or the administration of luteinizing hormone–releasing hormone (LH-RH) agonists (e.g., Lupron) or antiandrogens may slow disease progression. Radiation therapy can also be provided to patients with symptoms such as bone pain resulting from the metastases.

 KEY POINTS

- Prostate disease will affect over 90% of men during their lifetimes.
- Prostate cancer affects 1 in 10 men.
- History, prostate examination, pre- and post-massage UA with culture, and PSA levels are the cornerstones of evaluation for prostatic disease.
- Urologic consultation should be obtained for patients with prostate disease refractory to medical therapy or those suspected of having prostate cancer.

Sexually Transmitted Diseases

STDs are common infections; more than 8 to 12 million STDs are diagnosed annually in the United States. Although HIV is considered an STD, it is discussed in more detail separately in Chapter 45.

PATHOGENESIS

Sexually transmitted organisms enter through the mucosa or skin to cause disease. On mucosal surfaces, the organisms attach to the surface and cause an inflammatory reaction that enables the organism to penetrate. Organisms that produce skin ulcers usually gain access by small abrasions in the upper layers of the epidermis. These abrasions occur secondary to microtrauma associated with sexual intercourse, accounting for the fact that the most common locations for STD lesions are the penis, vagina, labia, and rectal surfaces.

Younger women are at a greater risk of STDs than older women because they have a more exposed transformation zone (squamous–columnar junction). Exposed columnar cells have a higher affinity for *Chlamydia trachomatis* and *Neisseria gonorrhoeae* than squamous cells and are also more vulnerable to infection by HPV. In addition, progesterone deficiency, commonly seen in younger women, results in a thinner protective mucous layer on the cervix, which facilitates the migration of pathogens to the upper genital tract.

CLINICAL MANIFESTATIONS

HISTORY

Most individuals with STDs seek care because of genitourinary symptoms or because they notice a genital lesion. The most commonly encountered symptoms in men are related to urethritis and epididymitis. In women, urethral symptoms and vaginal discharge are the most common presenting complaints. Both men and women can develop genital lesions such as ulcers and genital warts.

Some patients are asymptomatic but seek care because of exposure to a partner with a STD or because of a high-risk sexual contact. A sexual history inquiring about numbers of partners, sexual practices, history of

STDs, and any high-risk sexual contacts identifies individuals at risk.

PHYSICAL EXAMINATION

Careful examination of the genitalia is critically important for evaluating a patient with a suspected STD. The examination should focus on detecting skin lesions, rashes, lymphadenopathy, ulcers, and mucosal lesions. Specific clinical syndromes are listed below and summarized in Table 52-1.

■ TABLE 52-1 Clinical Characteristics of STDs	
Disease	**Characteristics**
Urethritis	Urethral discharge, dysuria, periurethral irritation
Hepatitis B	Flu-like prodrome, nausea, vomiting, arthralgias, rash, jaundice
Hepatitis A	Nausea, vomiting, diarrhea, jaundice
Human papillomavirus	Genital warts, abnormal pap smear
Herpes simplex	Painful genital vesicles and ulcers, dysuria, fever (primary infection), recurrences
Chancroid	Painful ulcer and inguinal lymphadenopathy
Syphilis	Primary: nontender, painless ulcers; secondary: rash, flu-like illness; tertiary: aortic insufficiency, aortic aneurysm, peripheral neuropathy, meningitis, psychiatric disease
Cervicitis	Vaginal discharge, dysuria
Bacterial vaginosis	Malodorous vaginal discharge, pruritus
Epididymitis	Testicular pain and swelling, urethral discharge

Urethritis

In men, the most common symptom of a gonococcal infection is a urethral discharge. Typically, the discharge from gonococcal urethritis is more purulent than that from a nongonococcal urethritis (NGU). NGU is usually caused by a chlamydial infection but may occur also due to *Ureaplasma* or *Mycoplasma* infections.

Hepatitis B

Sexual transmission accounts for 30% to 60% of hepatitis B cases. Common signs and symptoms of hepatitis B infections include jaundice, nausea, vomiting, arthralgias, fever, and abdominal pain.

Hepatitis A

Hepatitis A infection is usually transmitted by the fecal–oral route. However, the most frequent source of hepatitis A infection is household or sexual contact with an infected person.

Genital Warts

The HPV causes anogenital warts (condylomata acuminata). The lesions are typically cauliflower-like but can be smooth and either flesh-colored or pigmented. The lesions are usually asymptomatic and discovered by the patient or physician upon examination. The HPV strains most closely associated with cervical cancer are discussed in Chapter 57.

Genital Ulcers

Herpes simplex virus (HSV) and chancroid cause painful ulcers, whereas the ulcers of syphilis are painless. HSV is the most common cause of genital ulceration. Primary genital herpes usually presents 2 days to 2 weeks after exposure, with widespread vesicles and ulcers on the genitalia. Symptoms such as dysuria and fever are common and can be mistaken for a urinary tract infection (UTI). The initial infection is usually more severe than recurrences, presumably because of the body's immune response. Reactivation triggers include sunlight, skin trauma, cold or heat, stress, concurrent infection, and menstruation.

Chancroid is caused by *Haemophilus ducreyi* and is associated with inguinal lymphadenopathy and painful genital ulcers. Chancroid ulcers are deep and tender, with irregular borders and a purulent base.

Syphilitic chancres are caused by the spirochete *Treponema pallidum* and are painless, nontender, indurated ulcers with a clean base. The chancre develops about 3 weeks after exposure. Even without treatment, the primary lesion usually resolves within 4 to 6 weeks. The secondary stage of syphilis typically presents with a generalized maculopapular rash, often involving the palms and soles. Other symptoms include general malaise, fever, rhinorrhea, sore throat, myalgias, headaches, and generalized lymphadenopathy. Secondary syphilis may evolve into a latent asymptomatic stage with no symptoms but with positive serology testing. One-third of these patients eventually develop tertiary syphilis, which can cause significant morbidity and a shortened life span due to the associated cardiovascular and neurologic complications.

Cervicitis and Pelvic Inflammatory Disease (PID)

Either *C. trachomatis* or *N. gonorrhoeae* most commonly causes cervicitis. Many women with cervicitis are asymptomatic, while others may experience a vaginal discharge, dysuria, or vaginal spotting. Pharyngeal and anorectal gonorrheal infections can develop in patients who engage in oral or rectal sex. PID, often marked by the development of abdominal pain and fever, can occur if the upper female genital tract is involved. Physical examination may reveal pain with cervical motion, adnexal tenderness, and rebound tenderness. Table 52-2 lists the diagnostic criteria for PID. Although PID is most commonly caused by *N. gonorrhoeae* and *C. trachomatis*, other pathogens including anaerobes, gram-negative facultative bacteria (e.g., *Bacteroides fragilis*), and streptococci may play a role. Perihepatitis, also known as Fitzhugh–Curtis syndrome, is a rare complication of PID. Long-term complications of PID include tubal scarring, which

■ **TABLE 52-2** Criteria for the Diagnosis of PID	
Minimal criteria	Lower abdominal pain, adnexal tenderness, cervical motion tenderness
Additional criteria	Oral temp >101°F (38.3°C), abnormal cervical or vaginal discharge, elevated ESR, C-reactive protein, documented *N. gonorrhoeae* or *C. trachomatis* infection
Definitive criteria	Histopathologic evidence of endometritis on endometrial biopsy transvaginal US or other imaging modes showing thickened fluid-filled tubes with or without free pelvic fluid or tubo-ovarian complex, laproscopic abnormalities c/w PID

can cause infertility, chronic pain, and an increased risk of ectopic pregnancy.

Approximately 1% to 2% of patients with gonorrheal infections develop bacteremia. These individuals can develop septic arthritis and petechial or pustular skin lesions, which are found primarily on the dorsal aspect of the distal extremities, ankle, or wrist joints.

Bacterial Vaginosis (BV)

Although BV is associated with multiple sexual partners, it is still uncertain whether BV is transmitted sexually. BV is discussed in Chapter 62.

Vaginitis

Trichomonas is usually asymptomatic in men and is passed to women. *Candida* may be harbored under the foreskin in men and can be found in asymptomatic women. Candidal infections are not generally considered STDs. Vaginitis is discussed more fully in Chapter 62.

Epididymitis

Epididymitis is most common in young, sexually active men and is usually caused by gonorrhea or chlamydial infection. On examination, the epididymis, which is located on the posterior aspect of the testis, is tender and swollen. Infection with gram-negative bacilli can also cause epididymitis and this infection is generally associated with lower risk, older patients.

DIFFERENTIAL DIAGNOSIS

Lesions that can mimic condyloma acuminata (HPV infection) are seborrheic keratosis, nevi, molluscum contagiosum, pearly penile papules, and condyloma latum (syphilitic lesions). Urethral symptoms such as dysuria can be present in UTIs, prostatitis, and vaginitis. The differential diagnosis for PID includes appendicitis, ectopic pregnancy, ovarian torsion, ruptured ovarian cyst, endometriosis, IBS, and somatization disorder.

DIAGNOSTIC EVALUATION

Evaluation of STDs begins with a clinical assessment. In male patients with urethritis, a gram stain of the discharge looking for neutrophils and the presence of organisms is helpful. A urethral swab can also be sent for culture, DNA analysis, and either culture or immunofluorescence testing for *Chlamydia*. Finding intracellular gram-negative diplococci on the gram stain is diagnostic for gonorrhea. In women with urethral symptoms, it is important to rule out a UTI or vaginitis. Vaginal discharge can also be a sign of cervicitis or PID, and swabs of the discharge should be sent for culture, DNA analysis, or immunofluorescent testing. Gram stains are less valuable in women. A wet mount, KOH, pH determination, and whiff test are useful in characterizing a vaginal discharge.

Painful genital ulcers suggest HSV or chancroid. Painless ulcers suggest syphilis. The presence of multinucleated giant cells on a smear or a positive viral culture can diagnose HSV, while *H. ducreyi* can be isolated by cultures. Spirochetes seen on a dark-field examination from a scraping of an ulcer or direct immunofluorescent microscopy can confirm the diagnosis of syphilis.

The common serologic screening tests for syphilis—a RPR or a VDRL test—turn positive as early as 4 to 7 days after a chancre appears. The VDRL or RPR titer can be used to determine disease activity following treatment. False-positive tests for syphilis may occur in conditions such as antiphospholipid syndrome, advancing age, narcotic use, chronic liver disease, HIV, tuberculosis, and acute herpetic infection. Generally higher titers (>1:8) are more likely to represent true disease. A fluorescent treponemal antibody absorption (FTA-Abs) test should be used to confirm a positive RPR or VDRL result. The FTA-Abs will remain positive indefinitely and therefore cannot be used to determine disease activity.

HPV is commonly diagnosed by its appearance, but if necessary the diagnosis can be confirmed by tissue biopsy. Pap smears can detect cervical changes associated with HPV infection.

TREATMENT

Primary prevention, by encouraging condom use and avoiding high-risk sexual activity, is an important part of STD management. Vaccination for hepatitis B remains the most effective measure to prevent this disease. Hepatitis B immune globulin can be used in conjunction with the vaccine series in unimmunized individuals who have been exposed to the virus.

The treatment for genital warts depends on the number, size, morphology, and anatomic sites of the warts. Treatments include patient-applied therapies such as podofilox and imiquimod and provider-applied therapies such as cryotherapy, trichloroacetic acid, bichloroacetic acid, and surgical removal. Podofilox is not recommended for perianal, vaginal, or urethral warts and should not be used during pregnancy. Imiquimod directly eradicates HPV but has not been studied in pregnant women. Cryotherapy with liquid nitrogen eradicates warts by thermally induced cytolysis. Generally, two to three sessions are required for treating the warts.

Acyclovir, valacyclovir (Valtrex), and famciclovir (Famvir) are used to treat HSV. Treatment shortens the course of the infection and reduces the length of time that the virus is shed. Suppressive therapy is indicated for patients who have frequent recurrences.

Uncomplicated chlamydial infections can be treated with doxycycline for 7 days or with a single 1-g dose of azithromycin. Uncomplicated gonorrhea can be treated with intramuscular ceftriaxone or single oral doses of cefixime, ciprofloxacin, levofloxacin, or ofloxacin. Fluoroquinolone resistance is as high as 15% in some areas and for this reason, preferred therapies for gonorrhea are cefixime or intramuscular (IM) ceftriaxone. Treatment for gonorrhea should generally be followed by a regimen effective against *Chlamydia*. Erythromycin, ceftriaxone, or azithromycin are each active against chancroid.

Two regimens of oral antibiotics are recommended for mild PID: (1) ofloxacin plus metronidazole for 14 days or (2) an IM dose of ceftriaxone (better coverage against *N. gonorrhoeae*) or cefoxitin (better coverage against anaerobes) with concurrent probenecid plus oral doxycycline. The indications for hospitalizing patients with PID include pregnancy, failed outpatient therapy, the inability to follow or tolerate an outpatient oral regimen, severe illness, high fever, a tubo-ovarian abscess, immunodeficiency, or in the cases when the diagnosis is uncertain. Again, therapy should keep in mind local fluorquinolone resistance rates and generally, the ceftriaxone or cefoxitin along with doxycycline would be the preferred therapy.

Recommended regimens for women with BV include oral metronidazole and topical metronidazole or clindamycin. Penicillin is the treatment of choice for syphilis. For individuals with penicillin allergy, doxycycline or tetracycline can be used.

KEY POINTS

- Both hepatitis A and B are considered STDs because sexual transmission accounts for the majority of reported incidences.

- HSV and chancroid cause painful ulcers, whereas the ulcers of syphilis are painless.

- Either *C. trachomatis* or *N. gonorrhoeae* most commonly causes cervicitis. PID, often marked by the development of abdominal pain and fever, can occur if the upper tracts are involved.

- The differential diagnosis for PID includes appendicitis, ectopic pregnancy, ovarian torsion, ruptured ovarian cyst, endometriosis, IBS, and somatization disorder.

- The treatment for genital warts depends on the number, size, morphology, and anatomic sites of the warts. Treatments include patient-applied therapies such as podofilox and imiquimod and provider-applied therapies such as cryotherapy, trichloroacetic acid, bichloroacetic acid, and surgical removal.

- Uncomplicated chlamydial infections can be treated with doxycycline or a single 1-g oral dose of azithromycin. Uncomplicated gonorrhea can be treated with intramuscular ceftriaxone or single oral doses of cefixime, ciprofloxacin, or ofloxacin.

Chapter

53 Skin Infections

Skin serves as a barrier to fluid loss and protects internal organs against mechanical injury, infections, temperature changes, noxious agents, and trauma. When the skin's defenses are altered or destroyed, bacteria, viruses, fungi, and parasitic organisms can infect or infest it.

PATHOGENESIS

Clinical infection results from breaks in the skin (i.e., abrasions, needle punctures, and catheters), loss of local immunity, and changes in the skin flora. Although more than 100 bacteria are known to cause cellulitis, two gram-positive cocci, *Staphylococcus aureus* and group A beta-hemolytic streptococcus, account for the majority of skin and soft tissue infections. *S. aureus* can cause folliculitis, cellulitis, and furuncles (abscess/boil). Toxins elaborated by *S. aureus* can result in bullous impetigo and staphylococcal scalded skin syndrome. *Streptococci* are usually secondary invaders of traumatic skin lesions and can cause impetigo, erysipelas, cellulitis, and lymphangitis.

Viruses damage host cells by entering the cell and replicating at the host's expense. HSV infections can occur anywhere on the skin and are caused by two types of the virus: HSV-1 and HSV-2. HSV-1 is usually seen in oral infections, while HSV-2 is associated with genital infections. HSV infections have two phases: the primary phase representing infection transmitted by respiratory droplets or by direct contact with an active lesion or infected secretions, and the secondary phase representing a reactivation of latent virus from dorsal root ganglia.

The varicella virus, which causes chickenpox, is a highly contagious viral infection transmitted by airborne droplets or vesicular fluid. Patients are contagious from 2 days before onset of the rash until all lesions have crusted. Varicella can lay dormant in the dorsal root ganglion for many years. It reactivates and presents as herpes zoster (shingles) typically involving a painful vesicular rash that only involves a single dermatome. Warts are benign skin tumors confined to the epidermis resulting from HPV, which is transferred by touch and commonly occurs at sites of trauma. Molluscum contagiosum is caused by a poxvirus and produces an umbilicated skin lesion that is spread by autoinoculation, scratching, or touching a lesion.

The dermatophytes, or ringworm fungi, infect and survive only on dead keratin, namely, the top layer of the skin (stratum corneum), the hair, and the nails. Dermatophyte infections are clinically classified by body region with varying disease responses. "Tinea" means "fungus infection," so the term "tinea capitis" refers to a fungal infection of the scalp.

The yeast-like fungus *Candida albicans* and other *Candida* species live normally in the mouth, vaginal tract, and gut. They may become pathogenic and produce budding spores, pseudohyphae (elongated cells), or true hyphae. In individuals with altered defenses against yeast (e.g., due to pregnancy, oral contraceptives, antibiotics, diabetes, skin maceration, topical steroid therapy, and some endocrinopathies), *Candida* can infect the stratum corneum of mucous membranes (mouth, anogenital tract) and warm, moist intertriginous skin areas (axillae, groin, breast folds, digit spaces).

Scabies infestation begins when a fertilized female mite burrows through the stratum corneum to begin a 30-day life cycle of egg laying and deposition of fecal matter (scybala). After eggs have hatched, the mites can migrate to other areas such as the finger webs, wrists, extensor surfaces of the elbows and knees, axillae, breasts, waist, sides of hands and feet, ankles, penis, buttocks, scrotum, and palms and soles of infants, causing symptoms to intensify. The disease is transmitted by direct skin contact with an infected patient.

Three kinds of lice infest humans: *Pediculus humanus capitis* (head louse), *P. humanus corporis* (body louse), and *Phthirus pubis* (pubic or crab louse). Pediculosis capitis is most common in children. Live nits fluoresce and can be detected by Wood light. Pediculosis corporis is a disease of poor hygiene, where the lice live and lay their nits in the seams of clothing and return to the skin surface only to feed. Pediculosis pubis is an extremely contagious sexually transmitted disease and may involve not only the groin but also other hairy areas of the body. Eyelash infestation in a child may be a sign of sexual abuse by an infested adult.

CLINICAL MANIFESTATIONS

HISTORY

The onset of the skin lesions and associated symptoms—such as fever, warmth, or pruritus—should be part of the history. Tenderness, pain, mild paresthesias, or burning may occur at the site of inoculation with herpesvirus infections. A prodrome of localized pain, tender lymphadenopathy, headache, generalized aching, and fever may occur. Shingles may also present prior to the eruption with a prodrome of itching, pain, and burning in the affected dermatome. Associated underlying skin conditions or trauma should be noted. Local trauma or systemic changes like menses, fatigue, or fever may trigger a recurrence of herpes simplex infections. Known contact with cases of scabies, lice, viral, or fungal infection may suggest that transmission has occurred.

Medications and medication allergies may be important in identifying other potential causes for the rash and in determining therapy. An attack of chickenpox usually confers lifelong immunity to chickenpox, but a previous varicella infection can reactivate and cause shingles. Unlike chickenpox, an episode of shingles does not confer lifelong immunity.

PHYSICAL EXAMINATION

The lesions of impetigo are superficial and are characterized by honey-colored crusts. Erythema, warmth, edema, pain, and sometimes fever characterize cellulitis. Folliculitis is characterized by a pustule in association with a hair follicle. Furuncles are larger fluctuant erythematous lesions that also occur in association with hairy regions. Nikolsky sign aids in the diagnosis of staphylococcal scalded skin syndrome and is elicited when local skin separation occurs after minor pressure.

Herpes simplex appears as grouped vesicles on an erythematous base and is uniform in size, unlike the vesicles seen in herpes zoster or chickenpox. The chickenpox rash has a centripetal distribution, starting at the trunk and spreading to the face and extremities. Lesions appear as a **"dewdrop on a rose petal,"** with a thin-walled vesicle, clear fluid, and a red base; they appear as constellations of lesions in different stages at the same time. Warts are small tumors of the skin that obscure normal skin lines, have a mosaic surface pattern, and may have thrombosed vessels appearing as black dots on the surface. The lesions of molluscum contagiosum are discrete 2- to 5-mm slightly umbilicated flesh-colored, dome-shaped papules occurring on the face, trunk, axillae, and extremities in children and in the pubic and genital areas in adults.

Fungal infections are characterized by erythematous as well as hypo- or hyperpigmented lesions associated with scaling. They occur on various parts of the body. The classic ringworm lesion has a central clear area.

Lice are suspected when a patient itches without an apparent rash. Lice and nits may be identified on close visual examination. Scabies are associated with linear burrows on the distal extremities and occur as scattered pruritic papules on the rest of the body.

DIFFERENTIAL DIAGNOSIS

The differential diagnosis for bacterial infections includes other forms of dermatitis, such as eczema and contact or stasis dermatitis. Herpesvirus infections—including shingles, chickenpox, and herpes simplex—may be confused with eczema, impetigo, or contact dermatitis. The lesions of molluscum contagiosum may mimic warts or herpes simplex. Both warts and molluscum may be confused with skin tags, dermatofibromas, or nevi. The differential diagnosis for fungal infections includes pityriasis alba, pityriasis rosea, eczema, or in some instances psoriasis or seborrheic dermatitis. Scabies lesions may form vesicles, leading to the consideration of diagnoses such as herpes and contact dermatitis.

DIAGNOSTIC EVALUATION

Skin infections are commonly diagnosed clinically. Additional diagnostic measures obtained to assist with diagnosis include blood cultures, wound cultures, viral cultures of suspicious lesions, and microscopic examination of skin scrapings or suspected organisms (Table 53-1). Blood cultures are usually negative, but bacteremia can occur with extensive cellulitis. Wound cultures are in general not helpful, though some advocate obtaining "leading edge" cultures by injecting and aspirating from the edge of the infection. More helpful is a sterilely obtained culture from a purulent infection such as an abscess or furuncle. Viral culture is the most definitive method for diagnosing herpes infections. The diagnosis of fungal infections is made by KOH wet-mount preparations, which allow direct visualization under the microscope of the branching hyphae of dermatophytes in keratinized material. Culture is necessary for scalp, hair, and nail fungal infections to identify the true source of infection and determine proper treatment. Mycosel agar, dermatophyte test medium, and Sabouraud dextrose agar are the most common fungal culture media.

TREATMENT

Treatment generally involves use of a topical or oral medication directed at the offending organism. More extensive bacterial infections may require hospitalization and intravenous antibiotics. Furuncles are self-limited and usually respond to frequent moist, warm compresses followed by incision, drainage, and packing. Antibiotics are often prescribed but may not be necessary for furuncles that have been properly drained. For patients with recurrent impetigo or furuncles, nasal cultures for *S. aureus* and treatment of those with positive cultures with mupirocin

■ TABLE 53-1 Diagnostic Testing and Treatment of Common Skin Infections

Infection	Diagnostic Test	Treatment
Impetigo	Clinical exam	Topical mupirocin, oral dicloxacillin, cephalexin
Cellulitis	Clinical exam, blood or wound cultures	Oral or intravenous dicloxacillin, cefazolin, cephalexin
Furuncles	Clinical exam, culture of drainage	Incision and drainage, antibiotics
Herpes simplex	Clinical exam, Tzanck smear, culture	Antivirals: acyclovir, famciclovir, valacyclovir
Chickenpox, herpes zoster	Clinical exam, culture, serology	Antivirals as for herpes above
Warts	Clinical exam, biopsy	Electrocautery, cryotherapy, topical salacylic acid, imiquimod, or squaric acid immunotherapy
Molluscum contagiosum	Clinical exam, biopsy	Curettage, cryotherapy, Retinoin, salacylic acid

ointment administered intranasally helps to eradicate carriage of this bacterium and prevent recurrence. In addition, good hygiene and bathing twice a week with an antibacterial soap, such as Hibiclens or Dial, may aid with eradication and prevention.

Treatment for herpes simplex and varicella infections consists of measures to relieve discomfort, promote healing, and prevent recurrence. Antiviral agents decrease the duration of viral excretion, new lesion formation, and vesicles. Antipruritic lotions, antihistamines, and antibiotics for secondary bacterial infections are also recommended. Antiviral agents started within the first 48 to 72 hours may shorten the course of illness and, in the case of herpes zoster, may decrease the likelihood of developing postherpetic neuralgia. Systemic corticosteroids, either alone or along with antiviral agents, have also been shown to decrease the incidence of postherpetic neuralgia. Acyclovir and varicella zoster immune globulin (VZIG) are also indicated in immunocompromised patients.

Wart treatment depends on the site and severity of the wart; options include electrocautery, blunt dissection, topical salicylic acid or imiquimod, liquid nitrogen, or tape occlusion. Another effective option for home therapy of warts in children is treatment with squaric acid immunotherapy. Sensitization with 2% squaric acid on the forearm is followed with home application of 0.2% (a less potent dose than the initial sensitization dose) squaric acid to warts three to seven nights per week for at least 3 months. Success of eradication of the warts depends on educating parents and patients in safe application and use of the squaric acid. Studies are still pending to determine whether this immunotherapy can be utilized in the long-term prevention of warts.

In addition to topical or systemic antifungal agents, treatment of candidal infections should include keeping the infected skin area clean and dry. Scabies treatment with gamma benzene hexachloride

(Lindane) must be used exactly as directed to avoid potential neurotoxicity. Persistent itching may be treated with oral antihistamines or, if inflammation is present, topical steroids. To eradicate lice, nit removal is an important component of treatment, because the nits may hatch and reinfect the patient. Treatment with a cream rinse containing formic acid (Step 2 Cream Rinse), vinegar compresses, and use of a metal nit comb is effective. Petrolatum jelly, baby shampoo, manual plucking of lice, and fluorescein drops are methods of treating eye infestations (see Table 53-1).

KEY POINTS

- Clinical infection results from breaks in the skin (i.e., abrasions, needle punctures, and catheters), loss of local immunity, and changes in the skin flora.

- Although more than 100 bacteria have been identified as causing cellulitis, two gram-positive cocci, *S. aureus*, and group A beta-hemolytic streptococcus account for the majority of skin and soft tissue infections.

- HSV-1 is usually seen in oral infections, while HSV-2 is associated with genital infections.

- Wart treatment depends on the site and severity of the wart; options include electrocautery, blunt dissection, topical agents, liquid nitrogen, and tape occlusion.

- Oral antibiotics are usually effective for treating most cases of cellulitis; because of staphylococcal penicillin resistance, penicillinase-resistant antibiotics (cloxacillin or dicloxacillin) or cephalosporins (e.g., cephalexin) should be selected.

Chapter

54 Tobacco Abuse

Tobacco abuse is the leading preventable cause of death and disability in the United States. Each year in the United States, approximately 400,000 deaths are attributable to tobacco use. Although the percentage of smokers in the United States has declined to about 25%, millions of Americans continue to smoke, and the incidence of adolescent smoking has fallen very little since its peak in the 1970s. Smoking among teenage girls has even increased.

PATHOGENESIS

Smoking is a complex behavior that is still not completely understood. Pharmacologic and psychological models have been proposed. The psychological and behavioral models propose that smoking is a learned behavior that continues because the individual receives gratification from it. Smoking also becomes a habit, triggered by situations such as stress or alcohol. There also appears to be a link between depression and smoking.

The pharmacologic model emphasizes physical addiction to smoking. There is abundant evidence that nicotine is an addictive drug capable of creating tolerance and physical dependence as well as causing withdrawal symptoms. According to this model, smokers use tobacco to maintain their nicotine levels and avoid withdrawal. Withdrawal symptoms include craving for cigarettes, restlessness, irritability, poor concentration, headache, and nausea. Withdrawal varies greatly among smokers. Clinically, those who need to smoke shortly after rising, smoke at least one pack a day, or have difficulty abstaining for even a few hours are at greatest risk for withdrawal symptoms. Although withdrawal symptoms explain why many smokers fail to quit during the first week, they do not explain why many smokers have trouble abstaining for long periods of time.

Epidemiologic data clearly identify multiple benefits for smoking cessation. Box 54-1 lists some health consequences of smoking. Even older individuals benefit from stopping tobacco use after years of smoking or from quitting after a smoking-related illness. Lung cancer risk drops significantly 10 years after a smoker quits. Coronary risk reduction occurs much more rapidly; the excess risk of a second MI is cut in half within 1 to 2 years of quitting.

■ BOX 54-1 Health Consequences Associated with Smoking
Cancers
Lung cancer
Oral cancers
Larynx cancers
Pharyngeal cancers
Esophageal cancers
GU cancers—kidney, bladder, cervical
GI cancers—pancreas, stomach
Cardiovascular
Myocardial infarction
Cerebral vascular disease
Peripheral vascular disease
Pulmonary
Chronic obstructive pulmonary disease
Recurring respiratory infections
Secondhand Smoke–Related Problems
High incidence of respiratory tract infections
Asthma in children of smokers
High risk of lung cancer in household members of smokers
Pregnancy
Lower birth weight babies
Higher incidence of sudden infant death syndrome (SIDS)
Others
Osteoporosis
Peptic ulcer disease
Skin wrinkling
Discolored skin and teeth
Halitosis

CLINICAL MANIFESTATIONS

HISTORY

Smokers may present with symptoms of one of the smoking-related illnesses listed in Box 54-1. More commonly, smokers complain of cough, sore throat, shortness of breath, and frequent infections. The history should focus on when and why the patient began to smoke. Smoking can be quantified in pack-years by multiplying the average number of packs smoked per day by the number of years of smoking. Asking whether the patient has thought about quitting, tried to quit, or intends to quit helps assess readiness and motivation to quit. By understanding and accepting the patient's past failures or fears about quitting, the physician can help address barriers to smoking cessation.

PHYSICAL EXAMINATION

The physical examination may show signs of underlying smoking-related disease. The mouth and oral cavity should be examined for lesions that may represent cancer. The tongue in smokers often has a brownish discoloration due to exposure to the tar in smoke. Wheezing and diminished breath sounds may indicate COPD. Peripheral pulses may be diminished, suggesting vascular disease.

DIFFERENTIAL DIAGNOSIS

In general, laboratory tests are not helpful for the diagnosis but may be indicated to evaluate the consequences of smoking. Pulmonary function tests may help quantify pulmonary damage and provide evidence of the importance of smoking cessation. If the tests are normal, it is important to stress the importance of stopping smoking now to prevent future damage.

CLINICAL EVALUATION

By providing all smokers seen in the office with even brief advice, the physician can help to increase the proportion of smokers who quit. The National Cancer Institute lists four "A"s for office-based intervention:

1. **Ask**—about smoking at every opportunity. Ask those who smoke whether they are interested in stopping.
2. **Advise**—every smoker with a clear, unambiguous direct message. Tailor the advice to the patient's individual situation.
3. **Assist**—patients in their efforts to stop. If a smoker is ready to quit, ask him or her to set a quit date. Provide self-help material and offer pharmacologic therapy, such as nicotine replacement. Consider a referral to a formal smoking cessation program.

If the individual is not ready to quit, discuss the benefits and barriers to smoking cessation. Make the information as relevant to the individual as possible. Advise the smoker to avoid exposing family members to secondhand smoke. Indicate a willingness to help in the future, when the smoker is ready, and continue to ask about quitting in follow-up visits.

4. **Arrange**—a follow-up appointment, generally within 1 to 2 weeks after the quit date. Make sure you congratulate those who have quit and reinforce the benefits of giving up smoking. Discuss high-risk situations for relapse and review coping mechanisms. For those who fail to quit, provide positive reinforcement for taking the first steps toward quitting. Ask about what obstacles the patient encountered and discuss strategies to overcome these problems in the future. Encourage the smoker to set another quit date.

TREATMENT

The most effective approaches address nicotine addiction and behavioral dependence. Nicotine replacement mitigates some of the symptoms of withdrawal by continuing nicotine exposure, although at reduced and tapered doses. Nicotine delivery can be achieved with transdermal patches, nicotine-containing chewing gum, lozenges, or nicotine inhalers. All are ideally used for 2 to 3 months and then discontinued. They may be utilized for more extended periods of time if needed to ensure continued abstinence from smoking.

Nicotine replacement is not a panacea but does improve the quit rate. For example, nicotine patches double quit rates. They should be offered to smokers willing to set a quit date, who will not smoke while on the patch, and who ideally will follow a behavioral program either individually or in a group setting. The side effects of the patch are mild, generally being limited to skin irritation. Nicotine gum was the original form of nicotine replacement. Side effects of the gum are mostly related to vigorous chewing and the release of excess nicotine. These symptoms include sore jaw, mouth irritation, hiccups, nausea, dizziness, and headache. Data suggest that combined use of patches, to provide a continuous release of nicotine, along with rapid-release forms of nicotine (inhalers, gum, lozenges) is more effective in addressing vulnerable periods of increased desire for nicotine.

Bupropion, originally marketed as an antidepressant, also enhances quit rates. It is contraindicated with seizures. It is useful for people who do not want or have been unable to quit with nicotine replacement. It is generally started 1 week before the target quit date. Bupropion has been used in conjunction with nicotine replacement, and some evidence suggests that the combination of the two is more effective than either one alone. Varenicline is an agonist acting on a nicotinic receptor and has been shown to be an effective oral therapy. Varenicline is started at an escalating dose for 1 week while the patient is still smoking and the patient stops smoking during the second week of use. Nausea is the most common adverse effect.

The behavioral model has also stimulated a host of strategies to help manipulate the environment. The physician can work with the patients to develop strategies like spending time in places where smoking is not permitted or rewarding themselves with the money saved by not smoking. Organized group programs such as those sponsored by the American Cancer Society or the American Lung Association may also be of benefit. These societies sponsor telephone services that provide education, encouragement, advice, and referral.

KEY POINTS

- Tobacco abuse is the leading preventable cause of death and disability in the United States.

- There are benefits even for older individuals who stop smoking after many years or quit after a smoking-related illness.

- By providing all smokers seen in the office with even brief advice, the physician can help to increase the proportion of smokers who quit.

- Bupropion, varenicline, and nicotine replacement are medication options.

Urinary tract infections (UTIs) affect women more often than men. Bacteriuria is present in 1% of infants of both genders, 1% to 2% of school-age girls, and 3% to 4% of women of childbearing age, while males have a prevalence of bacteriuria of 0.3% after infancy. With increasing age, the occurrence of bacteriuria increases for both genders to about 15% of the geriatric population.

PATHOGENESIS

Normal urine is sterile due to the antibacterial properties of the bladder mucosa and of the urine itself and because of the removal of bacteria through voiding. In most UTIs, bacteria gain access to the bladder via the urethra. Women are vulnerable to UTIs because bacteria can access the bladder through the shorter female urethra. Further ascent of bacteria from the bladder is the pathway for most renal parenchymal infections.

UTIs can be divided into lower tract infection (urethritis, cystitis, and prostatitis) and upper tract infection (acute pyelonephritis and intrarenal and perinephric abscesses), which may occur together or independently. Infections of the urethra and bladder are usually superficial, while prostatitis, pyelonephritis, and renal suppuration signify tissue invasion.

Gram-negative bacilli are the most common cause of infection. *Escherichia coli* is the most common pathogen and accounts for 70% to 80% of cases of UTI. Other gram-negative rods—such as *Proteus*, *Klebsiella*, *Enterobacter*, *Serratia*, and *Pseudomonas*—account for a smaller proportion of infections and are associated with urologic manipulation, calculi, obstruction, and catheter-associated infections. *Proteus* species, by virtue of urease production, and *Klebsiella* species, through the production of extracellular slime and polysaccharides, predispose individuals to form stones.

Although gram-positive cocci are less common, *Staphylococcus saprophyticus* accounts for 10% to 15% of acute symptomatic UTIs in young women. Enterococci frequently cause infection in geriatric patients, and enterococci and *Staphylococcus aureus* cause infections in patients with renal stones or previous instrumentation. Isolation of *S. aureus* from the urine should arouse suspicion for a bacteremia seeding the kidneys.

Sexual intercourse increases the likelihood of cystitis. In addition, the use of a diaphragm and/or a spermicide has been associated with increases in vaginal colonization with *E. coli* and in the risk of urinary infection. Any impediment to the free flow of urine—such as tumor, stricture, stone, neurologic disease, or prostatic hypertrophy—is associated with an increased frequency of UTI. Urinary infections are detected in 2% to 8% of pregnant women, and 20% to 30% of pregnant women with asymptomatic bacteriuria subsequently develop pyelonephritis. This predisposition to upper tract infection during pregnancy results from decreased ureteral tone and peristalsis and temporary incompetence of the vesicoureteral valves.

Vesicoureteral reflux is associated with UTIs in children and can lead to renal scarring and chronic renal disease. Vesicoureteral reflux occurs during voiding or with elevation of pressure in the bladder. Reflux of urine from the bladder predisposes individuals to upper tract infections. Vesicoureteral reflux is common among children with a family history of vesicoureteral reflux and those with anatomic abnormalities of the urinary tract.

CLINICAL MANIFESTATIONS

HISTORY

Patients with dysuria, frequency, urgency, and suprapubic pain usually have cystitis. The urine often becomes grossly cloudy and malodorous and is bloody in about 30% of cases. Symptoms of acute pyelonephritis include fever (>101°F or 38.3°C), shaking chills, nausea, vomiting, diarrhea, and flank pain. Symptoms of cystitis may or may not precede an upper tract infection. Patients should be asked about previous UTIs, renal disease, kidney stones, and recent surgical procedures or antibiotic use. Other medical problems, such as diabetes, should be noted. The patient should be asked about sexual activity and contraceptive use.

Older children experience UTI symptoms similar to those found in adults. In infants and younger children, irritability, fever, nausea, vomiting, bed-wetting, and diarrhea may be presenting symptoms of a UTI. Elderly patients may also present with nonspecific symptoms, such as change in mental status, malaise, incontinence, and poor appetite.

PHYSICAL EXAMINATION

The physical examination should include temperature, an abdominal examination, and checking for costovertebral angle tenderness. For individuals who are unable to distinguish between the "internal" dysuria associated with urethritis and cystitis and the "external" dysuria that may occur with vaginitis, a genital examination can be helpful.

DIFFERENTIAL DIAGNOSIS

The differential diagnosis of dysuria includes UTI, vaginitis, and urethritis. Approximately 30% of patients with acute dysuria, frequency, and pyuria have midstream urine cultures with either no growth or insignificant bacterial growth. Clinically, these patients cannot be readily distinguished from those with cystitis. In this situation, sexually transmitted pathogens— such as *Chlamydia trachomatis*, *Neisseria gonorrhoeae*, and HSV—or a low-count *E. coli* or staphylococcal UTI may account for the symptoms. Chlamydial or gonococcal infection should be suspected when there is a gradual onset of illness, no hematuria, no suprapubic pain, and more than 7 days of symptoms. A new sex partner or exposure to chlamydial or gonococcal urethritis should heighten suspicion for a sexually transmitted infection. Infection with *C. trachomatis*, *N. gonorrhoeae*, *Trichomonas*, *Candida*, and HSV should be considered in patients with vaginal discharge, mucopurulent cervicitis, genital lesions, and urethritis symptoms but negative cultures.

Noninfectious causes such as urethral or bladder irritation from conditions such as trauma or exposure to chemical irritants (e.g., coffee, spicy foods, citrus) may also cause dysuria. A negative culture and a normal UA characterize interstitial cystitis, which is most common in young women. Cystoscopy may reveal inflammation and mucosal hemorrhage. Bladder tumors, instrumentation, and trauma may also cause cystitis symptoms.

Dysuria is less common in men. In younger sexually active men, urethritis is the usual etiology. Older men usually have a UTI or irritative symptoms secondary to BPH. Other considerations in men include prostatitis or epididymitis.

Patients with upper tract infection usually experience back pain. Noninfectious causes of flank pain include renal stones, renal infarction, and papillary necrosis.

DIAGNOSTIC EVALUATION

Many experts recommend treating healthy young women with characteristic symptoms of acute uncomplicated cystitis and pyuria without doing an initial urine culture. The absence of pyuria suggests an alternative diagnosis. The leukocyte esterase "dipstick" method is less sensitive than microscopy in identifying pyuria but is a useful alternative when microscopy is not available. Pyuria in the absence of bacteriuria (sterile pyuria) may indicate infection with organisms such as *C. trachomatis*, *Ureaplasma urealyticum*, *Mycobacterium tuberculosis*, and fungi or noninfectious urologic conditions such as calculi, anatomic abnormality, nephrocalcinosis, or polycystic disease. WBC casts suggest upper tract involvement.

A urine culture is indicated if the diagnosis is uncertain, in males, in patients with suspected upper tract infections, and in those with complicating factors such as pregnancy or diabetes.

Growth of more than 100,000 organisms per milliliter from a properly collected midstream clean-catch urine sample indicates infection. In urine specimens obtained by suprapubic aspiration or catheterization, colony counts of 100 to 10,000/mL generally indicate infection. In some circumstances (antibiotic treatment, high urea concentration, high osmolarity, low pH), relatively low bacterial colony counts may still indicate infection. Dilute urine or recent voiding also reduces bacterial counts in urine.

TREATMENT

Table 55-1 outlines treatment for UTIs in adults. The following principles underlie the treatment of UTIs:

1. A UA, Gram stain, or culture is indicated to confirm infection before starting treatment. If a culture is obtained, antimicrobial sensitivity testing should be used to direct or modify therapy.
2. Factors predisposing to infection, such as obstruction and calculi, should be identified and corrected if possible.
3. In general, uncomplicated infections and lower tract infections respond to shorter courses of therapy, while upper tract infections require longer treatment. Early recurrences usually mean relapse. Recurrences more than 2 weeks after completing therapy nearly always represent reinfection with a new strain.
4. Community-acquired infections, especially initial infections, are usually due to antibiotic-sensitive strains.
5. In patients with repeated infections, instrumentation, or recent hospitalization, the presence of antibiotic-resistant strains should be suspected.

Cystitis usually responds to shorter courses of antibiotics. Single doses of fosfomycin and short courses (3 days) of fluoroquinolones (norfloxacin, ciprofloxacin, ofloxacin) have been used successfully to treat acute uncomplicated episodes of cystitis, but a higher relapse rate makes longer courses (5 to 7 days) more desirable.

TABLE 55-1 Urinary Tract Infections in Adults

Category	Diagnostic Criteria	Principal Pathogens	First-Line Therapy	Comments
Acute uncomplicated cystitis	Urinalysis for pyuria and hematuria (culture not required)	• *Escherichia coli* • *Staphylococcus saprophyticus* • *Proteus mirabilis* • *Klebsiella pneumoniae*	• Fosfomycin • Nitrofurantoin • TMP/SMX DS (Bactrim, Septra) • Trimethoprim (Priloprim) • Ciprofloxacin (Cipro) • Ofloxacin (Floxin) • Norfloxacin (Noroxin)	• Quinolones, fosofomycin and nitrofurantoin are first-line agents in areas of TMP/SMX resistance or in patients who cannot tolerate TMP/SMX
Recurrent^a cystitis in young women	Symptoms and a urine culture with a bacterial count of more than 100,000 CFU/mL of urine	• Same as for acute uncomplicated cystitis	• If the patient has more than three cystitis episodes per year, treat prophylactically with postcoital, or continuous daily therapy (see text)	• Repeat therapy for 7–10 days based on culture results and then use prophylactic therapy^a
Acute cystitis in young men	Urine culture with a bacterial count of 1000 to 10,000 CFU/mL of urine	• Same as for acute uncomplicated cystitis	• Same as for acute uncomplicated cystitis	• Treat for 7–10 days
Acute uncomplicated pyelonephritis	Urine culture with a bacterial count of 100,000 CFU/mL of urine	• Same as for acute uncomplicated cystitis	• If gram-negative organism, oral fluoroquinolone • If gram-positive organism, amoxicillin • If parenteral administration is required, ceftriaxone (Rocephin) or a fluoroquinolone • If *Enterococcus* species, add oral or IV amoxicillin	• Switch from IV to oral administration when the patient is able to take medication by mouth; complete a 14-day course

(continued)

TABLE 55-1 Urinary Tract Infections in Adults (continued)

Category	Diagnostic Criteria	Principal Pathogens	First-Line Therapy	Comments
Complicated urinary tract infection	Urine culture with a bacterial count of more than 10,000 CFU/mL of urine	• E. coli • K. pneumoniae • P. mirabilis • Enterococcus species • Pseudomonas aeruginosa	• If gram-negative organism, oral fluoroquinolone • If Enterococcus species, ampicillin or amoxicillin with or without gentamicin (Garamycin)	• Treat for 10–14 days
Asymptomatic bactiuria in pregnancy	Urine culture with a bacterial colony count of more than 100,000 CFU/mL of urine	• Same as for acute uncomplicated cystitis	• Amoxicillin • Nitrofurantoin (Macrodantin) • Cephalexin (Keflex)	• Avoid tetracyclines and fluoroquinolones • Treat for 3–7 days
Catheter-associated urinary tract infection	Symptoms and a urine culture with a bacterial count of more than 100 CFU/mL of urine	• Depends on duration of catheterization	• If gram-negative organism, a fluoroquinolone • If gram-positive organism, ampicillin or amoxicillin plus gentamicin	• Remove catheter if possible, and treat for 7–10 days • For patients with long-term catheters and symptoms, treat for 5–7 days

aPatient is given a prescription for an antibiotic to take if symptoms develop.
TMP/SMX, trimethoprim/sulfamethoxazole; CFU, colony forming unit; IV, intravenous.
Adapted from Stamm WE, Hooton TM. Management of urinary tract infections in adults. N Engl J Med. 1993;329:1328–1334.

TMP/SMX can be utilized in areas where known resistance of *E. coli* is less than 20%. Males with UTI often have urologic abnormalities or prostatic involvement and should receive a 7- to 14-day antibiotic course.

With upper tract infections, the majority of cases respond to 10 to 14 days of therapy. Longer periods of treatment (2 to 6 weeks) aimed at eradicating a persistent focus of infection may be necessary in some cases. In women, acute uncomplicated pyelonephritis without accompanying clinical evidence of calculi or urologic disease is due to *E. coli* in most cases. A 14-day course of a fluoroquinolone or a third-generation cephalosporin is usually adequate. Ampicillin, amoxicillin, or TMP/SMX should not be used as initial therapy because 20% to 30% of strains of *E. coli* are now resistant to these drugs.

Acute cystitis in pregnancy can be treated with amoxicillin, nitrofurantoin, or cephalosporin. All pregnant women should be screened and, if positive, treated for asymptomatic bacteriuria. Acute pyelonephritis in pregnancy usually requires hospitalization and parenteral antibiotic therapy, generally with cephalosporin or extended-spectrum penicillin. After treatment, a culture to document clearing of the infection is indicated, and cultures should be repeated monthly thereafter until delivery. Continuous low-dose prophylaxis with nitrofurantoin is indicated for pregnant women with recurrent infections.

In a child or infant who is toxic, dehydrated, or unable to tolerate oral intake, initial antimicrobial therapy should be given parenterally, and hospitalization considered. Re-evaluation and repeat urine testing are indicated in children who do not improve after 2 days of antibiotic therapy.

Intravenous pyelography and cystoscopy is indicated in women with relapsing infection, a history of childhood infections, stones, painless hematuria, or recurrent pyelonephritis. Most males with a single UTI require investigation. Men or women presenting with acute infection and signs or symptoms suggestive of an obstruction or stones should undergo US or CT scan. Girls with recurrent UTI, boys with a single UTI, and children with pyelonephritis should undergo evaluation including renal US and voiding cystourethrogram (VCUG). The VCUG is generally performed after completing a course of antibiotics and sterilizing the urine, since infection itself may cause reflux.

Patients with frequent symptomatic infections may benefit from long-term administration of low-dose antibiotics to prevent recurrences. Daily or thrice-weekly administration of a single dose of TMP/SMX (80/400 mg), TMP (100 mg), or nitrofurantoin (50 mg) is effective. Prophylactic antibiotics and voiding after sexual intercourse reduce recurrences in women whose infections are temporally related to intercourse. Other patients for whom prophylaxis appears to have some merit include men with chronic prostatitis; patients undergoing prostatectomy, both during the operation and in the postoperative period; and pregnant women with asymptomatic bacteriuria. Asymptomatic bacteriuria in older women is common and does not require therapy.

KEY POINTS

- UTIs affect women more often than men.
- Gram-negative bacilli are the most common cause of infection. *E. coli* is the most common pathogen and accounts for 70% to 80% of cases of UTI.
- The differential diagnosis of dysuria includes UTI, vaginitis, and urethritis.
- Pyuria is present in almost all urinary infections; its absence suggests an alternative diagnosis.
- In general, uncomplicated infections and lower tract infections respond to shorter courses of therapy, while upper tract infections require longer treatment.

56 Urticaria

Urticaria, also known as hives or wheals, is a pruritic, immune-mediated skin eruption consisting of well-circumscribed lesions on an erythematous base; it can affect any part of the body. Angioedema is a related condition that affects deeper layers of the skin and often involves the face, tongue, extremities, or genitalia. Urticaria and angioedema can occur together. Urticaria affects 10% to 20% of the population and is classified as acute (less than 6 weeks' duration) or chronic (more than 6 weeks). Urticaria and angioedema can be a manifestation of many conditions, and determining the underlying cause can be challenging.

PATHOGENESIS

A number of stimuli, such as medications or foods, may serve as antigens that bind to IgE receptors on mast cells, causing them to degranulate. In other cases, physical or chemical stimuli may directly cause mast cell degranulation. Hypersensitivity to acetylcholine triggers mast cell degranulation in the physical urticarias. Autoimmune diseases associated with immune complex formation are additional causes of urticaria. These various stimuli trigger release of chemical mediators that increase blood flow and capillary permeability, causing leakage of protein-rich plasma from the local postcapillary venules and resulting in hive formation. Angioedema occurs with massive transudation of fluid into the dermis and subcutaneous tissues. Pruritus is usually present, but to a milder degree in angioedema, because there are fewer mast cells and sensory nerve endings in the deeper tissues.

CLINICAL MANIFESTATIONS

HISTORY

The history is a critical element in trying to establish the cause of urticaria. Having the patient keep a log of activities may be helpful for identifying triggers in chronic cases. All medications taken within 2 weeks of onset should be considered as a potential cause of urticaria or angioedema. Foods and food dyes may also cause urticaria. Occasionally a patient may have urticaria or angioedema with a seasonal pattern due to a seasonal allergen that is inhaled, ingested, or contacted. Such patients may have other manifestations of atopy, such as allergic rhinitis or asthma, in reaction to the same allergens.

Viral infections, such as infectious hepatitis and infectious mononucleosis, and parasitic infections may also cause urticaria. The physical urticarias result from environmental factors such as a change in temperature or by direct stimulation of the skin from pressure, stroking, vibration, or light. In exercise-induced urticaria, pruritus, urticaria, angioedema, wheezing, and hypotension occur as a result of exercise.

Systemic vasculitides (e.g., with Sjögren syndrome, rheumatoid arthritis, hepatitis, and SLE either with or without cryoglobulinemia) are associated with lesions that are visually indistinguishable from urticaria. There is an increased incidence of urticaria in association with thyroid disease (hyper- and hypothyroidism) that may resolve with the control of the thyroid disease. Urticaria with carcinoma of the colon, rectum, or lung and with lymphoid malignancies such as Hodgkin disease and B-cell lymphomas has been reported. Hereditary complement deficiencies may also result in severe angioedema, with symptoms including laryngeal edema and abdominal pain.

PHYSICAL EXAMINATION

At the time of the office visit, the patient may be free of lesions. Skin lesions that are present should be examined; their characteristics and distribution may help to identify possible causes. For example, typical urticarial lesions will be erythematous plaques that blanch with pressure. Nonblanching purpuric lesions raise the possibility of an underlying vasculitis. Swelling that involves the face, lips, and periorbital region suggests angioedema.

A thorough examination looking for other associated or underlying diseases is warranted. The examination should include the ears, pharynx, sinuses, teeth, and lungs for signs of underlying infection. Examination of the abdomen should note the presence of hepatosplenomegaly or tenderness.

Lymphadenopathy and joint swelling, effusion, or warmth should be documented.

DIFFERENTIAL DIAGNOSIS

In addition to idiopathic urticaria, the differential diagnosis includes underlying systemic diseases such as the connective tissue diseases, infections, neoplasm, and thyroid disease. Studies examining the frequency of the different forms of urticaria and underlying causes vary depending on the study population. However, food and medications are thought to account for a significant percentage of cases, with physical and contact urticarias occurring less often. Underlying thyroid disease was found in 12% of one study population and sinus disease in 17% in another study. In up to 90% of cases of chronic urticaria, no cause is identified. The differential diagnoses for urticaria are outlined in Box 56-1.

DIAGNOSTIC EVALUATION

For patients with acute urticaria, the history and physical examination will direct any further evaluation. In patients with chronic urticaria, diagnostic testing may include a CBC, liver and renal function tests, UA, and ESR. Thyroid function should be tested in those with chronic urticaria, including testing for antithyroglobulin and antimicrosomal antibodies. For those with elevated antibodies but normal function, annual thyroid function testing is recommended. Further workup is directed by clinical history and physical examination, keeping in mind the differential diagnosis listed in Box 56-1. In patients with chronic urticaria and no apparent cause, referral to an allergist for allergy testing is warranted. In addition to testing for the standard allergens, evaluation of patients with urticaria or angioedema may include the procedures outlined in Table 56-1. Despite evaluation, many patients remain undiagnosed.

TREATMENT

Underlying diseases—such as connective tissue diseases, thyroid disease, and infections—should be treated and any identified triggers avoided. Medications that may be causing urticaria or angioedema, such as an ACE inhibitor, should be replaced by alternatives. For those patients with an acute attack, the severity of the attack and the presence or absence of respiratory or mucosal involvement dictates treatment measures. Those with mild symptoms are treated with H_1 receptor blockers. These medications include the classic antihistamines such as diphenhydramine and the newer nonsedating antihistamines such as loratadine. Those with severe symptoms should receive subcutaneous epinephrine, antihistamines, and a tapering course of corticosteroids. Many patients with severe reactions are hospitalized for observation and therapy.

Therapy for chronic urticaria is often empiric, since only a fraction of cases have any identifiable cause. Therapy includes antihistamines. In refractory cases, H_2 blockers, such as cimetidine, to block the H_2 receptors present in the skin, can be used in combination with antihistamines. Doxepin, a tricyclic antidepressant, has strong antihistaminic effects and can be useful in treating chronic urticaria. Leukotriene antagonists, such as montelukast, have also been shown to be helpful. Steroids in 7- to 14-day tapering courses are sometimes used for acute control of exacerbations and in those patients requiring repeated or chronic use of steroids, studies suggest that cyclosporine or sulfasalazine may be useful as steroid-sparing agents to suppress chronic urticaria. Patients with hereditary angioedema who have frequent, recurrent, or severe disease may benefit from the use of anabolic steroids, such as danazol, which is thought to increase levels of C1 esterase inhibitor and thus lessen severity of the disease. Other medications that have been studied and found beneficial to varying degrees for chronic urticaria include dapsone, hydroxychloroquine, colchicine, tacrolimus, mycophenolate, and the new antiallergy monoclonal antibody omalizumab. Most cases of chronic urticaria or angioedema resolve within 1 year, and only 10% to 20% of patients will have long-term symptoms.

■ **BOX 56-1** Differential Diagnosis for Urticaria

Idiopathic
Food and food additives
Medications
Infections (e.g., sinusitis, vaginitis, hepatitis, infectious mononucleosis)
Environmental allergens
Insect stings
Physical urticarias (heat, cold, pressure, exercise, vibration, sunshine)
Connective tissue disease
Malignancy
Hereditary C1 inhibitor deficiency
Hyperthyroidism

TABLE 56-1 Testing Procedures for Urticaria and Angioedema

Food and drug reactions	Elimination of offending agent, challenge with suspected foods, lamb and rice diet, special diets eliminating natural salicylates and food additives
Inhalant allergens	Skin tests, in vitro histamine release from human basophils, radio-allergosorbent test
Collagen vascular diseases and cutaneous vasculitis	Skin biopsy, CH_{50}, C4, C3, factor B, immunofluorescence of tissue
Malignancy with angioedema	CH_{50}, C1q, C4, C INH determinations
Cold urticaria	Ice cube test
Solar urticaria	Exposure to defined wavelengths of light, red cell protoporphyrin, fecal protoporphyrin, and coproporphyrin
Dermographism	Stroking with narrow object (e.g., tongue blade, fingernail)
Pressure urticaria	Application of pressure for defined time and intensity
Vibratory angioedema	Vibration with laboratory vortex for 4 minutes
Aquagenic urticaria	Challenge with tap water at various temperatures
Urticaria pigmentosa	Skin biopsy, test for dermographism
Hereditary angioedema	C4, C2, C INH by protein and function
Familial cold urticaria	Challenge by cold exposure, measurement of temperature, white blood cell count, sedimentation rate, and skin biopsy
C3b inactivator deficiency	C3, factor B, C3b inactivator determinations
Idiopathic	Skin biopsy, immunofluorescence (negative), autologous skin test

 KEY POINTS

- Urticaria is extremely common, affecting up to 10% to 20% of the population.
- In addition to allergens as triggers of urticaria, the differential diagnosis should include consideration of the presence of systemic disease, most notably the connective tissue diseases, infections, neoplasm, and thyroid disease.
- Despite evaluation, many patients remain undiagnosed.
- For those patients with an acute attack, the severity of the attack and the presence or absence of respiratory or mucosal involvement dictate treatment measures. Therapy for chronic urticaria is often empiric, since only a fraction of cases have any identifiable cause.

Chapter 57

Abnormal Pap Smear

The Papanicolaou (Pap) smear was developed as a screening tool for cervical cancer in the late 1940s. Its widespread use has been associated with a decrease in cervical cancer from 14.2 cases per 100,000 in 1973 to 7.8 cases per 100,000 in 1994. False-negative rates for Pap smears vary between 15% and 45%. Errors occur from poor sampling and fixation technique and the cytologist's failure to recognize abnormalities. Despite these limitations, regular Pap smear screening and the natural history of cervical cellular changes leading to cancer make Pap smear testing an extremely effective cancer prevention tool. More recently the ThinPrep method, which collects cells in a fluid medium to minimize background and drying artifact, has been introduced to improve Pap smear results.

PATHOGENESIS

The cervix is covered by squamous and columnar epithelium. As the cervix matures, columnar cells are replaced by squamous cells in a process known as squamous metaplasia. It is the squamocolumnar junction—where squamous metaplasia is most active—that is vulnerable to injury and the area where the development of abnormal cells usually begins.

The observation that the immature squamous cell epithelium at the squamocolumnar junction is particularly sensitive to injury correlates with the epidemiologic observation that this is the most common site of cervical cancer. Immature cells are also more common at menarche and during the postpartum period, which may explain why early sexuality and multiple pregnancies place women at high risk for cervical cancer. The natural history of cervical cancer should be viewed as a progression from mild dysplasia to carcinoma in situ to invasive carcinoma. The slow progression of these changes and the availability of effective early treatment make the Pap smear one of the most effective cancer screening tools.

HPV is the major cause of most abnormal Pap smear results. DNA fragments of HPV have been found in over 90% of cervical cancer cells. Serotypes 16, 18, 31, 52, and 58 are most closely associated with cervical cancer. Recent improvements in testing for these viral serotypes are becoming an important adjunct to the traditional Pap smear.

CLINICAL MANIFESTATIONS

HISTORY

A good history can identify risk factors for cervical cancer and facilitate decision making about how frequently to obtain Pap smears. Risk factors include early age of initiating sexual activity, multiple sexual partners, history of STDs, smoking, HIV, current or prior history of condyloma, and previously abnormal Pap smears. Pap smear screening should begin 3 years after onset of sexual activity or at age 21, whichever comes first. The frequency of Pap smears is controversial. Since there is a long asymptomatic period and early cervical intraepithelial neoplasia is easily treated when detected, the American Cancer Society (ACS) no longer recommends annual Pap smears for women at low risk for cervical cancer. Starting at age 25, the ACS recommends obtaining Pap smears in low-risk women every 3 years after two negative smears 1-year apart. Screening may be discontinued after age 65 provided that previous testing has been normal.

PHYSICAL EXAMINATION

During the 24 hours prior to the examination, the patient should not douche, have sexual relations, or use tampons. Most physicians recommend rescheduling Pap smears if a woman is menstruating. To sample the cervix correctly, a cytobrush is rotated in the cervical canal and a wooden or plastic spatula rotated over the cervix at the squamocolumnar junction. The physical examination may be normal, but occasionally genital warts or a lesion may be visible. Bleeding and cervical friability can be a sign of cervical disease or infection. When the cervix appears abnormal, a Pap test alone may not be sufficient for evaluation. In other words, a normal Pap smear should not prevent the clinician from proceeding to colposcopy if there is a suspicious lesion.

DIFFERENTIAL DIAGNOSIS

Box 57-1 lists the descriptive changes for Pap smears. The Bethesda system is the preferred system and interprets specimen adequacy as satisfactory, satisfactory but limited, or unsatisfactory. If the reading is limited then the reason (e.g., lack of endocervical cells) should be given. Next, the smear may be classified as normal or other. "Other" interpretations include benign cellular changes (e.g., infection or reactive changes, as from inflammation). The Bethesda system also uses the term "squamous intraepithelial lesions," which includes two grades: low-grade squamous intraepithelial lesion (LSIL) and high-grade squamous intraepithelial lesion (HSIL). LSIL is consistent with mild dysplasia. HSIL includes moderate and severe dysplasia.

DIAGNOSTIC EVALUATION

The first step is to evaluate the adequacy of the Pap smear. If there are no endocervical cells present, this indicates inadequate sampling of the squamocolumnar junction. Often these smears have to be repeated unless this is expected (i.e., pregnancy, menopause). However, for a low-risk individual with previously normal Pap smears, a physician may exercise discretion and defer a repeat examination for 1 year. Cervical inflammation from infections such as *Chlamydia* or yeast may cause cells to appear abnormal; in such instances the Pap smear should be repeated after the infection has been treated.

Atypical squamous cells can fall into two categories: atypical squamous cells of undetermined significance (ASCUS) which are changes in cells beyond the normal reactive process but that lack the criteria for a squamous intraepithelial lesion (SIL) and atypical squamous cells that cannot exclude HSIL (ASC-H). Follow-up of patients with ASCUS can include either testing for HPV, repeat cytology at 6-month intervals, or colposcopy. If HPV testing is negative, then repeat cytologic testing is recommended in 12 months. If repeat cytologic testing is negative, then yearly Pap smears may be resumed. Follow-up testing after colposcopy should include either HPV testing in 12 months or repeat cytologic testing every 6 months times two. A subsequent abnormal smear is an indication for

■ BOX 57-1 Bethesda System
Adequacy of Specimen
Satisfactory for evaluation
Satisfactory for evaluation but limited by (SBLB): no endocervical cell, inadequate history provided
Unsatisfactory for evaluation, specify reason
Descriptive Diagnosis
Within normal limits
Benign cellular changes:
Infection: *Trichomonas vaginalis, Candida, Coccobacilli* c/w shift in vaginal flora, *Actinomyces* species, HSV
Inflammatory changes, except cellular changes of HPV infections
Epithelial cell abnormalities
Squamous cell
ASCUS: borderline changes more reactive than definitive
LSIL: borderline changes including HPV, mild dysplasia, CIN I
HSIL: moderate dysplasia or CIN II, severe dysplasia or CIN III, and CIS, +/–HPV changes
Squamous cell carcinoma: cancer or invasive
Glandular cell
Endometrial cells, cytological benign in a postmenopausal woman—endometrial hyperplasia or cancer
AGCUS (atypical glandular cells of undetermined significance): borderline cells between reactive changes to premalignant/malignant process
AIS: adenocarcinoma in situ
Adenocarcinoma: endocervical suggesting adenocarcinoma or ACIS, endometrial suggesting possible endometrial cancer, extrauterine that could be from vagina, ovary, tube, or metastatic
Other malignant neoplasms: small cell carcinoma, melanoma, lymphoma, sarcoma, etc.
Hormonal evaluation (vaginal smears only): hormonal pattern compatible or incompatible with age and history
Hormonal pattern incompatible with age and history: specify
Hormonal evaluation not possible due to: specify

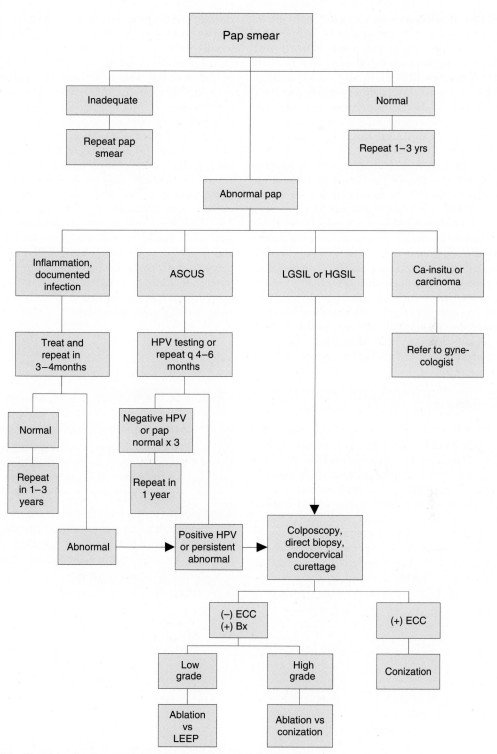

Figure 57-1 • Algorithm for the management of an abnormal Pap smear.

colposcopy. If adherence to more frequent monitoring is a concern or the patient is at high risk, immediate colposcopy is indicated. Patients with LSIL follow similar recommendations to those with ASCUS. Patients with HSIL should usually undergo colposcopy-directed cervical biopsy and endocervical curettage (ECC). If the assessment is inadequate (i.e., the lesion cannot be fully visualized), conization or loop electroexcision procedure (LEEP) are indicated.

Occasionally atypical glandular cells of undetermined significance (AGUS) are noted on a Pap smear. Colposcopy with ECC is recommended for all patients with AGUS because of the risk of adenocarcinoma in situ (AIS) and adenocarcinoma. If the AGUS is classified as favoring a neoplasia, then the risk of AIS or adenocarcinoma is about 20% and cone biopsy is indicated even if colposcopy and ECC are negative. Most authorities also recommend evaluation of the upper genital tract with an endometrial biopsy for woman over age 35 or those with abnormal bleeding. On occasion, endometrial cells are noted. A postmenopausal woman with this finding is at risk for endometrial carcinoma and should have an endometrial biopsy.

TREATMENT

Since abnormal Pap smears are associated with HPV, other STDs should be considered in evaluating these patients (Figure 57-1). Approximately 60% of Pap smears with ASCUS/LSIL regress spontaneously. Low-risk patients may be followed with repeat Pap smears every 6 months until 2 consecutive negative smears are obtained. Patients with an abnormal smear on follow-up require colposcopy to rule out a high-grade lesion. Most experts recommend that patients with HSIL should undergo colposcopy and directed biopsy. Therapy is based on the histologic readings and ECC findings. Since dysplasia is

thought to be a precursor to cervical cancer, destruction or excision of the abnormal area of the cervix is usually performed. Higher-grade lesions or positive ECC generally require conization or an LEEP. Lower-grade lesions may be treated with observation, laser, cryotherapy, or LEEP depending on the size and location of the lesion. Carcinoma in situ is generally referred to a gynecologist and requires conization. Procedures such as conization or LEEP involve removal of a portion of the cervix and thus place patients at risk for preterm labor, incompetent cervix, or cervical stenosis in future pregnancies. After treatment for dysplasia, women need Pap smears every 6 months for 1 year and if negative, may revert to yearly screens. In pregnancy, ASCUS and LSIL should be followed up with colposcopy and repeated again postpartum. HSIL should undergo colposcopy performed by an experienced colposcopist during pregnancy and at 6 weeks postpartum. In either situation, ECC is always contraindicated during pregnancy.

KEY POINTS

- HPV is the major cause of abnormal Pap smears. Serotypes 16, 18, 31, 52, and 58 are most closely associated with cervical caner.

- ASCUS may be followed with repeat smears in a low-risk individual. High-risk individuals, HPV-positive patients, or patients whose repeat smear is abnormal should undergo colposcopy.

- Individuals with HSIL on Pap smear should undergo colposcopy, endocervical curettage, and directed cervical biopsy. Conization or LEEP may be indicated to fully evaluate and treat these higher risk patients.

Abnormal Vaginal Bleeding

The normal menstrual cycle ranges from 21 to 35 days. Day 1 of the cycle is the first day of bleeding. The menstrual flow usually lasts from 2 to 7 days and the average amount of blood loss is 30 to 40 mL; less than 80 mL is considered normal. The volume of blood loss is subjectively assessed and not clinically important. Important factors to consider are presence of anemia and interference with lifestyle as manifested by disruptions in schedules, activities, and passage of blood clots or use of an excessive number of pads or tampons.

Abnormal vaginal bleeding is subdivided into (1) menorrhagia—irregular cycles with excessive flow, duration, or both; (2) metrorrhagia—irregular bleeding between cycles; (3) menometrorrhagia—excessive bleeding in amount, duration, or both at irregular intervals; (4) polymenorrhea—regular bleeding at intervals of less than 21 days; (5) oligomenorrhea—regular bleeding at intervals of more than 35 days; and (6) intermenstrual bleeding—uterine bleeding between regular cycles.

PATHOGENESIS

A normal menstrual cycle consists of a proliferative and a secretory phase. During the proliferative or follicular phase, follicle-stimulating hormone (FSH) released by the pituitary stimulates a primary ovarian follicle to release estrogen, which stops menses and stimulates the endometrium. At midcycle, a LH surge triggers ovulation. After ovulation, the luteal or secretory phase begins, the corpus luteum develops, and progesterone levels increase. Normal menstruation occurs if fertilization does not take place and estrogen and progesterone levels drop, resulting in the sloughing off of endometrium. Normally, this cycle recurs with a regular periodicity, with menstruation generally occurring 14 days after ovulation. Cycle-length variability is primarily due to variability in the time for follicle development during the proliferative phase.

An imbalance between estrogen and progesterone in the proliferative phase, at ovulation, or in the secretory phase can cause abnormal vaginal bleeding. Persistently low levels of estrogen are associated with a thin endometrium and intermittent spotting with light bleeding. Excess estrogen stimulates the proliferation of endometrium; but without sufficient progesterone, the endometrium becomes abnormally thick. Eventually the endometrium outgrows its vascular support, becomes friable, and sloughs off irregularly, resulting in estrogen breakthrough bleeding. A sudden estrogen withdrawal after ovulation may trigger self-limited vaginal bleeding (midcycle spotting).

The most common form of abnormal vaginal bleeding is dysfunctional uterine bleeding (DUB). DUB is caused by hormonal imbalances from a functionally abnormal hypothalamic–pituitary–ovarian axis resulting in abnormal follicle development and anovulation. The corpus luteum does not develop and a progesterone-deficient state ensues. In DUB, the vaginal bleeding occurs irregularly (metrorrhagia) because of a progesterone-deficient secretory phase. In contrast, progesterone breakthrough bleeding can occur in patients taking oral contraceptives with a high progesterone-to-estrogen ratio or receiving IM progesterone. The endometrium in this instance becomes atrophic and ulcerated, causing metrorrhagia.

Abnormal vaginal bleeding can be due to structural abnormalities, such as uterine fibroids, polyps, or endometrial hyperplasia. Systemic illnesses—such as coagulation disorders, platelet abnormalities, and renal or hepatic disease—may affect coagulation as well as the metabolism and excretion of estrogen and progesterone. Obesity increases peripheral estrogen production, which interferes with the hypothalamic–pituitary axis. Thyroid disease, adrenal disease, and prolactin disorders alter the normal hormonal feedback mechanisms, thus again leading to alteration of menstrual flow.

CLINICAL MANIFESTATIONS

HISTORY

The menstrual history should include onset of menarche and duration of the menstrual period as well as the frequency of menstruation, flow, and bleeding pattern. In contrast to ovulatory cycles, anovulatory cycles lack regular cycle length and a biphasic temperature curve. Women are also less likely to experience premenstrual symptoms, dysmenorrhea, breast tenderness, and a change in cervical mucus. A history of liver, renal, or thyroid disease may suggest a potential etiology. Use of anticoagulants, oral contraception, or hormone replacement therapy (HRT) is a potential cause of abnormal bleeding. Review of systems—particularly regarding weight change, hirsutism, exercise, increased stress, and the presence of galactorrhea or visual changes—may help to determine the cause of abnormal bleeding.

PHYSICAL EXAMINATION

The physical examination should include vital signs, including orthostatic blood pressure and pulse, signs of pregnancy, assessment for systemic disease, and a sterile speculum and bimanual exam-

TABLE 58-1 Symptoms Associated with Different Patterns of Vaginal Bleeding

Type	Associations	Causes	Ovulation
Midcycle spotting	Pelvic pain (*mittelschmerz*)	Ovulatory bleed	+
Menorrhagia	von Willebrand dz, platelet disorder, structural lesion	Thrombocytopenia, uterine fibroids adenomyosis endometrial polyps	+
Metrorrhagia	Situational stress, weight loss, exercise training, hypo- or hyperthyroidism, hyperprolactinemia, infertility, hirsutism, obesity, or amenorrhea	Hypothalamic dysfunction with progesterone-deficient state	+
		Polycystic ovarian syndrome	–
Menometrorrhagia	Menstrual cramps	Uterine fibroids	+
Oligomenorrhea	Frequency >35 days	Prolonged follicular phase	+
Polymenorrhea	Frequency <21 days	Inadequate luteal phase or a short follicular phase	+
Intermenstrual bleed		IUD cervical disease	+
Postcoital bleed	Cervix ulcerations	Cervical cancer	+
	Spotting b/w menses	Cervical polyps, erosions, vaginal lesions	+
	Fever, pelvic pain, cervical discharge	Pelvic inflammatory diseases	+
Pregnancy	Amenorrhea, vaginal spotting, unilateral pelvic pain	Ectopic pregnancy	NA
	Painless vaginal bleeding	Placenta previa	NA
	Vaginal bleed w/clots, abdominal pain	Placenta abruption	NA
Perimenopausal bleed	Metrorrhagia, vasomotor symptoms	Estrogen withdrawal	–
Postmenopausal bleed	>40 years	Endometrial cancer Cervical cancer Cervical or vaginal lesions	–
	Continuous combined estrogen w/progesterone cyclic: 3 week on and 1 week off, estrogen	Breakthrough bleed or spotting	–

NA, not applicable.

ination. Orthostatic changes indicate significant blood loss and a more acute course. Patients with PCOS and anovulatory bleeding often have hirsutism in conjunction with irregular menses and obese body habitus. A cushingoid appearance may indicate an adrenal abnormality, whereas the presence of a goiter and hyporeflexia may indicate thyroid disease. Characteristics of hyperprolactinemia include visual field changes and milky nipple discharge. A bleeding diathesis can present with petechiae and ecchymoses, along with menorrhagia. A sterile speculum examination can identify vaginal or cervical lesions and directly visualize the amount of bleeding. The bimanual examination can assess cervical motion tenderness and detect uterine and adnexal masses.

DIFFERENTIAL DIAGNOSIS

Malignancy, trauma, and sexual abuse or assault are potential causes of abnormal bleeding. Table 58-1 lists some other causes of abnormal vaginal bleeding. Establishing the pattern of bleeding as ovulatory or anovulatory helps narrow the differential diagnosis. For example, anovulatory bleeding is common in DUB, obese patients, and those suffering from infertility. Pregnancy-related bleeding can be due to an ectopic pregnancy, miscarriage, threatened abortion, trophoblastic disease, and placenta previa or abruption. Abnormal bleeding can be a side effect of oral contraception or other hormonal therapy and of systemic disorders, particularly thyroid, adrenal, pituitary, and hypothalamic conditions. PID, coagulopathies, and anatomic lesions (e.g., cervical erosions) are other causes of premenopausal bleeding. Perimenopausal bleeding is typically irregular. The likelihood of cervical and endometrial cancer and endometrial hyperplasia is greater in those over age 35, particularly peri- and postmenopausal patients. Fibroids and polyps are benign neoplasms that can cause abnormal bleeding. In postmenopausal women, vaginal bleeding is most commonly associated with endometrial carcinoma or HRT.

DIAGNOSTIC EVALUATION

Figure 58-1 outlines the evaluation of the patient with abnormal vaginal bleeding. The initial evaluation should include a Pap smear (unless there is a record of a recently documented normal smear), a CBC, and—in peri- and premenopausal patients—a pregnancy test. If a genital lesion is detected, appropriate treatment or referral for evaluation and treatment should be advised. If the uterus is enlarged, an US to assess the uterus should be obtained. Cervical culture may be helpful in patients at high risk for infection and those with symptoms of infection. Thyroid tests may be helpful in addition to testing for any systemic diseases suggested by the history and physical (e.g., prolactin levels in a patient with galactorrhea and abnormal bleeding).

In younger patients with menorrhagia, coagulation disorders should be considered if there are other signs or symptoms of a bleeding disorder. Adolescents and young women with anovulatory patterns should have their TSH and prolactin levels checked. Those with suspected PCOS may warrant measuring the LH, FSH, dehydroepiandrosterone sulfate (DHEA-S), and free testosterone levels on the third day of the menstrual cycle. An LH:FSH ratio greater than 2:1 is consistent with PCOS.

Women over the age of 35 require an approach that considers the possibility of endometrial cancer. Thus, in this age group, US and endometrial biopsy are recommended. Saline infusion sonohysteroscopy and hysteroscopy are more invasive diagnostic tests that may be helpful if bleeding persists and further testing is warranted. The exception to this may be in those postmenopausal women who have recently been started on HRT. Bleeding occurs commonly in the first 6 months of HRT, and adjustment of the progesterone dosage followed by observation may be tried. If abnormal bleeding persists, further evaluation is indicated.

Vaginal bleeding more than 12 months after menopause is considered postmenopausal bleeding. Postmenopausal bleeding is abnormal and merits investigation because of the risk of cancer in this age group.

TREATMENT

Management depends on the degree of bleeding, presence of anemia, and results of the evaluation. In hemodynamically unstable patients, hospitalization, transfusion, and stabilization of the bleeding with intravenous estrogen or surgical management are necessary. For patients with DUB who are not anemic, observation may be sufficient, or oral contraceptives can be used to regulate the menstrual cycles and provide contraception. Supplemental iron is indicated for anemic or iron-deficient individuals. Patients with DUB who are unresponsive to medical therapy warrant referral.

In oligomenorrhea and PCOS, induction of menses at least every 3 months with progesterone is indicated to prevent endometrial hyperplasia and its risk for progression to cancer. Progesterone used in this manner will not prevent pregnancy; therefore, oral contraceptives are indicated for those patients with oligomenorrhea desiring contraception. Progesterone-releasing intrauterine devices (IUDs) are another option that combines lessened menstrual flow with reliable contraception. Clomiphene is useful for inducing ovulation in those desiring pregnancy.

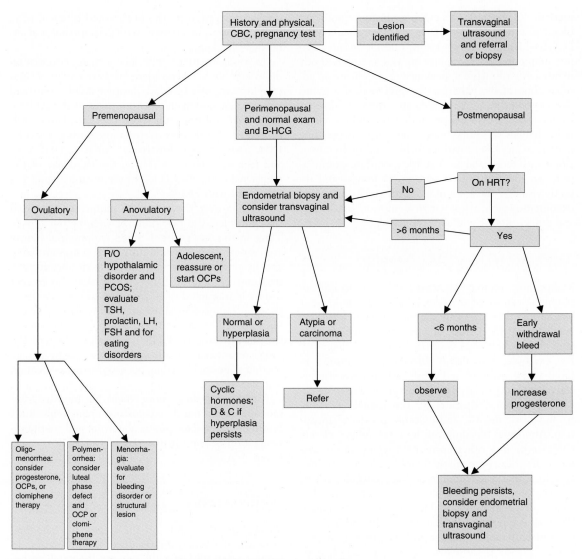

Figure 58-1 • Algorithm for the evaluation of abnormal vaginal bleeding.

Perimenopausal and postmenopausal women without surgical conditions can be treated with cyclic hormonal therapy or adjustment of previously prescribed doses of hormones. Lesions of the vulva and vagina should be biopsied. Patients with surgical causes or those who are not responding to medical therapy warrant referral to a gynecologist. Surgical options include endometrial ablation or hysterectomy.

KEY POINTS

- The most common cause of abnormal vaginal bleeding in a premenopausal patient is DUB secondary to anovulation; in a perimenopausal patient, endometrial hyperplasia and carcinoma; and in a postmenopausal patient, endometrial carcinoma and hormone replacement therapy.

- DUB is not associated with pelvic pathology, medications, systemic disease, or pregnancy.

- Because of the high likelihood of cancer in peri- or postmenopausal patients, endometrial biopsy and transvaginal ultrasound ought to be done early in the investigation.

Chapter

59 Amenorrhea

Amenorrhea is the absence of menstrual periods in a woman of reproductive age. Physiologic amenorrhea occurs when a woman reaches menopause, becomes pregnant, or breast-feeds. Primary amenorrhea is defined as the absence of menarche by age 16 years with normal pubertal development or by age 14 years without the onset of puberty. Secondary amenorrhea is defined as absence of menses for 6 months in a woman who previously had menses or for at least 6 cycles or 12 months in a woman with previously irregular menses. Excluding physiologic causes, secondary amenorrhea has a prevalence rate of about 4%. Primary amenorrhea is less common, with about 99% of women having menses by age 16.

PATHOGENESIS

The hypothalamus, anterior pituitary, ovary, and uterus orchestrate the menstrual cycle. The pulsatile release of gonadotropin-releasing hormone (GnRH) from the hypothalamus stimulates the anterior pituitary gland to release LH and FSH into the bloodstream. FSH stimulates the ovarian follicles, which produce estrogen and later progesterone. Estrogen stimulates the endometrial lining. An LH surge and ovulation occur midcycle, triggered by the positive feedback between FSH and the hypothalamus–pituitary axis. The dominant follicle develops into a corpus luteum and secretes progesterone. If the oocyte fails to be fertilized, the progesterone production of the degenerating corpus luteum decreases and the endometrial lining of the uterus begins to slough off. If there are no anatomic anomalies that inhibit outflow, menstruation occurs. Amenorrhea reflects an interruption of the mechanisms of normal menstruation and may result from abnormalities in the hypothalamus, anterior pituitary, ovaries, or uterus.

Stress, chronic infection, systemic illness, anorexia nervosa, and excessive exercise can suppress hypothalamic GnRH secretion through neuronal pathways in the arcuate nucleus and cause amenorrhea. Pituitary failure secondary to Kallman syndrome, where the GnRH neurons fail to migrate from the olfactory bulb, results in amenorrhea. Trauma, hypotension, infiltrative or inflammatory processes, pituitary adenoma, or craniopharyngioma can impair pituitary function.

Ovarian failure can result from chromosomal abnormalities, radiation, chemotherapy, and premature menopause. Hypothyroidism and hyperprolactinemia can suppress the secretion of GnRH, FSH, and LH.

CLINICAL MANIFESTATIONS

HISTORY

The history should include a menstrual history (presence of menarche, menstruation duration and flow, dysmenorrhea), a review of development (growth and sexual development), chronic illnesses, and medications. It is also important to discuss a teenager's sexual history and substance abuse while reassuring her, in a private setting, of the confidentiality of the conversation. Emotional stress or pronounced weight loss may be a clue to hypothalamic dysfunction. It is useful to ask about visual changes, headache, galactorrhea, presence of goiter, fatigue, palpitations (thyroid disease); presence of abdominal pain, bloating, and normal pubertal changes (vaginal outlet obstruction). In female athletes, discussion of nutrition, physical activity, weight changes, dieting, and body image may give clues to an underlying eating disorder.

PHYSICAL EXAMINATION

The physical examination begins with vital signs, including weight and height, followed by a careful funduscopic examination, thyroid gland palpation, breast examination with attempts to elicit galactorrhea, abdominal examination, and a bimanual pelvic examination. In patients with primary amenorrhea, evaluation of the secondary sexual characteristics and possible signs of virilization and uterine or vaginal abnormalities is important. A pale vaginal mucosa lacking normal rugal folds suggests estrogen deficiency. Short stature (<60 inches) in a patient with primary amenorrhea merits evaluation for Turner syndrome. Hirsutism, obesity, and acanthosis may be signs of PCOS.

DIFFERENTIAL DIAGNOSIS

Table 59-1 lists common causes of primary and secondary amenorrhea. The causes of primary amenorrhea include hormonal aberrations, congenital defects, chro-

■ TABLE 59-1 Causes of Amenorrhea

Primary	Helpful Tests
Physiologic	
Pregnancy	B-HCG
Hypothalamic/pituitary	
Thyroid disease	TSH
Pituitary adenoma	Prolactin, MRI, or CT scan
GnRH deficiency (Kallman syndrome)	LH, FSH
Polycystic ovarian syndrome	LH, FSH, progesterone challenge
Chronic medical disease	LH, FSH, estradiol, prolactin
Stress, eating disorders	LH, FSH, estradiol, prolactin
Medications	Trial off medication
Ovarian	
Gonadal dysgenesis	LH, FSH, karyotype
Congenital adrenal hyperplasia	17-Hydroxyprogesterone
Testicular feminization	Karyotype
Outflow tract	
Imperforate hymen	Physical examination
Rokitansky–Kuser–Hauser syndrome	Physical exam, karyotype, pelvic ultrasound
Secondary	**Helpful Tests**
Physiologic	
Pregnancy	B-HCG
Lactation	History
Menopause	History/age, FSH
Hypothalamic/pituitary	
Thyroid disease	TSH
Pituitary adenoma	Prolactin, MRI or CT scan
Polycystic ovarian syndrome	LH, FSH, progesterone challenge
Sheehan syndrome	LH, FSH
Stress, eating disorders	LH, FSH, estradiol, prolactin
Chronic medical disease	LH, FSH, estradiol, prolactin
Medications	Trial off medications
Ovarian	
Premature ovarian failure	FSH, estradiol; karyotype, age 30
Uterine	
Asherman syndrome	Hysterosalpingogram, estrogen/progesterone

mosomal abnormalities, and hypothalamic or pituitary dysfunction. In patients with primary amenorrhea and normal secondary sexual characteristics, the most likely cause is an anatomic abnormality, such as the failure to develop a normal uterus or vagina. In contrast, the lack of secondary sexual characteristics suggests a hormonal problem. The most common hypothalamic etiology is Kallman syndrome, while a tumor or compression from a Rathke pouch cyst may cause pituitary gland dysfunction. Ovarian function may be defective due to gonadal dysgenesis, as seen in Turner syndrome.

Many of the causes of secondary amenorrhea overlap with the causes of primary amenorrhea. After pregnancy, the most common causes are hypothalamic amenorrhea due to stress or illness, hyperprolactinemia, hypothyroidism, or PCOS, which accounts for 30% of secondary amenorrhea. In a few women, Turner syndrome may present as premature ovarian failure. Abrupt rapid onset of virilization suggests a serious underlying problem.

DIAGNOSTIC EVALUATION

The evaluation of a patient with primary amenorrhea is driven by the clinical examination (Figure 59-1). If secondary sexual characteristics such as breast development are present, anatomic abnormalities or testicular feminization syndrome should be suspected. For patients with a uterus but no breasts, gonadal dysfunction or a hypothalamic–pituitary axis problem is likely. The absence of both a uterus and breasts indicates the need for a chromosomal analysis. Consultation with a specialist is often useful in a patient with primary amenorrhea.

The evaluation for secondary amenorrhea starts with a pregnancy test. If the pregnancy test is negative and no obvious explanation exists for the amenorrhea, a prolactin level and a TSH should be obtained. About 20% of the cases of secondary amenorrhea are caused by hyperprolactinemia. If these tests are normal, a progesterone challenge test determines whether a woman produces estrogen.

Medroxyprogesterone acetate (Provera) in an oral daily dose of 10 mg for 7 days is a commonly used method of progesterone challenge. Any bleeding, even a small amount, in the week after completing the progesterone indicates that the major components of the hypothalamic, pituitary, ovarian, and uterine pathways are at least minimally functional and that the patient is anovulatory. The most common cause of anovulatory periods is PCOS or a functional abnormality in the hypothalamus. An elevated LH is highly suggestive of PCOS in a woman with clinical evidence of PCOS such as mild hirsutism, infertility, and obesity. If the LH is normal, an LH:FSH ratio of 2.5 is consistent with PCOS. Functional hypothalamic amenorrhea is a diagnosis of exclusion, but a history of anorexia nervosa, stress, or extreme exercise suggests the diagnosis. In anovulatory patients with evidence of hyperandrogenism (e.g., hirsutism), testosterone and DHEA-S levels should be obtained. Testosterone levels greater than 200 mg/dL and/or DHEA-S levels greater than 7 mg/dL require a CT scan to rule out an adrenal or ovarian tumor. In PCOS, DHEA-S is often mildly elevated. An increased ratio of testosterone to DHEA-S suggests an adrenal cause and the need to obtain a 17-hydroxyprogesterone level to rule out late-onset congenital adrenal hyperplasia and Cushing syndrome.

The absence of withdrawal bleeding indicates that either an estrogen deficiency or an anatomic abnormality is present. If an estrogen deficiency is suspected, assessment of the FSH level is the next step. An elevated FSH level indicates ovarian failure. Patients below 30 years of age with ovarian failure should undergo karyotyping. If the FSH is low or normal, a MRI scan of the hypothalamus and pituitary is indicated to rule out a CNS lesion such as a craniopharyngioma, meningioma, pituitary adenoma, or granulomatous disease. If an outflow problem is suspected, a combination of estrogen and progesterone can be given. Estrogen is given daily for 3 weeks and progesterone is added the last 5 days. Failure to bleed after a combined estrogen and progesterone challenge indicates an outflow abnormality.

TREATMENT

Management depends on the underlying cause. Patients with congenital anatomic abnormalities usually require referral for surgery. Patients with primary amenorrhea with an absent uterus and no breast tissue can be treated with estrogens to promote breast development and prevent osteoporosis. Patients with breast tissue and an absent uterus may not require treatment.

Patients with hypothyroidism need replacement therapy. Those with a pituitary macroadenoma need evaluation for possible surgery, while patients with microadenomas may be treated with bromocriptine and close follow up.

Management of patients with anovulatory periods depends on whether they currently desire pregnancy or contraception. Those patients desiring contraception may elect to take birth control pills. For patients with anovulatory periods desiring pregnancy, drugs such as clomiphene are used to induce ovulation. For patients who do not respond to clomiphene, gonadotropins can be used to stimulate ovulation. If patients are not sexually active or do not want birth control pills, progesterone should be given on a regular basis to induce withdrawal bleeding and prevent endometrial hyperplasia. Patients with premature ovarian failure need HRT to treat menopausal symptoms and atrophic vaginitis. HRT or medications such as the bisphosphonates should be provided to prevent bone loss and osteoporosis. Formerly, HRT was felt to reduce the risk of heart disease. However, the Women's Health Initiative study found that one type of HRT, Prempro, a combination of estrogen and progesterone, not only does not prevent heart disease but also increases its risk during the first 2 years of therapy.

In patients with PCOS, normal periods may return with weight loss. In addition to amenorrhea, PCOS is associated with obesity, insulin resistance, impaired glucose tolerance, hypertension, hyperlipidemia, and

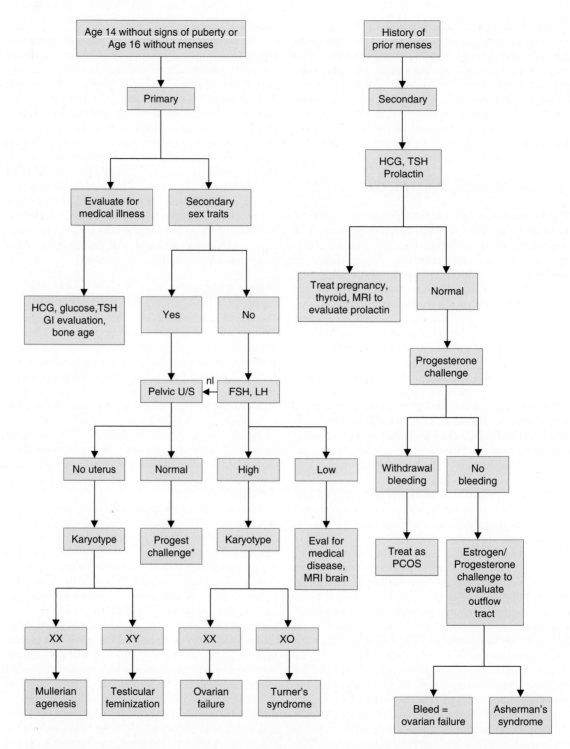

Figure 59-1 • Algorithm for the evaluation of primary and secondary amenorrhea.

*Complete work-up as for secondary amenorrhea and if negative bleed with estrogen and progesterone, then consider imperforate hymen or transverse vaginal septum as causes since Asherman's is a result of prior uterine surgeries (i.e D + C).

premature vascular disease. Medications such as met-formin and thiazolidinediones are being used to address the underlying metabolic defect with PCOS.

No data support the usage of HRT in treating amenorrheic female athletes, who are typically treated by the use of OCP initially, proper nutrition, and adjusted training regimens.

KEY POINTS

- Primary amenorrhea is the absence of menarche by 16 years of age with normal pubertal development or no pubertal development by the age of 14 years. Secondary amenorrhea is the absence of menses for 6 months or 6 previous cycles after establishing normal menses.
- Concealed pregnancy remains the most likely cause of primary or secondary amenorrhea in an otherwise normal adolescent.
- History taking should include a careful menstrual and medical history, including all medications, sexual history, a review of systems and history of drug abuse.
- Management of amenorrhea depends on the underlying causes. The most common treatment is restoring the menstrual cycle with either a progesterone withdrawal method or combined estrogen-progesterone therapy such as OCP.

60 Breast Masses

Discovery of a breast mass is a relatively common occurrence. In the United States, a woman's lifetime risk for developing breast cancer is 8% to 10%, with over 50% of cancers occurring in patients over age 65. Proper evaluation and treatment of breast masses are essential, since breast cancer is the most common malignancy in women. Although far less common, 1% of breast cancers occur in men.

PATHOGENESIS

Breast tissue contains epithelium, which forms the acini and ducts; fat; and fibrous tissue, which provides structural support. The hormones of the menstrual cycle also cause progression and regression of the ducts, and many normal women experience some breast tenderness around their menstrual periods. Under hormonal influence, breast tissue may be overstimulated, leading to the development of fibroadenomas, ductal dysplasia, and breast cysts. Cysts are collections of fluid, such as colostrum or dissolved cellular debris, that result from stricture and fibrosis of the small ductules.

Most breast cancers arise from malignant transformation of ductal or epithelial cells. The exact causes of breast cancer have not been determined for the vast majority of cases. Approximately 5% of cases are thought to be attributable to inheritance of the *BRCA1* or *BRCA2* genes. Breast cancer is not considered a consequence of fibrocystic disease.

Breast cancers are commonly divided into epithelial or nonepithelial (stromal) malignancies. The epithelial cancers are most common and are further classified as lobular or ductal carcinomas. Lobular carcinomas are more common in younger patients and ductal carcinomas more frequent in older patients. Ductal carcinomas are more invasive than lobular lesions. The first site of metastases is usually the axillary lymph nodes, although metastases are found in less than 10% of patients with breast tumors less than 1 cm in diameter.

CLINICAL MANIFESTATIONS

HISTORY

The history should include questions about how long the mass has been present, how it was discovered, and whether any change has occurred. Additional helpful

information includes the presence of pain or discharge, weight loss, or bone pain. Past personal or family history of breast cancer, menstrual history, and use of any hormonal therapies should also be obtained.

PHYSICAL EXAMINATION

The physical examination includes both inspection and palpation of the breast. One should inspect for masses, skin changes such as inflammation or edema, and skin dimpling or nipple retraction. Palpation of the axillary and supraclavicular regions can be done while the patient is seated by feeling for enlarged lymph nodes. Careful and methodical palpation of each quadrant of the breast should be performed, along with areolar pressure around the nipple to assess for breast discharge.

DIFFERENTIAL DIAGNOSIS

The most common causes for breast masses are fibrocystic changes, fibroadenomas, and breast cancer. Less common causes for breast masses include hamartomas, adenomas, abscesses, lipomas, intraductal papillomas, and fat necrosis. Mastitis and abscess formation are rare in nonlactating women.

Cancer typically presents in a postmenopausal woman as an isolated, painless, hard mass usually larger than 2 cm discovered on self-examination. The mass often does not have discrete borders but may be mobile. Over time, cancerous masses will enlarge, become fixed, and may be associated with palpable axillary lymph nodes. Other signs of breast cancer include skin dimpling, nipple inversion, nipple discharge (especially bloody discharge), and skin edema or inflammation.

Fibroadenomas commonly present in younger women as discrete, mobile, painless, rubbery masses. After an initial several-month period of growth, fibroadenomas generally stabilize in size, remain mobile, and do not spread to adjacent structures or lymph nodes.

Diffusely lumpy, tender breasts may indicate fibrocystic change. Fibrocystic changes will vary with the menstrual cycle and are most commonly found in younger women. Cysts that persist throughout the menstrual cycle and fail to resolve with aspiration or those with a bloody aspirate may be malignant and should be investigated.

DIAGNOSTIC EVALUATION

Most women presenting with a breast mass should have a mammogram. The exception is women under age 30, in whom mammograms may be more difficult to interpret because of the density of the breasts. In this case, clinical suspicion and US will help direct the evaluation. Easy mobility, regular borders, and a soft, squishy, or cystic feel suggest a benign mass. If the mass is accessible, fine-needle aspiration should be performed. If no mass can be palpated after aspiration and the aspirated fluid is not bloody, the patient may be followed clinically by re-examination. A persistent mass or bloody fluid mandates excisional biopsy to rule out malignancy. In addition to utilizing US to evaluate lesions and differentiate cystic from solid masses, it can also be used to direct biopsy. Solid masses with no fluid found on fine-needle aspiration generally require core-needle or excisional biopsy for evaluation.

In postmenopausal women, breast lumps should be regarded as cancer until proven otherwise. Mammography is typically the initial study performed. For best results, the radiologist should be informed of the suspicious area and special views obtained to fully evaluate the abnormal area. However, a normal mammogram or a reading suggesting a benign lesion in a patient with a dominant breast mass on examination does not rule out cancer. Some 9% to 22% of palpable breast cancers are not seen on mammography. In these instances, US can be used to characterize the mass and to help direct biopsies. Any palpable mass in a woman over the age of 40 should be biopsied.

Mammography is still useful even if a palpable mass is present that will need biopsy, since it can help locate the mass, guide needle biopsy, or find nonclinically evident lesions in the ipsilateral or contralateral breast. In addition, an initial mammogram provides a baseline for comparison with future mammograms and can help plan the surgical approach if a lesion requires surgery for accurate diagnosis. Fine-needle aspiration biopsy of a solid breast mass provides an adequate specimen in 60% to 85% of cases. Sensitivity is greater than 80% and specificity is greater than 99%. Thus, negative cytology does not preclude breast cancer. Solid lesions that have negative or suspicious cytology and cystic lesions with serosanguinous fluid require excisional biopsy. Some experts recommend that lesions appearing to be benign based on examination, mammogram, and a negative needle biopsy can be followed with serial mammograms and clinical evaluation. For cysts that are aspirated, resolve, have negative cytology, and do not return on breast examination, mammography or breast examination can be used for follow-up depending upon patient's age and risk.

Nipple discharge warrants thorough breast examination. It should be noted whether the discharge is unilateral or bilateral, bloody or milky, spontaneous or expressible, or localized to one duct. Guaiac testing and cytologic testing are helpful. Mammography is essential in evaluating these patients. If nipple discharge is unexplained, a surgeon will have to evaluate the ducts for early ductal cancer.

TREATMENT

Individuals with fibroadenomas may elect to do nothing or to undergo excision of the lesion. Women with fibrocystic change should be informed about the benign nature of the disease and that fibrocystic disease without atypical cells does not increase breast cancer risk. Treatment options include a supportive bra, vitamin E supplements, and avoidance of chocolate and caffeinated beverages. More severe cases may be treated with medications such as spironolactone or short trials of cyclic progesterone, danazol, or tamoxifen.

Management of the patient with breast cancer incorporates a team approach involving the family physician along with the surgeon and oncologist. Assessment for metastatic disease initially involves checking the CBC, liver enzymes, a chest x-ray, tumor markers (CA15-3), and in some cases a bone scan. A CT scan of the liver is indicated if liver enzymes are elevated. Surgery generally involves either a lumpectomy or modified radical mastectomy and assessment of lymph nodes, commonly with a sentinel node biopsy or axillary dissection. Postoperatively, after the patient has healed, radiation therapy and possibly chemotherapy may be provided depending upon the patient's age and lymph node and estrogen-receptor status. Co-ordination of care will require communication and involvement between the various members of the health care team and the patient to determine the best treatment for the patient's medical and psychological well-being.

KEY POINTS

- Fibrocystic change is common in women under 50 years of age and is hormonally mediated and benign.
- Fibroadenomas are common benign solid breast masses found in women under age 30.
- Malignant breast tumors are seen in approximately 20% of all dominant breast masses evaluated.
- Ultrasonography, mammography, fine-needle aspiration biopsy, and open biopsy are all methods of evaluating solid breast masses.

Chapter

61 Contraception

More than half of all pregnancies in the United States are unintentional, and about half of these pregnancies end in abortion. Contraceptive methods have been developed in order to limit the number of unintended pregnancies. Methods of birth control include natural family planning, barrier methods, IUDs, steroid medications, and surgical sterilization. Each birth control method has its disadvantages and advantages.

The theoretical efficacy rate of a birth control method is the number of unintended pregnancies per 100 women when the method is used exactly as instructed. Actual efficacy rates reflect the rate of women actually using the method for a year. Table 61-1 lists the efficacy rates of common forms of birth control. Birth control methods that require minimal patient involvement, such as surgical sterilization, have actual rates that approach theoretical rates, while actual rates may be much lower than theoretical rates for methods that require active patient involvement, such as barrier contraception.

NATURAL FAMILY PLANNING

This form of birth control includes several different methods based on abstinence or abstinence at selected times during the menstrual cycle. With natural family planning, one must keep track of the normal menstrual cycle and abstain from sexual intercourse during the period (7 to 10 days) surrounding ovulation. Measuring cycle length (calendar method), changes in cervical mucus, and changes in temperature can accomplish this. With the calendar method, ovulation is targeted as occurring 14 days before the onset of menses and requires that women abstain from sexual relations for several days before and after ovulation. In assessing cervical mucus, the woman inserts her fingers into the vagina to determine the amount and consistency of the mucus. Intercourse should be avoided when the mucus is thin and copious. The temperature method requires the woman to measure her temperature first thing in the morning before getting out of bed. At ovulation, the temperature will rise by 0.4 to 0.8 °C. Again, sexual intercourse should be avoided during the period surrounding ovulation.

The recent availability of home hormonal assays has also come to play a part in natural family planning. Some couples combine barrier methods with natural planning.

Natural methods are not effective directly after childbirth because it may take several months for the resumption of normal menstrual cycles, especially if the mother is breast-feeding. Natural methods should not be recommended for women with irregular menses. Candidates for this type of contraception must be highly motivated, since prolonged periods of abstinence are necessary. Studies have found the failure rate for this form of contraception to be approximately 20% per year.

BARRIER METHODS

Commonly used barrier methods are diaphragms and condoms. Since both require active patient participation, patient motivation must be taken into account in choosing this method.

Diaphragm use requires instruction and experience and is more effective in older women who are familiar with it. The failure rate is estimated at 2.4 to 19.6 per 100 woman-years. In users over 25 years of age and with at least 5 months' experience, the failure rate was 2.4 per 100 woman-years. The diaphragm is placed into the vagina along the anterior vaginal wall and should cover the entire cervix, thus preventing passage of semen into the cervix. Diaphragms come in different sizes. After an initial fitting, patients must be refitted after pregnancy, pelvic surgery, or a weight change of more than 10 pounds. The diaphragm must be used together with a spermicidal lubricant containing nonoxynol-9. It must be inserted no longer than 6 hours prior to coitus and left in the vagina for at least 6 hours but not longer than 24 hours after coitus. Additional spermicide should be placed intravaginally without removing the diaphragm for each episode of intercourse. Women using this form of contraception may be more prone to develop UTIs.

There are two general types of condoms—one for the male and one for the female. The male condom is a sleeve made of latex, polyurethane (for latex-sensitive individuals), or lambskin that prevents pas-

TABLE 61-1 Failure Rates for Various Contraceptive Methods

Method	Percent of Women Who Become Pregnant	
	Theoretical Failure Rate	*Actual Failure Rate*
No method	85.0	85.0
Periodic abstinence	—	20.0
Calendar	9.0	
Ovulation method	3.0	
Symptothermal	2.0	
Postovulation	1.0	
Withdrawal	4.0	18.0
Lactational amenorrhea	2.0	15.0–55.0
Condom		
Male condom	2.0	12.0
Female condom	6.0	21.0–26.0
Diaphragm with spermicide	6.0	18.0
Cervical cap	6.0	18.0
Sponge		
Parous women	9.0	28.0
Nulliparous women	6.0	18.0
Spermicide alone	3.0	21.0
IUDs		
Progestasert	2.0	2.0
Paraguard copper T	0.8	0.7
Combination pill	0.1	3.0
Progestin-only pill	0.5	3.0–6.0
Norplant	0.09	0.09
Depo-Provera	0.3	0.3
Tubal ligation	0.2	0.4
Vasectomy	0.1	0.15

Adapted from Speroff L, Darney P. *A Clinical Guide for Contraception.* 2nd ed. Baltimore: Williams & Wilkins; 1996:136.

sage of semen into the vagina. The condom must be placed on the erect penis before penetration. The female condom is placed in the vagina before intercourse and also prevents passage of semen into the vagina. Condoms can be used with other forms of contraception (e.g., spermicide), and latex condoms are recommended to prevent transmission of STDs. The pregnancy rate for condoms is approximately 1.6 to 12 per 100 woman-years, depending on age and the motivation of the patient.

STEROID CONTRACEPTIVE MEDICATIONS

Oral contraceptives (OCs), specifically estrogen and progestin preparations, are among the most reliable form of birth control. Pregnancy rates are less than 0.5 per 100 woman-years with perfect use and about 3% with typical use in the general population. OCs containing estrogen (most frequently ethinyl estradiol) together with one of several different progestin components inhibit gonadotropin secretion and ovarian function and induce changes in the cervical mucus and endometrial lining that inhibit sperm passage and ovum implantation.

Box 61-1 lists some noncontraceptive benefits of OCs. Women with a history of ovarian cysts or dysmenorrhea will benefit from the effects of OCs in ovarian suppression and thinning the endometrium.

OC use is contraindicated in women 35 years of age and older who smoke because of the increased risk of venous thrombosis and cardiovascular complications. Additional contraindications for OC use include history of venous thromboembolic disease, known cardiovascular disease, undiagnosed vaginal bleeding, breast cancer, and active liver disease. Relative contraindications include depression, diabetes, gallbladder disease, lactation, and obesity.

Abnormal bleeding and nausea are the most common side effects. Nausea is usually related to the OC's estrogen content; decreasing the dose of estrogen to 20 µg may help relieve nausea but increases the risk of breakthrough bleeding. Other side effects include weight gain, headache, breast tenderness, acne, fluid retention, and depression. Multiphasic pills that vary the dose of progestin were developed to decrease the incidence of progestin-related side effects and breakthrough bleeding, although there is no convincing evidence that multiphasics reduce side effects. However, women who have acne or hirsutism may benefit from a pill containing one of the less androgenic progestins (e.g., desogestrol or norgestimate). Another progestin called drospirenone (Yasmin) is a derivative of spironolactone and partially blocks the effects of mineralocorticoids; it may cause less bloating, weight gain, breast tenderness, and swelling than other preparations.

Many women experience side effects of OCs at first, but encouragement to continue the same regimen for 3 months is important, since many of these annoying but benign side effects will resolve with time. Some women prefer an extended-cycle regimen, where they take 84 active pills in a row and reduce menses to four times per year. Women desiring pregnancy after discontinuation of the pill should be counseled that there might be a several-month delay in resumption of ovulation. Postpartum OCs can be started as early as 2 to 3 weeks in non-breast–feeding individuals; however, many providers advise waiting until 6 weeks due to risks of venous thromboembolism. Lactation can be suppressed by OCs containing more than 50 mg of estrogen, and progestin-only pills are generally indicated for nursing mothers.

Progestin-only hormonal contraception is available orally, by injection, and as a subdermal implant. These agents may be used in patients who are unable to tolerate estrogenic side effects or with contraindications to estrogen use (e.g., cardiovascular disease, venous thromboembolic disease). The oral progestin-only contraceptive, also known as the "mini-pill," is slightly less effective than the combination pill. The injectable form of steroid contraception, depot medroxyprogesterone acetate, is 99% effective in preventing conception. It is given as 150 mg IM every 3 months. The subdermal hormone implant is also an effective form of reversible contraception. The major disadvantages are the expense and occasional difficulty in removing the implants, which are placed under the skin. Side effects of progestin-only contraception include acne, headache, weight gain, and irregular bleeding. Spotting and bleeding are the most common and troublesome side effects of these agents. Progestin-only agents do not affect lactation.

A recent addition to the steroid contraceptive medications is the monthly injectable combination of medroxyprogesterone acetate and estradiol cypionate, which has a 1-year cumulative pregnancy rate of 0.2%. Return to fertility is rapid when injections are stopped. Ovulation occurs during the third-month post-treatment. The most frequent reasons for discontinuation are weight gain, excessive bleeding, breast pain, menorrhagia, and dysmenorrhea. A birth control patch containing both estrogen and progesterone (Ortho-Evra) is also available. The patch is changed weekly and menses occurs during the "off" week. Its efficacy and side effects are similar to those of OCs.

Hormone-releasing vaginal rings (NuvaRing) provide low-dose release of 120 µg of etonogestrel and 15 µg of ethinyl estradiol per day. The ring is "one size fits all," stays in place for 3 weeks, and is taken out for the fourth week. Data for efficacy are comparable to other combined hormonal forms of contraception. Disadvantages include not wishing to have a foreign body in the vagina and the fear of expulsion.

■ **BOX 61-1** Noncontraceptive Benefits of Oral Contraceptives
Reduce the risk of the following conditions
Ovarian cancer
Endometrial cancer
Ectopic pregnancy
Pelvic inflammatory disease
Anemia
Dysmenorrhea
Functional ovarian cysts
Benign breast disease
Osteoporosis

INTRAUTERINE DEVICES

The IUD works by interfering with sperm mobility and fertilization. IUDs have an efficacy rate of two to three pregnancies per 100 women-years. This form of contraception is independent of the act of intercourse, highly effective, inexpensive, and reversible. Thus, women who use IUDs are among the most satisfied of all contraceptive users.

Two main types of IUDs are the copper-containing T-shaped devices and the progesterone-releasing devices. Copper-containing IUDs can remain in place for 10 years, whereas progesterone-releasing devices must be changed more frequently. The copper-containing IUDs may cause irregular uterine bleeding, an effect that is less prevalent with the progesterone IUDs. The levonorgestrel intrauterine system (Mirena) releases low doses of levonorgestrel at 20 μg/day in the uterine cavity for 5 years. The 5-year cumulative failure rate is 0.71 per 100 women, nearly equal to that of sterilization.

IUDs must be inserted under sterile conditions. It is recommended that an IUD should be placed within 5 days of the menstrual cycle, but it may be inserted any time the patient is not pregnant. Contraindications to IUD insertion are pregnancy, undiagnosed vaginal bleeding, and PID. Relative contraindications include nulliparity, prior ectopic pregnancy, history of multiple sexual partners, history of a previous STD, an abnormal Pap smear that has not been fully evaluated, and uterine anomalies. The most common side effects are cramping and bleeding which usually diminish with time. These symptoms can be helped by NSAIDs. All of the IUDs are visible on x-ray.

Complications of IUD use include pelvic inflammatory disease, ectopic pregnancy, spontaneous abortion, dysmenorrhea, metrorrhagia, and uterine perforation. The risk of PID associated with IUD use is correlated to ascending contamination at the time of insertion. Nonetheless, IUDs are usually contraindicated in women at high risk of cervical STDs.

STERILIZATION

Approximately 1 million sterilizations are performed in the United States each year. The two forms of sterilization performed are vasectomy and tubal ligation. Of these two procedures, tubal ligation is performed more often than vasectomy and is the most commonly used birth control method in the world. In order to avoid postprocedure regret, it is extremely important to **stress the irreversibility** of these procedures. Risk factors for regret include depression, young age, low parity, unstable marriage, and having the procedure at the time of a cesarean section.

Tubal ligation is an invasive procedure that can be performed laparoscopically or at the time of a cesarean section. Tubal continuity is interrupted surgically, thus preventing passage of the sperm or ovum. A newer procedure, performed hysteroscopically, is placement of Essure coils within the fallopian tubes, leading to their occlusion. Confirmation of tubal occlusion is recommended 3 months after the procedure by performance of a hysterosalpingogram. Vasectomies can be performed as outpatient procedures under local anesthesia, with less time away from work and a more rapid recovery. The procedure involves incising the scrotum, identifying the vas deferens, and then surgically removing a portion of each vas, thus preventing the passage of sperm. Vasectomy does not result in immediate sterility. Clearance of sperm occurs after about 25 ejaculations and must be confirmed by semen analysis. Complications from either procedure are uncommon. Vasectomy failures can be picked up by postoperative semen analysis, whereas failures of tubal ligation are detected when the patient becomes pregnant. Each of these procedures is potentially reversible, although they are labeled as "permanent" sterilization. Tubal ligation can be reversed with a success rate of 40% to 85%. Success rates for reversal of vasectomy range from 37% to 90%.

POSTCOITAL CONTRACEPTION

Postcoital hormonal approaches include the use of Ovral or Lo-Ovral, with a dose of two Ovral pills taken within 72 hours of unprotected intercourse, followed by 2 more taken 12 hours later. A progestin-only product (Plan B) is now available for postcoital contraception. Antiemetic medication may be needed with these regimens. Bleeding should occur within 3 to 4 weeks. If pregnancy occurs, abortion should be discussed because of the possible teratogenic effects of the high-dose steroids. Emergency contraception prevents at least three of four pregnancies that would have occurred. Postcoital IUD insertion within 5 days after intercourse is also effective.

KEY POINTS

- More than half of the pregnancies in the United States are unintended.
- Natural family planning methods focus on abstinence around the time of ovulation but have a 20% failure rate.
- Barrier methods require significant patient motivation, but they can be effective.
- Condoms can be combined with other methods of contraception and can help prevent sexually transmitted disease.
- The most effective methods of contraception are IUDs, hormonal contraception, and surgical sterilization.
- The method of contraception should be tailored to the individual patient.

62 Vaginitis

Vaginitis is characterized by vaginal discharge that is unusual in amount, odor, or symptoms, such as itching or burning.

PATHOGENESIS

The normal vaginal environment includes secretions, cellular elements, and microorganisms. Normal physiologic vaginal secretions are typically clear to opaque, containing primarily mucus and exfoliated cells. Physiologic vaginal secretions vary with age, stage of the menstrual cycle, pregnancy, and use of oral contraceptives. Normal vaginal flora contains numerous bacteria, with **lactobacilli** being the most prevalent. The lactobacilli produce hydrogen peroxide, which is toxic to pathogens and maintains the normal vaginal pH between 3.8 and 4.5. Vaginitis occurs when the vaginal flora is altered by the introduction of pathogens or changes in the vaginal environment.

Antibiotics, contraceptives, sexual intercourse, douching, and the introduction of sexually transmitted organisms are common factors that can disrupt the normal vaginal environment. These events can change the acidic pH of the vagina, leading to an overgrowth of different organisms. The most common organisms causing symptoms include *Candida*, *Trichomonas*, and *Gardnerella*, which is associated with BV.

CLINICAL MANIFESTATIONS

HISTORY

Most women with vaginitis complain of vaginal discharge, itching, or burning. The patient should be asked about the onset and duration of symptoms, previous episodes of vaginitis, and treatments. A general medical review, dermatologic review, and contraceptive history can be helpful. Illnesses such as diabetes and HIV and medications such as antibiotics or corticosteroids are associated with candidiasis. It is important to inquire about pelvic pain, fever, and possible pregnancy.

A sexual history can help identify patients at risk for STDs. Inquiry about the use of bubble baths, douches, deodorants, and spermicide preparations may help identify individuals with irritant or contact vaginitis.

The amount, consistency, color, or odor may suggest the cause. *Candida* usually produces itching, with a thick white discharge, sometimes described as cottage-cheese-like. Other typical symptoms include vulvar and vaginal itching, burning, dysuria, and dyspareunia. Symptoms of *Trichomonas* also include itching and often a profuse, frothy discharge with an unpleasant odor. The discharge can vary in color and may be yellow, gray, or green. Patients with BV may be asymptomatic or have a slight increase in discharge. Some patients will complain of profuse discharge often associated with a fishy odor but have only minimal itching.

Dysuria is also a common symptom of vaginitis and usually occurs when the urine touches the vulva. In contrast, internal dysuria, defined as pain inside the urethra, is a sign of cystitis.

PHYSICAL EXAMINATION

Inspection of the external genitalia for inflammation, masses, lesions, enlarged lymph nodes, and abnormal tissue is important. The pooled vaginal discharge should be assessed for color, consistency, volume, and adherence to the vaginal wall. Typically, *Candida* produces a thick discharge that adheres to the vaginal wall, while BV or *Trichomonas* causes a thin discharge that pools in the vaginal vault and is easily swabbed off the vaginal wall. A bimanual examination is important to check for uterine or ovarian tenderness or enlargement.

DIFFERENTIAL DIAGNOSIS

Approximately 90% of vaginitis cases are secondary to BV, candidiasis, or *Trichomonas*. Viral infections, such as HSV and HPV, sometimes cause vaginal irritation and discharge. Cervicitis, related to a chlamydial or gonorrheal infection, can also cause a vaginal discharge.

If no infection is identified, other causes of vaginitis—such as an allergic reaction, topical irritation, hormonal changes, and foreign bodies such as a forgotten tampon or condom—should be considered. Other noninfectious causes of vaginitis include skin conditions such as lichen sclerosis or early vulvar cancer. Atrophic vaginitis is common in menopausal women.

DIAGNOSTIC EVALUATION

A speculum examination is necessary to rule out neoplasm or foreign bodies and to determine whether the discharge is from vaginitis or cervicitis. A mucopurulent discharge from the cervix and cervical bleeding induced by swabbing the endocervical mucosa suggest cervicitis. Risk factors for cervicitis include age less than 24 years and a new sexual partner within the past 2 months. If cervicitis is suspected, tests for *Chlamydia* and *Neisseria gonorrhoeae* should be obtained.

If the history and physical examination are consistent with vaginitis, a sample of the discharge should be obtained. Standard office examinations include a wet mount preparation, a pH measurement, a whiff test to detect amines, and a slide prepared with 10% KOH. A positive whiff test is seen in BV when a fishy odor develops after 10% KOH is added to a slide. The odor results from the liberation of amines and organic acids produced by the alkalinization of anaerobic bacteria. A KOH preparation also dissolves most cellular material except filamentous hyphae and budding forms of yeast, aiding the detection of fungal tangles and spores. A Gram stain of vaginal secretions is even more sensitive for identifying yeast infections.

The wet mount is useful for detecting clue cells, *Trichomonas*, and polymorphonuclear leukocytes. Clue cells are vaginal epithelial cells that are coated with coccobacilli and are seen in BV (greater than 20% of epithelial cells). They have a sensitivity and specificity up to 98% for the detection of BV. Scanning several microscopic fields for *Trichomonas* has a sensitivity of 60% and a specificity of up to 99%. The *Trichomonas* protozoon is slightly larger than a WBC and has three to five flagellae. A wet mount may also detect fungal hyphae, increased numbers of polymorphonuclear cells (seen in *Trichomonas* infection), or round parabasilar cells (seen in atrophic vaginitis).

The pH can be determined by placing litmus paper in the pooled vaginal secretions or against the lateral vaginal walls. A pH greater than 4.5 is found in 80% to 90% of patients with BV and frequently in patients with *Trichomonas* vaginosis. The pH level is also high in atrophic vaginitis.

A vaginal culture for candidiasis using Saboraud or Nickerson medium is helpful if microscopy is negative and *Candida* is still suspected. Alternatively, many clinicians will use a trial of antifungal therapy. Culture for *Trichomonas* increases the sensitivity of diagnosis. Since BV is a polymicrobial infection, culturing vaginal secretions is usually not recommended for suspected cases.

TREATMENT

Treatment for candidal vaginitis includes topical therapy with one of the azole agents, such as miconazole or terconazole. Miconazole (Monistat) is available as an OTC preparation. Nystatin suppositories and gentian violet are also effective. Fluconazole, given as a single 150-mg oral dose, is as effective as a topical regimen. Colonization with yeast is present in 20% of women, and the incidental finding of yeast on a Pap smear does not necessitate treatment if there are no symptoms. Recurrent yeast infections may respond to ketoconazole for 1 to 2 weeks or fluconazole weekly.

Trichomonas can be treated with a single 2-g dose of metronidazole or with 250 mg of metronidazole three times a day for 7 days. Metronidazole has the potential for an Antabuse-like reaction, so patients should be cautioned about drinking alcohol while they are taking it. The most common side effects of metronidazole include nausea, abdominal cramps, and an unpleasant metallic taste. Treatment of the sexual partner is important, since 70% of sexual partners will be asymptomatically colonized with *Trichomonas*. Treatment for BV usually consists of either 500 mg of metronidazole three times a day for 7 days or 300 mg of clindamycin three times a day for 7 days. Single-dose therapy with 2 g of metronidazole can be considered when compliance may be a problem. Both clindamycin and metronidazole are available as intravaginal preparations and offer an effective alternative.

 KEY POINTS

- Most cases of vaginitis in women of childbearing age are due to infection from *Candida*, *Trichomonas*, or BV.
- Laboratory evaluation of vaginal discharge consists of a wet mount, KOH preparation, whiff test, and pH determination.
- A thick, cottage-cheese-like discharge suggests *Candida*, while a profuse, malodorous, gray–green frothy discharge is more consistent with *Trichomonas*.
- BV is a polymicrobial infection.
- Metronidazole is effective for *Trichomonas* and bacterial vaginitis.

Chapter 63
Preconception Counseling and Prenatal Care

Preconception counseling should ideally begin before a woman of childbearing age desires pregnancy. Opportunities for preconception counseling exist during routine office visits, especially for pregnancy or STD screenings. Since many pregnancies are unplanned, starting early folate supplementation, counseling about avoiding dangerous environmental exposures or medications, and curbing harmful habits like smoking may result in a healthier pregnancy and baby.

GENETIC COUNSELING

For a history of prior pregnancies with known neural tube defects (NTDs), folic acid supplementation is critical to decrease the risk with the current pregnancy. For otherwise healthy pregnancies with no prior history of NTD, daily supplementation of 400 µg of folate for at least 1 month prior to conception and at least 3 months into the pregnancy is recommended. For women with diabetes or epilepsy, a 1-mg daily supplement is advised; for those with a history of prior NTDs, 4 mg daily is recommended.

Screening for genetic diseases such as sickle cell anemia, cystic fibrosis, thalassemia and Tay–Sachs disease depends on the parents' ethnic background, medical history, family history, and desire to have this information in advance. A family history of cystic fibrosis or congenital hearing loss also merits an offer of genetic testing. An important component of genetic counseling is presenting parents with options to continue or terminate a pregnancy based on the information given. Parents who do not wish to terminate for any reason may forego genetic testing or may use the information from genetic tests to prepare for the possibility of having a child with special needs.

MEDICAL ASSESSMENT

A woman with a medical condition such as diabetes, hypertension, DVT, seizures, depression, or anxiety is at particular risk for complications to herself and/or her fetus. Optimal preconception control of blood sugar with diet, exercise, and possibly insulin helps decrease the risk of congenital anomalies and spontaneous abortion as pregnancy progresses. Optimal BP control helps decrease the risk of pre-eclampsia, renal insufficiency, and fetal growth retardation in hypertensive women. Methyldopa and calcium channel blockers are routinely used as antihypertensive medications in pregnancy. It is important to avoid ACE inhibitors, ARBs, and thiazide diuretics in the first and second trimesters because of the risk of congenital anomalies.

If possible, women with epilepsy should optimize seizure control with the lowest dose of a single medication. No single agent is the drug of choice for seizures in pregnancy. Pregnancy is a risk factor for DVT; women who are on warfarin (Coumadin) for a previous history of thrombosis should have anticoagulation therapy continued, but it should be switched to heparin (low molecular weight or unfractionated) because of the teratogenic effects of warfarin. If there is a personal or family history of thromboembolic disease, screening for a clotting disorder may be advised prior to conception. Women with depression or anxiety may continue antidepressant therapy with SSRIs if necessary, but benzodiazepines should be avoided because of their rare teratogenic effects.

SCREENING

High-risk patients should be evaluated for HIV and syphilis. Hepatitis B and, if necessary, rubella and varicella immunizations should be updated before a planned pregnancy. Pregnancy should be avoided for 1 to 3 months following rubella and varicella immunizations because they are live attenuated vaccines. The risk of toxoplasmosis decreases by avoiding cat litter, garden soil, and raw or undercooked meat. Frequent hand washing and universal precautions for child care and health care workers decreases the risk of contracting CMV and parvovirus B19 (fifth disease).

ENVIRONMENTAL TOXINS

Occupational exposures and household chemicals such as paint thinners, strippers, other solvents, and pesticides should be avoided. Smoking cessation, avoiding alcohol, limiting tuna and swordfish consumption, and screening for illicit drugs are also important to decrease risk to mother and fetus.

LIFESTYLE

Patients should be counseled to control weight, engage in regular moderate exercise, avoid overheating during pregnancy with the use of a hot tub or sauna, limit caffeine to two cups of coffee or six glasses of soda a day, and to avoid overuse of vitamins A and D. Nutritional screening includes assessment for iron, calcium, and protein deficiencies as well as lactose intolerance. Women should also be screened for domestic violence.

PRENATAL CARE

Prenatal care encompasses care for the pregnant mother, fetus, and family. The objectives of prenatal care include the following: reduction of maternal morbidity and mortality, reduction of fetal morbidity, enhancement of fetal health, and education about good parenting skills and infant care for the early childhood years. The timing of prenatal visits for low-risk pregnancies is listed in Box 63-1.

The EDD is established by Nägele rule, using the date of the patient's last menstrual period (LMP) minus 3 months plus 1 week and 1 year. This is based on assumptions of a 28-day menstrual cycle and normal length of gestation, which is about 280 days. When the cycle is irregular or the LMP is uncertain, US measurements between the 14th and 20th weeks of gestation provide an accurate determination of gestational age.

INITIAL PRENATAL VISIT

Often, the evaluation, education, and planning that should be discussed before pregnancy takes place during the first prenatal visit. A thorough physical examination of the thyroid, heart, breasts, and pelvis

BOX 63-1 Prenatal Visit Schedule for Low-Risk Pregnancies

| Preconception Visit |
| Up to 1 year before conception |
| First Prenatal Visit |
| 6–8 weeks after missed menses |
| Every 4 Weeks |
| Up to 28 weeks gestational age |
| Every 2 Weeks |
| Up to 36 weeks gestational age |
| Every Week |
| Until delivery |

is important. The pelvic examination should assess the bony architecture, uterus, adnexae, any abnormal vaginal discharge, and possible genital lesions. At this time, a Pap smear and cultures (for *Neisseria gonorrhoeae* and *Chlamydia*) should be obtained. Blood tests include a CBC, rubella titer, hepatitis B

BOX 63-2 Routine Prenatal Laboratory Tests

| Initial Visit |
| Pap smear, cervical culture, urine culture, CBC, rubella titer, hepatitis B surface antigen, ABO blood group, Rh type and antibody screen, serologic test for syphilis (VDRL), and HIV test. |
| 15th–20th Week of Gestation |
| Offer MSAFP/triple-marker screen to test for NTDs, Down syndrome as well as other genetic and congenital anomalies. |
| 26th–28th Week of Gestation |
| 1-hour glucose challenge test for gestational diabetes mellitus. |
| Hemoglobin to screen for anemia. |
| Rescreening for Rh antibodies for Rh-negative women; if the antibody screen remains negative, the mother should receive Rh_0 (D) immune globulin at 28 weeks. |
| 35th–37th Week of Gestation |
| Group B streptococcus anogenital cultures; if positive, treat with antibiotics during labor to prevent transmission to neonate. |

surface antigen, ABO blood group, Rh type and antibody screen, serologic test for syphilis (VDRL), and HIV test. A clean-catch urine specimen should be obtained to check for asymptomatic bacteriuria, which should be treated if present. The National Institutes of Health and the American College of Obstetricians and Gynecologists (ACOG) recommend offering all Caucasian women testing for cystic fibrosis status.

SUBSEQUENT PRENATAL VISITS

An interval history and physical examination are performed at each visit to determine mother's BP, state of physical and emotional health and nutrition, the presence of fetal movement, vaginal discharge or bleeding, and growth progress. A urine specimen should be obtained at each visit in order to check for proteinuria and glycosuria. Routine laboratory tests are listed in Box 63-2.

KEY POINTS

- Preconception counseling should cover genetic screening, medical assessment for chronic diseases, screening for infectious disease, and updating of immunizations; it should also provide advice on proper nutrition and exercise, help with quitting unhealthy habits, and advice on avoiding environmental hazards.

- Prenatal care includes care of the pregnant mother, the fetus, and the family and growing infant for up to 1 year. The aim of prenatal care is to decrease morbidity and mortality of the mother and fetus, enhance family bonding, foster parenting skills, and decrease family violence.

Common Medical Problems in Pregnancy

Pregnancy generally occurs during a healthy period of a woman's life. However, many women have medical concerns or develop acute medical conditions during pregnancy. In addition, women with chronic medical conditions may be at increased risk for complications of pregnancy. The most common medical problems that develop during pregnancy involve the digestive, cardiopulmonary, genitourinary, hematopoietic, and endocrine systems.

DIGESTIVE SYSTEM

Concerns about weight gain and diet are common during pregnancy. A balanced diet should be consumed; on average, a woman requires 300 calories/day over baseline. Recommended weight gain varies by prepregnancy weight; women of average weight should gain about 25 to 35 lb, overweight women 15 to 25 lb, and underweight women up to 40 lb during pregnancy. Daily folate supplementation of 400 µg is recommended to reduce the risk of neural tube defects. A calcium intake of 1200 to 1500 mg is recommended to preserve maternal bone structure as well as iron supplementation to prevent anemia. Caffeine intake of no more than two cups of coffee per day is recommended, and alcoholic beverages should be avoided. Multivitamins are often prescribed, but intake of vitamin A in excess quantities can be teratogenic.

Nausea and vomiting are common early signs of pregnancy, occurring in over half of the pregnancies. The exact cause is unknown. Typically early-morning nausea is common between 6 and 13 weeks, but nausea can occur any time of the day. Around 22 weeks, these symptoms normally resolve. Nonpharmacologic means such as avoiding offending foods, frequent small meals, drinking liquids apart from meals, and keeping dry crackers at the bedside generally suffice for treatment. In extreme cases, dehydration and weight loss may occur, requiring hospitalization and antiemetics.

Reflux is a common complaint during pregnancy because of hormonal changes and increases in abdominal pressure as the uterus enlarges. Behavioral advice should be provided (Chapter 17). Antacids can be used for symptom relief; in some cases medications such as famotidine may be necessary. Proton pump inhibitors (PPIs) may be required in cases refractory to H_2 antagonists.

Constipation—due to progesterone-induced alterations in bowel transit—is a common problem in pregnancy. Dietary management through an increase in the consumption of fluid and fiber is the initial means of treatment. Psyllium supplements can also be used, but chronic laxative use and regular use of enemas should be discouraged.

CARDIOPULMONARY SYSTEM

Dizziness, presyncope, and syncope are a common and usually benign occurrence. These symptoms arise in response to hormone-induced vasodilatation and alterations in venous return, resulting from mechanical compression by the uterus that limits venous return. Women with these symptoms should be evaluated to rule out more serious problems such as dehydration, anemia, or a cardiac etiology as the cause.

HTN and DVT are two serious conditions related to pregnancy. Each of these conditions can cause maternal morbidity and mortality as well as fetal compromise. HTN is present when the BP is greater than 140 systolic and/or 90 diastolic. HTN may be preexisting or gestational, with onset during pregnancy. Gestational HTN without proteinuria or symptoms follows a benign course. A subcategory of gestational HTN is termed pre-eclampsia and is present when the BP is elevated along with proteinuria (>300 mg/24 hours) and symptoms such as headache, visual changes, and abdominal pain. Maternal complications include seizures, renal compromise, hepatic injury, and thrombocytopenia. Fetal complications include growth restriction, oligohydramnios, abruption, and possibly fetal death. Patients with chronic HTN are at increased risk for superimposed pre-eclampsia. Patients with a prior history of pre-eclampsia may benefit from low-dose aspirin as a preventive measure in subsequent pregnancies. Patients with pre-eclampsia warrant close monitoring, and delivery is usually induced when complications arise or at 37 weeks' gestation. A full discussion of pre-eclampsia and its treatment is beyond the scope of this chapter.

Pregnancy causes venous pooling, changes in coagulation factors, and mechanical impedance to venous return. These factors contribute to the increased risk of DVT associated with pregnancy. In addition, patients with previously unrecognized hypercoaguable states such as factor V Leiden mutation, protein C or S deficiency, and antiphospholipid antibodies may first present during pregnancy. Diagnosis of DVT is generally made using venous duplex scans of the lower extremities. Patients suspected of pulmonary embolism may require CT scanning, V/Q scanning, or pulmonary angiography to establish the diagnosis. Warfarin crosses the placenta and is a known teratogen that is contraindicated during pregnancy. Pregnant patients should be treated with intravenous heparin followed by subcutaneous heparin or low-molecular-weight heparin until delivery. With unfractionated heparin, the dose is given every 8 to 12 hours and adjusted for a partial thromboplastin time 1.5 to 2.0 times normal. When low-molecular-weight heparin is used, antifactor Xa levels must be monitored and therapy is generally converted to unfractionated heparin in the last month of pregnancy.

Asthmatic patients may improve, worsen, or remain unchanged during pregnancy. Management generally follows the guidelines outlined in Chapter 38 for nonpregnant patients. Patients are at increased risk for preterm labor and pre-eclampsia. Fetal surveillance to monitor for fetal growth and well-being is recommended.

About one in five women smoke during pregnancy. Smoking can aggravate existing cardiopulmonary diseases and has been associated with a number of problems such as low birth weight, spontaneous abortion, premature delivery, intrauterine growth retardation, placental abruption, and placenta previa. Smoking cessation during pregnancy results in birth weights similar to those of nonsmoking women.

GENITOURINARY SYSTEM

A moderate increase in vaginal discharge is common with pregnancy and may not signify an underlying disorder. Evaluation for vaginitis and STDs should be performed, as discussed in Chapters 52 and 62.

UTIs occur in 10% to 15% of pregnant women because of urinary stasis, glycosuria, and vesicoureteral reflux. Up to 6% of pregnant women have asymptomatic bacteriuria and are at increased risk for pyelonephritis. Pyelonephritis is associated with increased risk for preterm labor. Evaluation should include US assessment for obstruction, along with UA and cultures. Treatment with empiric antibiotics such as amoxicillin or a cephalosporin, or nitrofurantoin in penicillin-allergic patients, should be initiated and then modified as necessary by culture results.

Fluoroquinolones and sulfa drugs in the last trimester are contraindicated. Follow-up cultures after therapy are warranted to document bacterial eradication. In those with persistent bacteriuria, retreatment followed by chronic suppressive antibiotics throughout pregnancy is warranted. In addition, suppressive therapy is generally recommended for those treated for pyelonephritis.

HEMATOPOIETIC SYSTEM

Anemia is the most common hematologic problem encountered during pregnancy. Hemodilution occurs during normal pregnancy; thus anemia during pregnancy is defined as a hemoglobin of less than 10 g/dL. Women are more susceptible to iron deficiency anemia during pregnancy because of the increased maternal RBC mass, fetal needs, and blood loss that occurs with delivery. During pregnancy, iron supplementation (ferrous sulfate) of 300 mg/day is recommended when the hemoglobin is greater than 10 g/dL; this dose may be taken two to three times daily by iron-deficient women. Evaluation of the pregnant woman with anemia should proceed as described in Chapter 36; it should include RBC indices and a peripheral smear. For those with megaloblastic indices, vitamin B_{12} and folate levels should be obtained; for those with microcytic indices, iron studies should be checked. In those with a history or family history of hemoglobinopathy, confirmation by hemoglobin electrophoresis is advised. In women at risk, genetic counseling and fetal diagnostic testing with chorionic villous sampling or amniocentesis may be warranted.

ENDOCRINE SYSTEM

Hypothyroidism is commonly present before pregnancy but may also develop during pregnancy. The most common cause of hypothyroidism during pregnancy is Hashimoto thyroiditis. The evaluation and treatment of hypothyroidism are discussed in Chapter 48. Of note, thyroid-binding protein levels increase during pregnancy and make it necessary to check TSH levels, since most women require higher dosages than in the nonpregnant state.

Hyperthyroidism is discussed in Chapter 47. Pregnancy affects treatment decisions, and medical therapy with PTU is preferred, since methimazole has been associated with aplasia cutis, a congenital defect of the scalp. Surgery is the second option for those not controllable with PTU. Radioactive iodine is contraindicated owing to risks of ablation of fetal thyroid tissue.

Gestational diabetes affects 2% to 5% of all pregnancies and is associated with hydramnios, preterm labor, macrosomia, hypertensive disease, fetal hypoglycemia, and hyperbilirubinemia. Risk factors for developing gestational diabetes include family history of type 2 diabetes, advanced maternal age, obesity, and non-Caucasian ethnicity. Screening for diabetes is recommended for all pregnancies between 24 and 28 weeks' gestation using a 50-g glucose load followed an hour later by measurement of the glucose level. A value greater than 140 mg/dL indicates the need for a 3-hour glucose tolerance test.

Patients diagnosed with gestational diabetes are counseled to monitor their diet, weight gain, and fasting and postprandial glucose values. Moderate exercise is safe in women without medical or obstetric complications. Absolute contraindications for exercise during pregnancy include significant cardiopulmonary disease, incompetent cervix, premature labor or ruptured membranes, placenta previa, persistent bleeding, pre-eclampsia, or pregnancy-induced HTN. Fasting glucose values greater than 95 mg/dL and postprandial values greater than 120 mg/dL indicate a need for insulin therapy or the initiation of oral hypoglycemics, such as sulfonylureas or metformin.

Fetal monitoring should begin at 32 to 34 weeks' gestation in poorly controlled patients or those with additional risk factors. US surveillance in the late second and third trimesters is also commonly used to monitor amniotic fluid volume and fetal weight. Patients with well-controlled gestational diabetes may be permitted to progress to term before induction of delivery is considered, whereas poorly controlled diabetics or those with abnormal testing (e.g., macrosomia) may require induction or cesarean section after 38 weeks or confirmation of fetal lung maturity.

Maternal glucose testing should be repeated postpartum, since hyperglycemia persists into the postpartum period in up to 10% of women with gestational diabetes. These women are also at increased risk for future diabetes and should be reassessed periodically.

KEY POINTS

- The most common medical problems that develop during pregnancy involve the digestive, cardiopulmonary, genitourinary, hematopoietic, and endocrine systems.

- Nausea and vomiting are common early signs of pregnancy, occurring most often between 6 and 13 weeks and resolving by 22 weeks' gestation.

- HTN and developing DVT are two serious conditions related to pregnancy. Each of these conditions can cause maternal morbidity and mortality as well as fetal compromise.

- UTIs occur in 10% to 15% of pregnant women due to urinary stasis, glycosuria, and vesicoureteral reflux.

- Hemodilution occurs during normal pregnancy; thus anemia during pregnancy is defined as hemoglobin of less than 10 g/dL.

- Gestational diabetes affects 2% to 5% of all pregnancies and is associated with hydramnios, preterm labor, macrosomia, hypertensive disease, fetal hypoglycemia, and hyperbilirubinemia.

65 Postpartum Care

The postpartum period, or puerperium, begins after delivery of the placenta and continues for 6 to 12 weeks. During this time, the physiologic changes of pregnancy revert to the nongravid state. Along with these changes, there are emotional and other psychosocial changes resulting from the delivery and the adjustment to caring for a newborn infant.

POSTPARTUM PHYSIOLOGIC CHANGES

Uterine changes begin immediately upon delivery. First, there is denudation of the endometrium when placental detachment occurs. Contraction of the uterus and thrombosis of vessels lead to hemostasis. Bleeding does occur following delivery but diminishes to a reddish-brown discharge by the third day postpartum. The endometrium is infiltrated by leukocytes and begins restoration. A mucopurulent discharge (lochia serosa) is present for up to 3 weeks, followed by a yellow-white discharge (lochia alba) that may persist for up to 6 weeks. A brief period of bleeding may occur about 14 days following delivery due to sloughing of the endometrial eschar. At term, the pregnant uterus is 10 times larger and heavier than in the nongravid state. Within 2 weeks of delivery, the uterus is within the pelvis; by 6 weeks, it has returned to its normal size.

Prolactin elevation leads to suppression of ovarian function in the postpartum period. In women who do not breast-feed, prolactin levels will return to normal by the third week and ovulatory function returns on average by 10 weeks postpartum. In women who breast-feed, prolactin levels remain elevated and ovulation is suppressed for 6 months or more in over 90% of those who exclusively breast-feed.

POSTPARTUM CARE

The usual postpartum hospital stay is 2 days for vaginal deliveries and 3 to 4 days for cesarean section deliveries. During this time, the mother is able to learn how to care for her infant. Breast-feeding should be encouraged and rooming in of the infant permitted so as to facilitate feeding and promote maternal–infant bonding. An experienced mother with an uncomplicated delivery

and good home support may be discharged earlier than 2 days. Typical follow-up in the office is in 1 to 2 weeks for evaluation of the infant and at 6 weeks for the mother. In many cases, physicians will arrange for earlier infant follow-up in the office if the mother and child are discharged early.

The patient should be counseled about the normal postpartum bleeding and discharge. If she has not had a laceration or episiotomy, she may use tampons with instructions to change them frequently. Patients who have had lacerations or episiotomies should be instructed to report any significant pain or fever. Care for the perineal wound should include use of laxatives, regular bathing or showering, and pain medication. For those with significant edema, sitz baths may provide added relief.

Physical activity will vary by the individual but can be according to patient tolerance. For patients who have had cesarean section deliveries, driving and physical activity should be restricted until pain subsides. Sexual activity may be resumed in uncomplicated deliveries when bleeding subsides and patient comfort permits. For those with lacerations or episiotomies, sexual activity should be avoided for at least 3 weeks.

POSTPARTUM COMPLICATIONS

Many patients experience one or more problems in the postpartum period. The most common problems are perineal pain, lactation-related problems, incontinence, bleeding, infections, or depression. The most common problems requiring readmission to the hospital are excessive bleeding and infection.

Normal blood loss following vaginal delivery is less than 500 mL; amounts exceeding this are considered to represent postpartum hemorrhage. Postpartum hemorrhage is described as early (<24 hours) or late (>24 hours). Almost three-quarters of postpartum hemorrhages are secondary to uterine atony. Other causes of postpartum hemorrhage include vaginal and cervical lacerations, retained products of conception, placenta accreta, and uterine rupture. A thorough examination must be performed at the time the bleeding is noted. While the cause is being determined, intravenous fluids should be administered and RBCs typed and cross-matched for possible transfusion. If no site of bleeding is identified and the patient is unstable, she should be taken to the operating room for further examination.

If a laceration is discovered, repair should be performed. For uterine atony, oxytocin, prostaglandins and methylergonovine are administered along with uterine massage. If bleeding continues, dilatation and curettage may be warranted. Dilatation and curettage is also indicated for suspected retained products of conception. Patients with suspected placenta accreta or uterine rupture require exploratory laparotomy and surgical repair.

Common causes of postpartum fever are UTI, endometritis, or mastitis. In patients with a perineal laceration or episiotomy repair, it is important to examine the site for infection. Patients with UTIs may complain of dysuria and suprapubic or back pain. A UA should be obtained along with urine culture. Antibiotics should initially cover gram-negative organisms and can be modified when culture results are available. Patients with endometritis most commonly present 2 to 5 days after delivery but can present a week or more following delivery with fever, malodorous vaginal bleeding, and uterine tenderness. Therapy includes use of broad-spectrum antibiotics until the patient has been afebrile for 48 hours and the WBC has normalized. Mastitis will present as a painful, tender breast with associated erythema, usually in the second or third postpartum week. The patient should be treated with antibiotics active against gram-positive organisms, including *Staphylococcus*, along with local moist heat and analgesics if needed. The patient may continue to breast-feed during therapy.

Urinary or fecal incontinence occurs in many women following delivery. Urinary incontinence occurs in up to 15% of women and anal incontinence in approximately 5%. Anal incontinence occurs more commonly after vaginal operative deliveries or deliveries associated with anal sphincter injury. Both conditions are generally self-limited and resolve within 6 months. Kegal exercises may be helpful in treating urinary incontinence. For those with persisting symptoms, further evaluation for neurologic or anatomic causes is warranted.

Lactation-related problems include breast engorgement, lactation failure, nipple confusion, and nipple soreness. Education of the patient in the prenatal and immediate postpartum periods can help to prevent these problems. Symptomatic breast engorgement occurs on the second to fourth days in those who do not breast-feed. In breast-feeding mothers, hot compresses before nursing may assist with the let-down of milk, and an increased frequency of feedings will resolve this problem. Lactation failure may be treated in a similar fashion, along with assessment of technique. If lactation failure occurs in association with excessive vaginal bleeding, the patient should be evaluated for retained products of conception. Nipple confusion will occur as a result of feeding infants from a bottle as well as the breast and can be prevented by breast-feeding exclusively. Nipple soreness requires a physical examination and evaluation of feeding technique. Proper positioning, frequent shorter feedings, and allowing the nipples to air-dry may assist with healing. Candidal infection can cause nipple soreness and can be treated with topical nystatin.

Many patients will complain of depressed mood following delivery. It is important to inquire about how the patient is adjusting to the newborn. During the initial 2 weeks, if the symptoms remain mild, observation and supportive care may be all that is necessary. This self-limited state is often referred to as the "postpartum blues." Up to 20% of women have more severe symptoms consistent with a major depression that requires treatment. If the patient has a past history of depression or of postpartum depression, the patient should be followed closely, being seen in the office 1 or 2 weeks after delivery. For those at risk, postpartum medication and/or psychotherapy have been shown to be effective therapies.

POSTPARTUM CONTRACEPTION

Contraception is discussed in Chapter 61. In women who are not breast-feeding, oral contraceptives can be started 2 to 3 weeks following delivery, though many physicians advise waiting for 6 weeks because of the associated thromboembolic risks. Combination oral contraceptives may suppress or diminish lactation and thus should not be started until the milk supply is established. Some authorities recommend progestin-only as the preferred method of hormonal contraception in those who wish to breast-feed. IUDs should not be inserted until 8 to 10 weeks following delivery so as to limit risk of perforation and expulsion of the IUD. Diaphragm fitting should be performed at the 6-week postpartum visit, since a previously used diaphragm may no longer fit properly. Recommendations for condoms and sterilization techniques are unaffected by the postpartum state.

KEY POINTS

- During the 6-week postpartum period, the physiologic changes of pregnancy revert to the previously nongravid condition.
- Postpartum complications of bleeding and infection are the most common causes of hospital readmission.
- Postpartum depression affects up to 20% of women.

Chapter 66

Preventive Care: Newborn to 5 Years

The American Academy of Family Physicians recommends a minimum of five visits from birth to 2 years of age and three visits for ages 2 to 6. Factors that determine the content of these visits are age-related disease prevalence, psychosocial behaviors, and development for the given age group.

During the ages between birth and 5 years, the most common causes of morbidity and mortality are perinatally acquired disease, congenital disease, SIDS, and accidents. Prior to the introduction of vaccines, infectious disease was also a significant contributor to infant and early childhood morbidity and mortality. The content of preventive health in this category involves physical examination and assessment of childhood development, administration of vaccines, screening for treatable congenital conditions, and counseling about safety issues.

NEWBORNS

Birth is a time of both joy and significant anxiety for parents. Most families, especially first-time parents, need education, reassurance, and encouragement. Ideally, education should begin during the prenatal period and continue during and after the hospital stay. Topics should include nutrition, sleeping, infant behavior, bathing, and elimination habits. At the first office visit, each newborn should receive a complete examination to detect abnormalities that might not have been apparent in the hospital.

NUTRITION

Either infant formula or breast milk can meet an infant's nutritional needs for at least 4 to 6 months. Breast-feeding is encouraged because of its low cost, convenience, and associated mother–infant bonding. Breast milk also contains all the nutrients required for good growth with the possible exception of vitamin D, which should be supplemented if there is a lack of sun exposure. Breast milk contains immunoglobulins such as immunoglobulin A (IgA), which result in fewer enteric and respiratory infections in breast-fed infants as well as a lower incidence of allergies and asthma as the child gets older. Working mothers can either pump their breasts and refrigerate or freeze the breast milk or breast-feed part time and formula-feed part time. Contraindications to breast-feeding are rare; they include metabolic diseases that require special formulas, maternal ingestion of medications transmissible in the breast milk that would be harmful to the infant, or maternal infectious disease such as HIV. The best way to determine whether breast-feeding is adequate is to monitor weights. Parents can also gauge adequate intake by monitoring the number of wet diapers per day (more than six).

Jaundice from breast-feeding peaks at 10 to 14 days of age. If jaundice is due to breast-feeding, holding breast-feeding for 12 to 24 hours often results in a significant drop in the bilirubin. In extreme cases, phototherapy or exchange transfusion may be necessary.

Formula provides adequate infant nutrition, and mothers who choose not to breast-feed should not be made to feel guilty. Iron-fortified formulas are recommended. Initially feeding the infant 1 to 2 oz of formula every 3 to 4 hours and on demand is appropriate.

SLEEP

Although sleep patterns vary among infants, a newborn often sleeps up to 20 hours/day. Infants should sleep on their backs, since the prone position has been associated with an increased risk for SIDS.

INFANT BEHAVIOR

All babies cry. Crying may be a sign of hunger, discomfort, a wet diaper, frustration, or a desire for attention. The average infant cries for 1 to 3 hours/day, and daily periods of crying can occur, often in the afternoon or early evening. Rhythm rockers, pacifiers, swaddling, and cuddling are common methods to reduce crying. Uncontrollable crying can be a sign of illness and merits medical evaluation. Infant colic is characterized by paroxysmal crying or irritability in the evening hours in an otherwise healthy infant. The crying episodes last for more than 3 hours/day and occur more than 3 days/week. Infantile colic generally has its onset by 3 weeks of age; almost 90% of cases resolve by 4 months of age.

In addition to inconsolable crying, the infant who feeds poorly, shows signs of respiratory difficulty, or exhibits skin color changes (e.g., cyanosis, jaundice) should be evaluated by a physician. Although infants may not mount a fever with infection, the presence of fever mandates physician evaluation. The parents should be instructed in proper methods for obtaining a rectal temperature in the infant.

BATHING

Sponge baths are recommended until the umbilical cord falls off (10 to 14 days of age). While the umbilical cord stump is still attached, the area around the cord can be cleaned with wipes at diaper changes. After the cord falls off, the child can be immersed in a small tub in up to 3 to 4 inches of water. Baths should be limited to every other day to avoid dry skin, and only baby soap should be used. The scalp should be washed once or twice a week. A mild shampoo can be used in children with cradle cap. Parents should be instructed never to place the infant in water warmer than 115°F (46°C) and never to turn their attention away while the infant is in the tub.

STOOLS

Breast-fed babies have between three and eight stools a day. Formula-fed infants generally have fewer. Many parents have concerns regarding infant constipation because of the grunting and facial redness associated with passage of bowel movements or due to lack of daily bowel movements. Infants and toddlers usually have visible straining for passage of normal bowel movements. After 2 weeks of age, infants may have less frequent bowel movements. If the infant is passing soft stools, having bowel movements every 3 to 7 days, is feeding adequately, and is otherwise well, the parents can be reassured.

Diaper rashes are common and usually respond to keeping the diaper area clean and dry. Harsh soaps should be avoided, and leaving the diaper area open to air is helpful for almost all types of diaper rashes.

Satellite lesions and involvement of the inguinal folds often identify a secondary infection with yeast. A yeast infection usually improves with topical antifungal preparations and frequent diaper changes.

SCREENING

In addition to a careful physical examination, infants require routine neonatal screening that differs from state to state but usually includes hypothyroidism, phenylketonuria, and galactosemia. Early recognition and treatment of these metabolic disorders can prevent irreversible damage. Neonates also receive prophylactic antibiotic eye ointment to prevent infections with *Neisseria gonorrhoeae* or *Chlamydia*, which may be acquired as the infant passes through the birth canal. Vitamin K is administered to prevent hemorrhagic disease of the newborn. Infants exposed in utero to HIV, syphilis, or hepatitis B need testing and appropriate treatment. Most states mandate a newborn hearing screen before discharge from the hospital, and abnormal tests will require follow-up. Many doctors recommend giving the first hepatitis B immunization prior to discharge from the hospital; however, in low-risk infants, this may be delayed until the first office visit.

1 TO 2 WEEKS

The first follow-up visit is commonly scheduled at 1 to 2 weeks of age. This visit should reinforce previous counseling and assess the adjustment of the parents and infant to the home environment. Questions regarding infant care and inquiry into infant feeding and elimination patterns should be part of this visit. Review of the perinatal congenital screening laboratory tests and examination of the infant with a focus on weight and the presence of jaundice are important. Newborns should regain their birth weight by 2 weeks of age. Intervention may be required for those with significant elevations in bilirubin level. Those infants who did not receive hepatitis B vaccine during hospitalization should receive the first of this three-shot series.

1 TO 18 MONTHS

Visits during this period will coincide with vaccine administration, with one extra visit at approximately 9 months of age. During this time, in addition to physical examination, the focus of the visits is on addressing parental concerns, reviewing the infant's growth and development, and administering vaccines. Counseling should also be provided regarding "childproofing" the home and safety measures such as storage of hazardous or poisonous materials in a

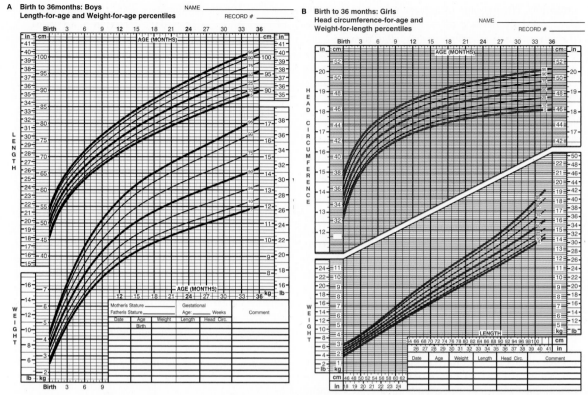

Figure 66-1 • A: Birth to 36 months: Boys—length-for-age and weight-for-age percentiles. Published May 30, 2000 (modified 4/20/01). **B:** Birth to 36 months: Girls—head circumference-for-age and weight-for-length percentiles. Published May 30, 2000 (modified 10/16/00). (Developed by the National Center for Health Statistics in collaboration with the National Center for Chronic Disease Prevention and Health Promotion (2000). http://www.cdc.gov/growthcharts.)

locked or out-of-reach cabinet, covering electric outlets, and providing the parents with a phone number for poison control.

Growth (height, weight, head circumference) should be plotted on a growth chart in order to assure that the rate of growth is proceeding normally (Figure 66-1A and B). Generally an infant should double its birth weight by 4 months and triple it by 1 year of age. Childhood development can be assessed through use of an instrument such as the Denver Developmental Screening Tool and by inquiring and observing the child's behavior in verbal, motor, and psychosocial skills (Table 66-1). A lead and hemoglobin level is generally obtained at 9 to 15 months of age. TB screening with an intradermal purified protein derivative (PPD) is recommended for all high-risk children at 12 to 15 months and is required by some preschools. Fluoride supplementation for infants living in areas with an inadequately fluorinated water supply should begin at 6 months of age. Solid foods should usually be introduced at 4 to 6 months of age. Prevention of bottle caries should be addressed and dental care of newly erupting teeth discussed. Most experts recommend that children be weaned from

the bottle by age 12 months to reduce the risk of dental decay.

As the child develops, additional topics in parental counseling will include window and stair guards and gates to prevent falls; storing of firearms, matches, and toxic substances in a locked or inaccessible place; and assuring that windowshade cords do not pose a risk. Even as a passenger on a bicycle, the infant or toddler should be provided with a helmet to prevent injury. Use of sunscreens and prevention of excessive sun exposure and sunburns to prevent future risk of skin cancer should begin at the infant stage and be reinforced frequently.

2 TO 5 YEARS

During this interval, there are usually no vaccinations to administer until the 5-year-old visit. Visits during this time are annual checkups where the child will have a physical examination, including BP measurement starting at age 3 years. Review of growth and development and reinforcement of safety measures are a focus of the visits. Prior to school entry, children should have their vision and hearing checked. TB screening (PPD) is required for

TABLE 66-1 Commonly Quizzed Developmental Milestones

Age	Gross Motor	Fine (Visual) Motor	Language	Social
1 month	Raises head slightly from prone	Follows with eyes to midline only; tight grasp	Alerts/startles to sound	Fixes on face
2 months			Smiles responsively	Recognizes parent
3 months	Holds head up, steady	Hands open at rest	Coos	Reaches for familiar objects or people
4–5 months	Rolls front to back, back to front; sits well supported	Grasps with both hands together	Orients to voice	Enjoys observing environment
6 months	Sits well unsupported	Transfers hand to hand; reaches with either hand	Babbles	Recognizes strangers
9 months	Crawls, cruises, pulls to stand	Uses pincer grasp; fingerfeeds	Begins to use "dada/mama"; understands "no"	Plays pat-a-cake
12 months	Walks alone	Throws, releases objects	1–8 words other than "dada/mama"; follows one-step commands	Imitates; comes when called; cooperates with dressing
15 months	Walks backward; creeps upstairs	Builds two-block tower; scribbles		
18 months	Runs	Feeds self (messily) with utensils	Points to body parts when asked	Plays around (not with) other children
21 months	Squats and recovers	Builds five-block tower	Two-word combinations	
24 months	Walks well up and down stairs	Removes clothing	Understands two-step commands; stranger understands half of speech	Parallel play
30 months	Throws ball overhand		Appropriate pronoun use	Knows first, last names
3 years	Pedals tricycle	Draws a circle	Three-word sentences; past tense; stranger uses plurals, understands three-fourth of speech	Group play; shares
4 years	Alternates feet going down stairs; skips	Catches ball; dresses alone	Knows colors	Imaginative play
5 years		Ties shoes	Prints first name	Plays co-operative games; understands "rules" and abides by them

Reprinted from Marino S, et al. *Blueprints Pediatrics*. 3rd ed. Malden, MA: Blackwell Publishing; 2004:44, with permission. Copyright 2004, Blackwell Publishing.

entry into most preschools, schools, and day care. The National Cholesterol Education Program recommends that children with a positive family history of premature CAD (<age 50 in men or <age 60 in women) or with parents with elevated cholesterol values undergo cholesterol screening beginning at age 2 years. A lead screening questionnaire can be used to determine which children in this age group need lead screening.

The 5-year visit is important for assessing school "readiness." The average child should be able to name four to five colors, know his or her age, and draw a person with a head, body, arms, and legs. Parents should make sure their child knows his or her name, address, and telephone number as well as how to deal with strangers.

KEY POINTS

- Preventive health care in children begins at birth.
- In addition to providing vaccinations and physical examinations, growth and development should be assessed.
- Counseling regarding infant and child care as well as safety measures is an important part of each health care visit.
- Breast milk contains immunoglobulins such as IgA, which result in fewer enteric and respiratory infections in breast-fed infants.
- Contraindications to breast-feeding are rare; they include metabolic diseases that require special formulas, instances where the mother takes a medication that is passed in the breast milk and is harmful to the infant, or if the mother has a contagious illness such as HIV.
- Infants should sleep on their backs, since the prone position has been associated with an increased risk of SIDS.

Health care visits during this time generally occur episodically in association with illness, summer camp physicals, or preparticipation clearance for sports activities. When children change schools, advance from elementary to middle school, or enter high school, they may be required to obtain physical examinations prior to entry. Thus, routine health care measures and counseling often have to be incorporated into visits for illness or preparticipation examinations.

The leading causes of morbidity and mortality in this age category are accidents along with homicide and suicide, which increase in prevalence as children enter adolescence. Also as children enter adolescence, increased risk-taking behavior and experimentation frequently lead to the use of cigarettes or other substances and high-risk sexual activities. In addition to the physical examination, review of immunization status, growth, and development and counseling are important to include during these health care visits (Table 67-1).

5 TO 6 YEARS

The health care visit at this age may be the last required visit until the child enters junior high school. Accidents continue to be the leading cause of morbidity and mortality at this age. In addition to reviewing the past medical history, including growth and development, preventive services should focus on updating any necessary vaccinations and providing counseling and anticipatory guidance. For children with chronic diseases, such as asthma, pneumococcal vaccine and annual influenza vaccination is recommended. For children who have not had chickenpox or have not been immunized, the varicella vaccine can be offered. The physical examination should include BP measurement, vision testing, and hearing screening. Screening for TB should be provided to those at risk, such as children living in poverty, those residing in areas where TB is prevalent, and those with history of TB exposure. Lipid screening should be encouraged in children with family history of premature CAD or with parents with cholesterol over 240 mg/dL. Routine UA is no longer recommended.

Counseling and anticipatory guidance are important parts of health care visits during childhood.

Safety issues to discuss include the routine use of seat belts and bicycle helmets, firearm safety, safe storage of toxic substances (including matches and lighters), and rules regarding encounters with strangers. Parents should be encouraged to provide good role modeling and a healthy environment that is smoke-free, includes a healthy diet, and incorporates exercise as part of the family routine. Protection from excess sun exposure should be encouraged for the entire family. Regular teeth brushing, flossing, and visits to the dentist should be encouraged. Television viewing should be limited, reading encouraged, and exposure to violence monitored. Children should be encouraged to participate in age-appropriate activities and praised liberally for their positive actions.

7 TO 12 YEARS

The child may have no routinely scheduled health care visits during this age range. Preventive care and counseling during this time may have to be incorporated into sick visits or preparticipation examinations. The physical examination should include BP measurement, assessment of growth and sexual development, and scoliosis screening. This last can be performed by having the child assume a diving position with the hands together and the trunk forward flexed. Asymmetry of the rib cage along the spine may be indicative of an abnormality. Immunization status should be reviewed and updated to ensure that the child is current with regards to MMR and hepatitis B vaccines. Pneumococcal vaccination and annual influenza shots should be administered to at-risk children. More recent immunization guidelines call for Tdap, and meningococcal vaccines for all 11- to 12-year olds and human papillomavirus vaccine for 11- to 12-year-old girls. Lipid screening can be offered for children with a strong family history of atherosclerosis. Vision and hearing screening should be performed if the history or physical examination suggests concerns about vision or hearing.

Counseling and anticipatory guidance should continue to emphasize accident prevention. Seat belt and bicycle helmet use should be reinforced. Water safety, along with encouraging the child to learn to swim, can be discussed during the visit.

■ TABLE 67-1 Preventive Care Ages 5 Years to 12 Years

Ages	Morbidity and Mortality	Testing/Vaccine	Counseling
5–6	Accidents	Blood pressure	Seatbelts
		Vision	Bicycle helmets
		Hearing	Firearms
		Tuberculosis (high risk)	Water safety
		Lipids (high risk)	Matches/poisons
		MMR	Exposure to violence
		IPV	Dental care
		DTaP	Exercise
		Pneumococcal[a]	Sun exposure
		Influenza[a]	
		Varicella[b]	
7–12	Accidents	Blood pressure	Seatbelts
		Scoliosis	Bicycle helmets
		Lipids (high risk)	Firearms
		Tuberculosis (high risk)	Water safety
		Hepatitis B	Matches/poisons
		MMR	Exposure to violence
		Pneumococcal[a]	Sun exposure
		Influenza[a]	Dental care
		Varicella[b]	Exercise
		Tdap	Diet
		Meningococcal	Tobacco/drugs/alcohol
		Human papillomavirus[c]	

[a]At-risk individuals.
[b]Offer in absence of prior disease.
[c]Recommended for 11- to 12-year-old girls.

Parents and their children should be educated regarding the importance of avoiding sunburns as well as the importance of using sunscreens and protective clothing in order to lower future risk of skin cancer. Additional questions to assess violence exposure, mood, and potential for engaging in high-risk behaviors should be incorporated into the visit. This portion of the interaction is best performed without the parents in the examination room. Reinforcement of healthful behaviors regarding exercise, sleep, and diet as well as abstinence from sexual activity, tobacco, drugs, and alcohol are important messages for the child to receive from the physician and his or her parents. Encouraging the parents to discuss these topics with their children is important, as is role modeling of the positive behaviors desired in the child.

KEY POINTS

- Accidents are a major cause of morbidity and mortality during childhood.

- As children enter adolescence, homicides and suicides are other leading causes of morbidity and mortality.

- In addition to accident prevention, counseling should be provided regarding risks associated with sun exposure, cigarette smoking, substance abuse, and sexual activity.

Adolescent Medicine

Adolescence is a period of rapid physical, cognitive, and emotional change. Physically, adolescent patients are generally very healthy. As a result, health care visits by adolescent patients are infrequent, generally occurring in association with illness or preparticipation evaluation for sporting activities. Problem-related visits are generally for respiratory, dermatologic, or musculoskeletal conditions. During the course of these examinations, many issues that might not necessarily fall within the scope of the visit should be addressed in order to provide comprehensive health care to this group of patients.

To obtain accurate information about the adolescent patient's habits and concerns, the patient and his or her parents must understand the need for confidentiality in all matters that do not pose an imminent threat to the patient's or others' lives. In order also to include the parents in their child's health care, the interview can be conducted in two phases, with the parents initially present and voicing their concerns, followed by a talk with the patient alone. Arrangements can be made with the parents that allow the patient to seek care when he or she feels it to be necessary, thus providing better access for care. In many states, adolescent patients can seek care on their own for STDs, pregnancy, contraception, and mental illness, including substance abuse. The ability to maintain this confidentiality may be compromised by the patient's limited resources and bills/insurance statements that are sent to the parents.

CLINICAL MANIFESTATIONS

HISTORY

In addition to eliciting parental concerns and the details surrounding these concerns, information regarding the past medical history, medication use, allergies, and family and social histories should be obtained. Immunization status should be reviewed. Additional history will have to be obtained directly from the adolescent patient without the parents' presence. Because of their increasing autonomy, emerging sexual identity, and the influence of peer groups, questions specific to adolescent patients are necessary (Box 68-1). Asking these questions in a nonthreatening way, such as "Some patients of mine ..." or "Do any of your

■ **BOX 68-1** Sample Questions for Adolescent Patients
Environment
Who lives in your home?
Who are you closest to at home?
Have there been any recent changes at home?
How do you get along with others at home?
Do you feel safe?
Education/Activities
How is school?
What grade are you in?
How are your grades?
What do you want to do after you graduate?
What do you and your friends do for fun?
What extracurricular activities are you involved with?
What are your hobbies?
Have you had a job?
How much do you exercise in an average day/week?
Body Image/Mood
How do you feel about your weight?
Has your weight changed recently?
What do you like or do not like about your body?
Do you ever feel sad or down?
How do you make yourself feel better?
Have you ever tried to hurt yourself or kill yourself?
Sexuality
Do you have a boyfriend or girlfriend?
Have you ever had sex?
Have you used condoms or other types of contraception?

(continued)

■ BOX 68-1 Sample Questions for Adolescent Patients (continued)

Have you ever been pregnant?
Have you ever had a sexually transmitted disease?
Drugs/Safety
Do you wear a seat belt?
Do you use a helmet for biking/rollerblading?
Do any of your friends smoke/drink/use drugs?
Have you ever smoked/drunk/used drugs?
Have you ever driven a vehicle after drinking/using drugs?
Have you ever ridden in a vehicle where the driver has used drugs or alcohol?

friends or the kids at school ..." may allow for more candid responses. Although adolescent patients do not openly show concern about their health, studies suggest that many do have such concerns. Many of these concerns may be related to the issues they are facing regarding their changing bodies, sexuality, substance use, or peer pressure. Nonthreatening questions about their concerns can help to provide any needed reassurance or counseling.

PHYSICAL EXAMINATION

The physical examination should include BP measurement, assessment of growth and development (including sexual maturity), scoliosis screening, and a general physical examination. A pelvic examination is indicated for sexually active teens and for teens with genitourinary complaints. For those with visual or hearing complaints, screening should be performed.

Assessment of cognitive and psychosocial development can be difficult. During adolescence, thought processes should change from concrete in nature to the ability to think abstractly. Another task of adolescence is developing autonomy and a sense of personal and sexual identity. Success in courses such as algebra and geometry indicates expected advancement from concrete to abstract thought processes. The development of increasing autonomy will be indicated by less interest in activities with parents/family and an increase in responsiveness to peer pressures and interest in peer-related activities. Advancing to the formation of a personal and sexual identity may be indicated by boyfriend/girlfriend relationships and the diminishing importance of the peer group.

Determining sexual maturity (Table 68-1) can assist in providing counseling regarding menarche and concerns about maturity. Pubertal changes occur earlier in girls than in boys and are heralded by the formation of the breast bud. The first sign of puberty in boys is testicular enlargement. In girls, the growth spurt generally occurs around Tanner stage 3, whereas in boys it does not occur until Tanner stage 4. Menarche occurs near the end of the growth spurt, which is on average at 12.8 years of age.

SCREENING

A tetanus booster shot, utilizing Tdap to include pertussis, and meningococcal vaccines are recommended at 11 to 12 years of age and should also be

■ TABLE 68-1 Tanner Stages of Sexual Maturity

Stage	Boys	Girls
1	Child-like penis No enlargement of testicles No pubic hair	No breast development No pubic hair
2	Penis unchanged Scrotum and testicles enlarge Small amount of fine, long pubic hair	Breast buds Small amount of fine, long pubic hair
3	Penis elongates Continued growth of testicles and scrotum Coarse and curly pubic hair	Breasts enlarge, areolas enlarge Coarse and curly pubic hair
4	Penis increased in diameter Darkening of scrotum Adult hair texture over pubic area	Continued breast growth Adult hair texture over pubic area
5	Adult penis, scrotum Pubic hair extends to thighs	Adult breast contours Pubic hair extends to thighs

provided for adolescents between the ages of 14 and 16 years who have not been previously vaccinated. For those individuals not currently on any vaccine or who have not had chickenpox, vaccination should be offered. Lipid screening should be encouraged in children with a family history of premature CAD or with parents whose cholesterol is above 240 mg/dL. A hemoglobin test is recommended for menstruating teenagers. Routine UA is no longer recommended.

Accidents continue to be the leading cause of death in the adolescent population. Other causes that increase in importance as the child enters adolescence are homicides and suicides. In addition, increased risk-taking behavior occurs during this period, leading to experimentation with tobacco, drugs, alcohol, and sexual activities. Since adolescence is often the time when adult behaviors develop, it is important to lay the groundwork for a healthy lifestyle. Thus, counseling during this age should include not only emphasis on accident prevention but also inquiries into these other high-risk behaviors.

The incidence of depression increases throughout adolescence to approximately 10% at age 18. Over half of adolescent girls and nearly three-quarters of adolescent boys will have sexual intercourse before they are 18 years of age. Thus, to have an impact on these common issues related to the adolescent period, identification of at-risk individuals, encouraging

dialogue on these matters between adolescent and parent, and referring those in need of further therapy is beneficial. Discussion of the risks associated with the use of the substances should be part of the counseling. In addition, counseling adolescents about birth control, STDs, and responsible sexual activity is important. For sexually active individuals, examination and screening for STDs are also recommended. Sexually active teenage women should have Pap smears beginning 3 years after onset of sexual activity or at age 21, whichever comes first. Vaccination against human papillomavirus should be provided to adolescent girls at ages 11 to 12 years and to older girls who have not been previously vaccinated.

KEY POINTS

- Parents can be included in the history but must respect the adolescent patient's need for confidentiality in receiving medical care.

- During adolescence, accidents, homicides, and suicides are leading causes of morbidity and mortality among adolescents; counseling should be provided regarding these risks.

- Over half of the 18-year-olds are sexually active and should be screened for STDs.

Common Medical Problems in Children

Many of the common medical conditions in children are covered in other chapters. Some additional conditions that are unique to children and that are discussed here include failure to thrive (FTT), stridor and croup, crying/colic, and seizure disorders (including febrile seizures).

FAILURE TO THRIVE

FTT is defined as failure of the child to grow and develop at an appropriate rate. This describes a condition and not a cause for the aberrant growth pattern. FTT should be suspected and evaluation undertaken when weight for height is less than 80% of predicted ideal weight, when the rate of growth is too slow (i.e., decreasing over two major percentile lines on growth chart), and when developmental or interactional milestones are delayed.

PATHOGENESIS

In order to grow and develop normally, children require oxygen, adequate nutrition/energy balance, hormonal balance, and love/nurturing. Energy needs must be met to satisfy basal metabolic requirements and support the child's growth. Conditions that lead to inadequate caloric intake, such as neglect or malabsorptive digestive disorders, will lead to slowed growth. Conditions that increase caloric expenditure or lead to less efficient use of calories, such as chronic infection or chronic pulmonary diseases, will make it difficult to meet caloric needs for growth. Finally, children who are neglected but provided with adequate calories and nutritional intake will not grow at a normal rate because their needs for emotional support and nurturing are unmet. The exact reason for this etiology of FTT is unknown but demonstrates the need for love and nurturing of children.

CLINICAL MANIFESTATIONS

History

The history should be focused and thorough, including events around birth, the social environment, family supports, and the types and amounts of foods offered to the child. A detailed review of systems should assess for respiratory, GI, and neurodevelopmental

milestones. The pregnancy history should be reviewed, including whether it was planned, any maternal conditions during pregnancy, substance abuse in the home, and whether the child was delivered at term or prematurely. Parental stature is also an important consideration in evaluating a child's growth.

Physical Examination

The physical examination will focus on growth parameters in addition to a thorough physical overview. Particular attention should be on the recognition of any dysmorphic features that may warrant referral for genetic evaluation. Any identified abnormalities, such as heart murmurs, should be evaluated. Social interactions with the examiner and developmental achievements should be noted.

DIAGNOSTIC EVALUATION

Laboratory evaluation should include a CBC, metabolic profile, UA with culture, and evaluation of the stool for reducing substances, occult blood, and ova and parasites. Additional studies are indicated as directed by the history and physical examination.

TREATMENT

Management includes a detailed psychosocial assessment of the home environment and frequently requires enlistment of social service assistance to uncover any social needs or parenting issues that should be addressed. Enrollment in public assistance programs, such as the Special Supplemental Nutrition Program for Women, Infants, and Children (WIC), may be of benefit. If there are concerns about neglect, Child Protective Services should be contacted to assess the suitability of the current home environment for the child. In cases where no cause is determined and the child continues to exhibit inadequate growth or in instances of severe malnutrition, hospitalization may be required for further assessment and to monitor growth and nutritional intake.

COLIC AND CRYING

Crying is a childhood form of communication that occurs commonly in infants. Crying may be normal or excessive. Normal infants at 2 weeks of age cry on average for 1¾ hours/day. Peak crying activity occurs at around 6 weeks of age and averages 2¾ hours/day. By 3 months of age, crying time in normal infants decreases to an average of 1 hour daily. Excessive crying is defined as crying more than 3 hours/day for more than 3 days/week. Excessive crying may be secondary to distress or disease or may be idiopathic. Idiopathic excessive crying is termed colic; it is generally self-limited and resolves by 3 months of age.

PATHOGENESIS

Many theories have been proposed to explain the causes of colic, but no data support one over another. Infants suffering from colic are thought to be more difficult and temperamental and more sensitive to environmental stimuli, hence respond by crying excessively. Parental responses to crying and anxiety are controversial contributing factors that may be primary or secondary to the excessive crying. Finally, many theories regarding GI motility, excess intestinal gas, or food or lactose sensitivity have been proposed. A combination of factors is probably contributory and no single cause has been delineated. Box 69-1 lists common causes of excessive crying.

CLINICAL MANIFESTATIONS

History

When parents bring their child in for evaluation of crying, a thorough history and physical examination are warranted. The birth history, prior history of any medical concerns, social history, and supports should all be noted. The onset of crying, parental responses, and specific parental concerns will help in evaluating the infant. Infant feeding, bowel movements, and sleep behaviors should be assessed.

■ BOX 69-1 Common Causes for Excessive Crying
Idiopathic (colic)
Anal fissure
Child abuse (fracture, shaken baby)
Constipation
Corneal abrasion/foreign body
Dermatitis
Gastroesophageal reflux
Otitis media
Urinary tract infection
Sickle cell disease
Stomatitis
Tourniquet injury to digit/penis (hair or fiber)

Physical Examination

The physical examination should be thorough and should evaluate for secondary causes of the infant's crying. Weight gain and growth are important parameters to monitor. Conditions noted in Box 69-1 should be evaluated. Laboratory evaluation may include UA and culture but otherwise is directed by identified factors in the history and physical examination.

TREATMENT

Physician reassurance that crying is a normal infant/child behavior, that crying does not harm the child, and that the behavior peaks at 6 weeks of age and wanes after 3 months of age is the first step. Management should then focus on parental strategies to respond to their infant or child and address the forms of distress that may be causing the crying. Parents may be armed with a set of responses to comfort the child. For example, they may cuddle and hold or rock the child initially. If crying persists, then changing and feeding the child may be tried. If crying persists, then changing the environment, such as going for a walk, may be attempted.

During the assessment of infants for colic or crying, parental frustration and child safety should be determined. Involving both parents or trusted friends or relatives may be important in providing respite for parents who are feeling particularly stressed.

STRIDOR AND CROUP

"Stridor" refers to audible, turbulent airflow due to narrowing of the larger airways. "Croup" refers to stridor in combination with hoarseness, a barking cough, and some degree of respiratory distress.

PATHOGENESIS

When the upper airways (subglottic region, vocal cords, pharynx) are affected, the harsh, adventitious respiratory sounds are noted during inspiration. When the obstruction occurs at the cricoid cartilage or below, stridor may be noted during expiration as well as during inspiration. Children are most commonly noted to have stridor because of the smaller caliber of their airways. Causes of stridor may be infectious, anatomic, functional, or due to foreign bodies. Common infectious etiologies include viral croup, bacterial epiglottitis, tracheitis, severe pharyngitis, and bronchitis. Anatomic causes may be congenital (vascular rings, laryngeal webs, choanal atresia) or secondary to airway trauma and scarring, as may occur from trauma, caustic ingestions, or intubation. Functional causes include laxity of the trachea or larynx (tracheomalacia, laryngomalacia) that resolve as the infant matures and the airways grow in diameter.

Croup generally affects children between 6 months and 3 years of age, with a peak incidence of 2 years of age. Croup is typically infectious in nature due to parainfluenza, respiratory syncytial, or influenza viruses. Spasmodic croup is a variant of croup that may be associated with viral upper respiratory infections or allergies and generally occurs at night, develops suddenly, and is recurrent.

CLINICAL MANIFESTATIONS

History

Assessment of children with stridor and croup should note the onset of the symptoms, any associated respiratory symptoms or fever, and the presence of respiratory distress. A foreign body should be suspected in stridor associated with a choking event. Abrupt onset associated with fever and drooling are characteristics of epiglottitis.

Physical Examination

The physical examination should include an assessment of the child's general appearance and vitals signs as well as throat and lung examinations. A child who is ill-appearing, leans forward, and is drooling may have epiglottitis. Throat examination should note size and appearance of the tonsils. On occasion, the epiglottis may be visible, but aggressive attempts at visualization should not be made, since they may upset the child and worsen any tissue trauma or airway edema that is present. Stridor may be heard on lung examination as a harsh inspiratory sound that is maximal over the laryngeal region and transmitted to the lungs. With significant airway narrowing, inspiratory and expiratory phases may be audible. Note should be made of the respiratory effort as evidenced by intercostal retractions and respiratory rate.

DIAGNOSTIC EVALUATION

When a bacterial cause is suspected, CBC, blood culture, and imaging may be helpful. The WBC is elevated with epiglottitis but generally normal or minimally elevated with viral causes. Soft tissue neck x-rays will reveal subglottic narrowing with viral croup, often referred to as the "steeple sign," whereas enlargement of the epiglottis supports the diagnosis of epiglottitis. Many foreign bodies are also visible on x-ray evaluation. CT of the neck and thorax and barium swallow studies may be helpful in evaluating children with stridor and suspected congenital anomalies.

TREATMENT

Treatment of children in respiratory distress often requires hospitalization. Patients with croup and stridor at rest, significant retractions, and decreased air movement warrant close monitoring. Treatment of croup includes the use of humidified oxygen or mist therapy for all patients. For children with mild to moderate symptoms who can be reliably followed up in the office and those who improve in the emergency department, oral dexamethasone has been shown to be effective. For those with more severe disease, dexamethasone can be provided orally or parenterally in the hospital. Racemic epinephrine can be given to those with severe disease, but patients who receive this treatment must be monitored for "rebound" after the effects of the medication wear off. For severe disease, monitoring in an intensive care unit (ICU) may be warranted, since up to 10% of these children require intubation.

Hospitalization is also advisable when epiglottitis or bacterial tracheitis is the suspected cause of stridor. Intravenous antibiotics, close monitoring, and—in many cases—intubation are required for successful treatment of these conditions.

Otolaryngology referral is recommended for those patients with stridor and congenital anomalies, foreign body, caustic ingestion, or trauma.

SEIZURE DISORDERS

Seizures occur due to abnormal discharges of neurons in the brain that occur locally (partial seizure), locally with propagation throughout the brain (complex partial seizure), or diffusely throughout the brain (generalized seizure). Seizures may occur as part of systemic condition such as a febrile illness, brain injury, or metabolic abnormalities, or they may be primary genetic disorders. Febrile seizures are generalized tonic–clonic seizures associated with a rapid rise in temperature due to viral or bacterial non-CNS infection and are the most common form of seizure. Febrile seizures affect up to 5% of children, most commonly between the ages of 6 months and 5 years. Nonfebrile seizures affect 0.5% to 1.0% of children and are classified as outlined in Box 69-2.

CLINICAL MANIFESTATIONS

History

In evaluating a child suspected of having had a seizure, an eyewitness description of the event is very helpful. Older children may be able to describe an aura preceding an event. The child's apparent level of alertness and associated motor activity can help to distinguish partial from generalized seizures. Recurrent episodes of staring or lack of attention may signify absence seizures. Incontinence, injury, and postictal drowsiness are characteristics associated with seizure activity. Review of systems should focus on thorough evaluation of neurologic or infectious diseases, including recent onset of fever.

Past history should be reviewed in detail, with focus on birth history, childhood development, and

BOX 69-2 Classification of Seizure Types

| Generalized |
| Absence |
| Myoclonic |
| Atonic |
| Tonic–clonic |
| Syndromes (e.g., infantile spasms, Lennox–Gastaut) |
| Partial |
| Simple |
| Complex |
| Partial with secondary generalization |
| Febrile |
| Neonatal |

history of CNS injury or infections. Family history of febrile and nonfebrile seizures is associated with an increased risk of seizures in those with affected first-degree relatives.

Physical Examination

The physical examination should note the child's alertness and activity following the event. Temperature elevation may suggest febrile seizure as the diagnosis. A complete physical examination should focus on sources of infection and include a neurologic examination searching for focal deficits. Appropriate developmental milestones should be determined as well.

DIAGNOSTIC EVALUATION

In children suspected of having had a simple febrile seizure (one generalized seizure, less than 15 minutes) who have an obvious source of infection and a normal postictal neurologic examination, no further workup is necessary. Complex febrile seizures are those that are focal or focal with generalization, last longer than 15 minutes, or occur repetitively. Complex febrile seizures require neuroimaging, lumbar puncture, and EEG to be fully evaluated. Patients with nonfebrile seizures should undergo neuroimaging and EEG

evaluation. Additional laboratory testing is dictated by the child's age and past medical history. Glucose testing is generally warranted, and infants with new-onset seizures should undergo screening for metabolic disorders.

TREATMENT

Treatment for febrile seizures consists of use of antipyretics with onset of illness to lessen the rapidity and extent of temperature rise and to prevent seizure activity. Parental education and reassurance are also very important aspects of care in these cases. Therapy for nonfebrile seizures consists of institution of anticonvulsant therapy, generally in consultation with a neurologist. Monitoring seizure control and childhood development are important aspects of care. Two-thirds of children with nonfebrile seizures have a good prognosis developmentally and in terms of seizure control. Some seizure types are associated with a poor prognosis for normal development regardless of success in controlling seizures (complex partial seizures, atypical absence), whereas in others prognosis may depend on the degree of seizure control (infantile spasms).

KEY POINTS

- In order to grow and develop normally, children require oxygen, adequate nutrition/energy balance, hormonal balance, and love/nurturing.

- Excessive crying is defined as crying more than 3 hours/day for more than 3 days/week. Excessive crying may be secondary to distress or disease or may be idiopathic.

- Causes of stridor may have an infectious, anatomic, or functional cause or be due to a foreign body. Common infectious etiologies include viral croup, bacterial epiglottitis, tracheitis, severe pharyngitis, and bronchitis.

- Febrile seizures affect up to 5% of children, most commonly between 6 months and 5 years of age. Nonfebrile seizures affect 0.5% to 1.0% of children.

Behavioral Issues in Children

Childhood is a critical time for the development of behavior and personality. It is therefore important for the family physician to understand normal behavioral development in children as well as how to respond to the challenges that parents of young children are likely to face.

BIRTH TO 2 MONTHS

BONDING AND ATTACHMENT

At birth, bonding occurs as unidirectional feelings of love from the parents to the child. Over the first year, parents and child develop reciprocal feelings toward each other, known as attachment. Strong bonding and attachment are essential for normal, healthy behavioral development and should be actively encouraged. It is important to encourage parents to interact with their children in positive ways and for them to allow time for themselves so that they will be more capable of positive interactions.

TEMPERAMENTS

Infants may display a wide range of temperaments that are partially hard-wired and partially environment-related. Understanding what constitutes a normal temperament helps physicians both to reassure parents and to monitor for truly abnormal behavior. Approximately 40% of infants are considered "easy." They sleep, eliminate, and feed on a relatively regular schedule; react positively to new stimuli; adapt well to new environments; and are generally happy. Some 10% of infants are classified as "difficult." Their sleeping, eating, and elimination schedules are irregular. These infants withdraw from new stimuli, adapt poorly, and are more often in a negative mood. "Slow-to-warm-up," cranky infants make up 15% of children and are known to have a low activity level. All other normal children display a mix of one or more of these temperaments.

CRYING

All infants have periods of crying. Most crying is the way in which infants communicate that they are wet, tired, hot, cold, hungry, need a diaper change, or just want to be held. However, many infants will still have periods of 15 minutes to an hour every day where they cry for no apparent reason. Encourage parents to continue to hold the crying baby to let them know that they are responding to their distress. Over time, parents will recognize these normal bouts of crying and be able to distinguish them from crying that signifies a true emergency. Crying for more than 2 hours straight that is not relieved by holding may be an indication of something more serious; the child should then be evaluated. Colic or unexplained bouts of crying for more than 3 hours a day more than 3 days a week can be very hard on parents. Physicians should let frustrated parents vent about the crying, educate them about normal crying patterns, and help them determine whether their child is truly colicky. They should also be reassured that colic typically resolves by 3 months of age.

2 MONTHS TO 1 YEAR

From 2 months to 1 year, a baby undergoes tremendous transformations and rapid development. At 2 months, the child learns to smile socially and respond to the parents. Prior to this, infants smile at random, and this can be frustrating to the parent. When social smiling appears, the parental response is generally positive and allows the parents to reinforce the behavior and the infant's learning.

As the infant learns to crawl and walk, its curiosity and desire to explore and learn can make parents anxious. Counsel parents on child safety but encourage them to allow their child to explore in a safe setting so that he or she can continue to learn and develop social and behavioral skills through interactions with the environment.

At the age of 8 to 9 months, children learn object permanence. This is also the time at which they will experience separation anxiety as they learn that parents still exist even though they cannot be seen. This realization of separation from the primary caregiver is very stressful for children. Parents should work to reduce this stress while continuing to encourage active exploration and the development of independence and identity.

1 YEAR THROUGH PRESCHOOL

DISCIPLINE

From 1 to 3 years of age, toddlers learn to walk and talk and become very much their own persons. They exert their independence by learning to say "no" and by exploring and testing new behaviors along with pushing their boundaries to see what they can get away with. Some parents may react negatively by scolding, threatening, or punishing the child physically by spanking, hitting, or other means. This kind of discipline is harmful to the child's self-esteem and sense of security.

Positive discipline is taught by setting boundaries while still allowing freedom of expression and exploration. Behaviors such as hitting, kicking, and biting must be dealt with quickly and appropriately so that they do not continue. The physician should help parents set up reasonable rules and also help them develop ways to present these rules and the consequences for disobedience clearly to their child. One way to modify behavior is with the "time-out" rule. When the child is breaking a rule, he or she should be removed from the situation and placed in a quiet place. The maximum time out should be 2 minutes per each year of age. Lecturing to or reasoning with the child is to be avoided, as it usually does not help. Temper tantrums will also peak between 2 and 5 years of age and must be dealt with calmly and consistently through the use of time-outs, ignoring the behavior, distracting the child with another activity, or holding the child calmly to help control the tantrum. While discipline should be started at an early age, the child will continue to act out and test boundaries throughout preschool, grammar school, and into adolescence.

TOILET TRAINING

One of the most significant milestones for a toddler is toilet training. The age of toilet training varies widely by culture, but in the United States it is generally accepted to be between 24 and 48 months of age. Parents need to be educated to look for signs of child "readiness" and not to initiate toilet training until then (Box 70-1). Power struggles between parent and child should be minimized, because these could lead to stool with holding by child and chronic constipation. Table 70-1 outlines an approach to toilet training that parents may take.

SLEEP DISTURBANCES

Children often have nightmares and may either wake up screaming or come to the parents' room crying. Such a child should be reassured that he or she is safe; then the parent should go back to the child's room and help the child to see that there are no dan-

■ **BOX 70-1** Signs of Readiness for Toilet Training
Developmental
Ability to ambulate
Stability while sitting
Ability to remain dry for several hours
Ability to pull up pants
Child can follow two-step commands
Child can communicate need to eliminate
Behavioral
Ability to imitate
Ability to put things in proper places
Demonstration of independence by being able to say "no"
Interest in toilet training
The desire to please
The desire for independence and control of functions of elimination
Diminished frequency of power struggles

gers such as monsters hiding under the bed or in the closet. It is acceptable to let the child stay in the parent's bed for a short time, but doing this continuously will make it difficult for the child to sleep alone and could disturb his or her regular sleeping pattern. Night terrors are events where a child partially awakens crying or screaming for a short period of time and is inconsolable. The child will then return to sleep and have no recall of the event. Night terrors are a variant of sleepwalking and occur during deep (stage 4) sleep, whereas nightmares occur during rapid-eye-movement (REM) sleep.

Children with chronic sleep disturbances should be evaluated for medical problems that interfere with sleep, such as obstructive sleep apnea and enuresis. Once medical conditions have been ruled out, the physician should encourage the parents to set up a nightly routine, limit vigorous activity in the evening, limit fluid intake after dinner, and limit television watching and video game playing before bedtime. If these measures do not alter the behavior, referral to a sleep specialist may be considered.

PRESCHOOL AND ELEMENTARY SCHOOL

Most elements of behavioral development that begin as toddlers continue into preschool and elementary school. However, some new behaviors and concerns also arise.

TABLE 70-1 A Sample Approach for Parents to Toilet Training

Vocabulary	Pick the words to use for elimination and then be consistent.
Buying the potty chair	Let the child pick out the chair or have him or her draw on it or write his or her name on the chair. Potty chairs are better than over-the-toilet covers.
Accessibility	Place the potty in an easily accessible location so that the child can see it and become comfortable with it.
Comfort level	Place child on the potty chair fully clothed at first, with toys to play with and books to read. Encourage the child to imitate you by having the child on the potty chair while using toilet yourself.
Making the connection	After a week of fully clothed potty sitting, encourage child to sit naked on the chair. Place soiled diapers in the potty chair to help the child make the connection. Once the child connects elimination with the potty chair, demonstrate disposal of feces in the adult toilet. The flushing of feces down the toilet can scare a child, so first let the child flush with pieces of toilet paper or wave bye-bye to feces.
Practice and encouragement	Praise the child each time he or she indicates the need to go potty. The child should be led to the chair and encouraged to eliminate. Also praise the child for successful potty attempts. Avoid punishing the child if potty attempts are not successful, as negative reinforcement can lead to numerous elimination problems later on.
Transition to toilet-training pants or underwear	After success with using the potty of at least 1 week, transition the child to training pants or cotton underwear. If the child cannot remain dry, return to diapers. Do not rush the child out of diapers. Continue positive reinforcement each time the child potties successfully.

ENURESIS

Children are often in the process of toilet training during their preschool years and should be toilet trained by the time they reach kindergarten or the first grade. However, many will still have enuresis. Enuresis is defined as urinary incontinence at any age at which urinary continence is considered normal. A child who has never been continent for more than a 3- to 6-month period is considered to have primary enuresis, while a child who was continent for 3 to 6 months and is now wetting again is considered to have secondary enuresis. The most common type of enuresis is primary nocturnal enuresis, or bedwetting.

A medical workup helps to rule out organic causes, such as infection. If organic causes are ruled out, behavioral enuresis is assumed. Treatment is usually not initiated until 6 years of age, owing to the high rate of spontaneous resolution. From 6 years of age onward, spontaneous cure rates are still high for both primary and secondary enuresis without organic cause. Still, treatment may be useful at this age. Common treatments are behavioral modification, bedwetting alarms, and medication with desmopressin acetate or imipramine. Behavioral modification works in part by getting the child involved. First, reassure parents that bedwetting has an excellent cure rate and talk to the child about the bedwetting experience and how he or she can help make it better. Have parents help the child to keep a calendar of wet and dry nights and urinate before bedtime; also have the child participate in changing the wet clothes and sheets. Parents should not give fluids after dinner or react angrily when child does wet the bed. Instead, they should offer praise or other positive reinforcement for each dry night.

SOCIAL PLAY

When infants and very young children engage in what is called "parallel play," each child plays in its own fantasy world alongside other children. They play together but not with each other. Children in preschool and grammar school play more and more with each other, developing friendships as well as learning valuable social skills. At this age, parents should teach their children about the value of sharing, as well as continuing to enforce limits and boundaries as deemed appropriate.

SPECIFIC BEHAVIORAL TOPICS

ATTENTION DEFICIT/HYPERACTIVITY DISORDER

Attention deficit/hyperactivity disorder, or AD/HD, is characterized by inattentiveness, impulsivity, and overactivity. The child is easily distracted and impulsive to a point where the behavior hampers him/her socially and academically. The inattentiveness is often picked up by teachers when the child fails to complete tasks once they are begun, fails to grasp directions, and makes mistakes because of inattentiveness as opposed to not understanding the task at hand. The impulsiveness manifests itself as shifting quickly from one activity to another and exhibiting the right behavior at the wrong time. Overactivity can be seen in children as they constantly move around and fidget in their seats.

The issue of AD/HD often first arises when a parent brings a child in proclaiming that the child's teacher has made a "diagnosis" of AD/HD. A careful examination of the history of the child's behavior, along with observation of the child in the examining room, is important in establishing the diagnosis. Physical examinations and neurologic workups are generally not fruitful and should be reserved for situations when seizures are suspected.

A combination of medical and behavioral interventions is necessary for appropriate treatment of AD/HD. Management is often complicated by concomitant learning disabilities, and children with AD/HD should be evaluated for these. Stimulants (e.g., dextroamphetamine and methylphenidate), nonstimulants (e.g., atomoxetine), antidepressant medications (e.g., bupropion), and antihypertensive medications (e.g., clonidine) are most commonly used in the treatment of AD/HD. A structured environment and regular schedules are also essential parts of treatment. Over time, neurologic maturity can result in improvement of symptoms. However, adolescents and young adults are often still depressed and unsure of how to function socially. Continued medical management may be necessary.

LEARNING DISABILITIES

Some 5% to 15% of school-age children are diagnosed with learning disabilities. These problems are usually not apparent until the child enters elementary school. Screening tests, such as the Ages and Stages Questionnaire, are useful tools in the primary care setting to help identify children needing further assessment. Children being assessed for learning disabilities should first have their hearing and vision evaluated. If those are normal, an extended neurologic examination along with an expanded neurodevelopment examination will be useful in describing the child's strengths and weaknesses. Teachers should be informed of the results of such an evaluation and should work with the parents and physician to develop an appropriate learning environment.

PARENTAL DIVORCE/DEATH OF A PARENT

The divorce rate in the United States is now estimated to be at 50% of all marriages. Divorce or death of a parent is extremely stressful for a child. Young children are often not aware that there is a problem between the parents until separation occurs and one parent leaves the home. Older children, on the other hand, may be aware of the tension and fighting for years before separation occurs. The departure of a parent is very disruptive to a child. In addition to the loss or decreased contact with a parent, there are financial consequences. The family may have to relocate, or stay-at-home moms may be suddenly forced to leave the home to work, causing the child to suffer an additional loss.

How a child initially responds to divorce depends mainly on his or her age. Children 2 to 5 years of age often regress, become irritable, or have trouble sleeping. The physician should encourage the stabilization of household and bedtime routines and restoration of contact with the absent parent, and encourage the parents to reassure their children that the divorce was not their fault. Children 6 to 8 years of age often grieve openly and feel rejected. In their case, reassurance and support of continued connection to both parents is important. At 9 to 12 years of age, children may be frightened or angry with one or both parents. The physician should be available to the children if they want to talk or vent. Adolescents likewise become angry as well as depressed. For them, the physician should encourage private discussion of the situation. Children who fare better are those who are given specific details about living arrangements and daily routines after the separation, are reassured repeatedly that the divorce is not their fault, are allowed to vent their sadness and frustration, and have the support of grandparents, family, and friends.

Death of a parent at a young age is less common, but the emotional fallout for a child is as serious or worse. The surviving spouse is grieving for the loss and may be emotionally unable to address the needs of the child. If the death was sudden, the family will likely be in a state of shock. The involvement of a social worker and psychological counseling are important aspects of helping the family grieve and adjust to life without the loved one.

KEY POINTS

- Positive discipline is taught by setting boundaries while still allowing freedom of expression and exploration.
- Some 5% to 15% of school-aged children are diagnosed with learning disabilities. These problems are usually not apparent until the child enters elementary school.
- In dealing with the issue of divorce, the physician should encourage the stabilization of household and bedtime routines and maintaining contact with the absent parent.

Normal body temperature varies between 97°F and 99.3°F (36.1°C and 37.4°C) rectally. Normal body temperature is usually lower in the mornings and higher in the evenings. Fever is defined as a rectal temperature greater or equal to 100.4°F (38.0°C). The majority of pediatric patients presenting with fever will have an obvious source for the temperature elevation, such as a viral upper respiratory infection, otitis media, or gastroenteritis. However, the source of infection is not always obvious and fever is not always due to infection. For example, fever can also occur with malignancies and connective tissue diseases. A thorough history and physical examination are necessary in evaluating children with fever. In children without an apparent source for fever after a complete history and physical examination, further evaluation is needed. Since the sources of fever, organisms causing infections, and the host immune responses to infection can vary by age, the clinical approach also varies by age. An age-dependent approach typically groups the children by the following categories: birth to 3 months, 3 months to 3 years, and 3 years and older. A fever that persists for longer than 14 days in a child without an identifiable cause is defined as a fever of unknown origin.

PATHOGENESIS

Fever is caused by the release of endogenous pyrogenic cytokines (e.g., interleukins, tumor necrosis factor, and interferons), in response to exotoxins from gram-positive organisms, endotoxins from gram-negative organisms, endogenous immunologic stimuli (e.g., malignancy), or medications. Monocytes, macrophages, and endothelial cells are the major cell types responsible for releasing these cytokines, which are also known as pyrogens. These pyrogens stimulate release of prostaglandins from the central hypothalamus, which then act on the preoptic and anterior hypothalamus to increase the thermoregulatory set point. Raising of this set point increases heat production and conservation, thus elevating the body temperature. Medications used to treat fever are active in either inhibiting prostaglandin production (NSAIDs) or blunting the hypothalamic response to alterations in the thermoregulatory set point (acetaminophen). Rigors

or shaking chills occur because the hypothalamic set point has risen rapidly. Cutaneous vasoconstriction occurs to help raise core temperature in fever, causing cold receptors in the skin to sense "cold." Hence many patients will bundle up with blankets despite having fever. Defervescence occurs when cutaneous vasodilatation occurs, which lowers fever and can result in sweats.

CLINICAL MANIFESTATIONS

HISTORY

Parents should be questioned regarding the onset of the fever, how the temperature was taken, and the height of the fever. In addition, associated symptoms—such as vomiting, diarrhea, rhinorrhea, respiratory difficulty, cough, and presence of rash—should be elicited. Inquiry into the child's behavior is an important part of the history. For example, pulling on an ear may indicate an ear infection, decrease in oral intake and number of wet diapers may indicate early dehydration, and refusal to walk may indicate a joint or extremity as the source of pain or infection. The child's activity level and oral intake are important in helping to assess the severity of illness. History of travel or exposure to illness and a thorough past medical history, birth history, immunization history, and review of systems should be included.

PHYSICAL EXAMINATION

The physical examination will often direct the intensity and direction of further workup of the febrile child. Temperature, vital signs, and weight should be recorded. Temperature in infants and toddlers should be obtained rectally. Older children may have their temperature taken orally. Tachycardia or tachypnea out of proportion to the temperature elevation suggest the presence of sepsis, dehydration, or a primary cardiac (e.g., myocarditis, pericarditis) or respiratory (e.g., pneumonia, bronchiolitis) condition.

Examination of the child should include an assessment of his or her general appearance, including alertness, irritability, and respiratory effort. Auscultation is often one of the initial parts of the examination and can be performed while the parent is holding the child. The abdomen, skin, and extremities—including range of motion—should be examined. Testing for meningismus and palpation of the fontanelles should be performed. Finally, inspection of the ears and oropharynx can be performed, usually after other parts of the examination that require the patient to be quieter or more cooperative.

DIFFERENTIAL DIAGNOSIS

The first and foremost consideration in the initial evaluation of the child with fever is an infectious etiology. The history and physical examination may help to determine the specific cause. For example, the parents may report a history of vomiting and diarrhea, suggesting gastroenteritis as the cause. The patient may have rhinorrhea or an erythematous, bulging tympanic membrane on physical examination, establishing the diagnosis of an URI or otitis media. However, it is not uncommon for a child to present without localizing symptoms, in which case a broader differential diagnosis must be entertained. The most common causes of fever in children are presented in Box 71-1. When the fever persists and is classified as fever of unknown origin (>14 days), additional diseases must be considered (Box 71-2).

DIAGNOSTIC EVALUATION

The approach to the child with fever varies depending on the child's age. For example, clinical assessment of infants between birth and 3 months of age cannot reliably distinguish those with serious infections from those with less serious causes of fever. The approach to infants in this age group often involves a full septic workup including a CBC, blood cultures, chest x-ray, UA, urine culture, and lumbar puncture.

Children between 3 months and 3 years of age are more likely to have an identifiable source of fever, and the clinical assessment is more reliable in establishing the severity of illness. Children without a source of their fever can be classified on the basis of their clinical appearance and the height of the temperature. Toxic-appearing children should be admitted to the hospital for evaluation and blood cultures, UA, urine culture, and chest x-ray. If the child has clinical signs of meningitis or appears seriously ill, lumbar puncture may be warranted. Empiric antibiotic coverage is usually provided pending culture results. Well-appearing children without a source of fever and a temperature below 102°F (39°C) may be followed clinically. Children with temperatures above 102°F (39°C) are at increased risk for occult bacteremia and an underlying bacterial illness. One approach to these children is to first obtain a CBC.

■ BOX 71-1 Common Causes for Pediatric Fever
Systemic Viral Infections
Fifth disease
Rubeola
Mumps
Measles
Rubella
Infectious mononucleosis
Occult Bacteremia
Respiratory Infections
Upper respiratory infections
Pharyngitis
Otitis media
Sinusitis
Bronchiolitis
Croup
Pneumonia
Gastrointestinal
Viral gastroenteritis
Bacterial gastroenteritis
Viral hepatitis
Nervous System
Viral meningitis
Bacterial meningitis
Encephalitis
Genitourinary
Pyelonephritis
Pelvic inflammatory disease
Musculoskeletal/Skin
Osteomyelitis
Septic joints
Cellulitis

Those with WBCs greater than 15,000 should be admitted and urine and blood cultures should be ordered. A chest x-ray is indicated in those with respiratory symptoms.

In children above age 3, occult bacteremia is significantly less common and clinical evaluation, including a thorough history and physical examination, can usually identify the source of fever. Laboratory evaluation in these older children is dictated by the clinical findings.

BOX 71-2 Causes for Fever of Unknown Origin

Infectious
Endocarditis
Sinusitis
Abscess
Tuberculosis
Infectious mononucleosis
Viral hepatitis
Cytomegalovirus
Malaria
Rheumatic fever
AIDS
Collagen Vascular
Juvenile rheumatoid arthritis
Lupus erythematosus
Vasculitis
Gastrointestinal
Ulcerative colitis
Crohn disease
Malignancy
Lymphoma
Leukemia
Neuroblastoma
Wilms tumor
Other
Drug-induced fever
Kawasaki syndrome
Hyperthyroidism
Environmental
Factitious

TREATMENT

For neonates (age birth to 1 month) and ill-appearing infants 1 to 3 months of age, hospitalization and empiric antibiotic coverage are indicated to cover the most common bacterial pathogens until culture results are available. Infants 1 to 3 months of age who appear well, have normal laboratory studies, and have a WBC between 5000 and 15,000 may be discharged with a follow-up visit in 24 hours. Empiric antibiotic coverage (e.g., ceftriaxone IM) is commonly provided pending follow-up and culture results.

Children in whom cultures are obtained should generally receive empiric antibiotic coverage until the culture results are available. Children between 3 months and 3 years of age with temperatures above 102°F (39°C) should have follow-up the next day.

KEY POINTS

- Fever is defined as rectal temperature of 100.4°F (38°C).
- The majority of children with fever will have a common identifiable source, such as upper respiratory infection, otitis media, or gastroenteritis.
- Important factors in evaluating febrile children without an apparent source include the age of the child, height of the fever, and appearance of the child.
- Febrile children from birth to 3 months of age warrant a laboratory evaluation including CBC, cultures, chest x-ray, and often lumbar puncture.
- The clinical appearance of the child and height of the fever dictate the workup of febrile children from age 3 months to 3 years.
- Clinical assessment will usually identify the source of fever in children over 3 years of age.

Otitis Media

The term "otitis media" encompasses four conditions: acute otitis media (AOM), recurrent otitis media (ROM), otitis media with effusion (OME), and chronic suppurative otitis media (CSOM). AOM is defined as a purulent infection involving the middle ear and is characterized by fever and ear pain. AOM is more common in the winter months, often occurring in association with URIs. The highest incidence of ear infection is seen in children who are between 6 and 36 months of age. Other risk factors include bottle-feeding, prematurity, Native-American ethnicity, exposure to passive smoke, and day care attendance. ROM is defined as three episodes of AOM within 6 months or four episodes within 1 year, with normal examinations between infections. OME is diagnosed when there are no signs and symptoms of infection but on the physical examination there is fluid behind the tympanic membrane (TM). This condition is often preceded by AOM. It is generally asymptomatic but may manifest as hearing loss. CSOM is characterized by foul-smelling otorrhea.

PATHOGENESIS

For anatomic reasons, children less than 2 years of age are more likely to develop OM. The eustachian tube in these children is shorter and is more horizontal than it is in adults, allowing easier passage of bacteria from the nasopharynx into the middle ear. Furthermore, the canal of the eustachian tube is very narrow and subject to occlusion by the surrounding adenoids and lymphoid follicles. Even mild URIs can cause these lymphoid tissues to enlarge and obstruct the drainage of fluid from the middle ear. URIs also damage the ciliated epithelium of the eustachian tube, which increases the likelihood of bacteria adhering to the wall and predisposes the individual to a superimposed bacterial infection. Ear pain results from increasing pressure due to fluid accumulation and inflammation.

The most common bacteria associated with otitis media are *Streptococcus pneumoniae*, followed by *Haemophilus influenzae* and *Moraxella catarrhalis*. About 30% of cases of AOM are due to viruses such as respiratory syncytial virus (RSV), parainfluenza, and rhinovirus. AOM is often followed by OME,

which usually resolves over 4 to 12 weeks. OME that is persistent or interferes with normal hearing requires evaluation and treatment.

CLINICAL MANIFESTATIONS

HISTORY

The presenting complaint of AOM can vary depending on the age of the child. Ear pain is the most common complaint in children able to complain of pain. Younger children may present with irritability, sleep disturbances, fever, excessive crying, or a history of pulling on the affected ear. Otitis media may also cause nausea, vomiting, and diarrhea. Older children may complain of hearing loss; in younger children, this may manifest itself as inattention, loss of balance, dizziness, or tinnitus. Clinical history alone, however, is poorly predictive of the presence of AOM, especially in younger children.

PHYSICAL EXAMINATION

AOM is usually associated with an upper respiratory infection. The examination of the ear should focus on the color and appearance of the TM and the presence of pus or air bubbles behind the TM. The affected TM may be dull or erythematous. Patients with AOM will also often have a bulging or retracted TM. Mobility of the TM, assessed with the pneumatic otoscope, is decreased in both AOM and OME. In OME, there is no fever or other sign of infection and the TM may appear dull or normal, but it is not erythematous. Children with CSOM will have otorrhea, which may be foul-smelling. They are also likely to have hearing loss, and examination of the TM will usually demonstrate a perforation.

DIFFERENTIAL DIAGNOSIS

Vigorous crying may cause a reddened TM and result in an abnormal examination. Infectious causes of a hyperemic tympanic membrane include AOM, ROM, or CSOM. Other causes of ear pain may include otitis externa, temporomandibular joint (TMJ) dysfunction, and pain referred from pharyngitis or a dental source.

DIAGNOSTIC EVALUATION

The diagnosis of OM is based on the history and physical examination and rarely requires laboratory studies. However, if the child is less than 6 weeks old and has a fever, a full sepsis workup is indicated. If symptoms persist despite the use of different antibiotics, tympanostomy to obtain fluid for culture and sensitivity may be needed to direct antibiotic therapy.

It is also important to differentiate otitis externa from OM. In otitis externa, the ear canal may appear red, with purulent material in the canal, and is usually tender to touch. The ear canal is neither erythematous nor tender to the touch with AOM. OME is diagnosed when there are no signs of infection but pneumatic otoscopy shows TM immobility indicating fluid behind the TM. Tympanometry can be a helpful diagnostic tool in confirming the presence of fluid in the middle ear. In addition, in children with OME, hearing evaluation may be warranted to document the impact of the fluid on the child's hearing. A chronic history of ear discharge along with the physical finding of perforated TM with visible discharge suggests the presence of CSOM.

TREATMENT

Many infections of the middle ear resolve spontaneously, requiring observation and supportive care only. Use of antibiotic therapy depends on the child's age, the certainty of the diagnosis, and the severity of illness (Table 72-1). The goals of treatment are to prevent recurrent infections that can lead to chronic otitis media and persistent OME. Persistent OME may affect a child's hearing and thus language development.

Children who are less than 6 months of age are at a higher risk of developing serious infections like meningitis or sepsis. Therefore such children should receive antibiotic therapy for AOM. Children above 6 months of age may be treated more conservatively. For less severely ill children, observation for 48 to 72 hours will give the child a chance to improve on his or her own as long as follow-up with the clinician is reliable. If symptoms worsen or do not improve after 48 to 72 hours, the drug of choice is amoxicillin (80 to 90 mg/kg/day) for 10 days. A different antibiotic should be prescribed if there is no response within 48 to 72 hours of starting amoxicillin or the patient is penicillin-allergic or at high risk for a resistant strain. Markers of high risk for resistance include a history of multiple infections, day care attendance, and recent therapy (3 to 6 months) with amoxicillin. Second-line choices of antibiotics include amoxicillin with clavulanic acid (Augmentin), second- or third-generation cephalosporins (e.g., cefixime, cefuroxime), and erythromycin with sulfasoxazole. Ceftriaxone may be used intramuscularly or intravenously in children who cannot take or keep down oral medicines. Children who have persistent symptoms despite multiple courses of antibiotics should have tympanocentesis with culture and sensitivity testing. Also, immunocompromised children may require a tympanocentesis before starting antibiotics.

Supportive therapy including antipyretics (acetaminophen or ibuprofen), topical anesthetic drops (Benzocaine), and local heat may be helpful for relieving pain. Parents should be advised not to expose children to passive smoking and to avoid supine bottle-feeding. Follow-up in 7 to 10 days is recommended to ensure symptom resolution, and subsequent follow-up should monitor for persistent OME.

TABLE 72-1 Criteria for Initial Treatment with an Antibacterial Agent or Observation in Children with Acute Otitis Media

Age	Certain Diagnosis	Uncertain Diagnosis
<6 months	Antibacterial therapy	Antibacterial therapy
6 months–2 years	Antibacterial therapy	Antibacterial therapy if severe illness; observation option[a] if nonsevere illness
>2 years	Antibacterial therapy if severe illness; observation option[a] if nonsevere illness	Observation option[a]

[a]Observation is an appropriate option only when follow-up can be ensured and antibacterial agents started if symptoms persist or worsen. Nonsevere illness is mild otalgia and fever <39°C (<102.2°F) in the previous 24 hours. Severe illness is moderate to severe otalgia or fever >39°C (>102.2°F). A certain diagnosis of acute otitis media meets all three of these criteria: (1) rapid onset, (2) signs of middle-ear effusion, and (3) signs and symptoms of middle-ear inflammation.
Reprinted from American Academy of Pediatrics and American Academy of Family Practice Subcommittee on Management of Acute Otitis Media Clinical Practice Guideline. *Pediatrics.* 2004; 113(5):1451–1465, with permission. Modified from the New York State Department of Health and the New York Region Otitis Project Committee. *Observation Option Toolkit for Acute Otitis Media.* Publication No. 4894. New York, NY: State of New York, Department of Health; 2002, with permission.

Patients who have ROM may benefit from prophylactic antibiotics such as amoxicillin 20 mg/kg at bedtime for 6 months or sulfasoxazole in penicillin-allergic patients. If this fails, the child should be referred to an otolaryngologist for possible tympanostomy tube placement. Children who have OME that persists for more than 4 to 6 months in spite of antibiotics may be candidates for myringotomy and tympanostomy tube placement. If there is significant hearing loss, tympanostomy may be performed earlier.

KEY POINTS

- AOM is diagnosed when there is a rapid onset of symptoms, middle-ear effusion, and a hyperemic tympanic membrane with decreased mobility.
- ROM is defined as three episodes within 6 months or four or more episodes within a year.
- The most common bacterial pathogens are *S. pneumoniae, H. influenzae,* and *M. catarrhalis.*
- The drug of choice is amoxicillin (80–90 mg/kg/day), unless infection with a resistant organism is suspected or the child is allergic to penicillin.
- Myringotomy and tympanostomy tube placement are indicated for recurrent infections despite antibiotic prophylaxis or for persistent effusion associated with hearing loss.

Preparticipation Evaluation

Over 30 million children participate in organized sports, and many more adults and children participate in unorganized sporting activities. Sports promote physical fitness, provide opportunities for psychosocial growth, promote self-confidence, and foster healthful lifetime habits and hobbies. The physician's role in sporting activities is to provide preparticipation health examinations (PPEs), counseling regarding appropriate participation, and care for injuries and illnesses. The purpose of the PPE is to identify medical conditions that may interfere with athletic performance as well as possible life-threatening conditions that may prevent an athlete from safely participating in his or her sport. The PPE also gives the physician a chance to evaluate healthy individuals who may not otherwise seek medical care, thus providing an opportunity to assess an athlete's general health and offer counsel about preventive issues such as tobacco avoidance and safe sex practices. Recently, emphasis has been placed on the PPE's role in identifying athletes at risk for sudden cardiac death. This is defined as a nontraumatic, nonviolent, unexpected event resulting from sudden cardiac arrest within 6 hours of a previously witnessed state of normal health. The incidence of sudden cardiac death among high school and college athletes is estimated at 1 in 200,000, with about 50 such deaths occurring annually. Although sudden cardiac death occurs infrequently, it can devastate the community, family, and medical personnel associated with such an event.

PATHOGENESIS

Physicians generally recommend that individuals participate in some form of physical exercise. However, physical exertion stresses the body and can exacerbate an underlying medical condition and place the participating individual at risk for harm. For example, the risk of injury to a solitary kidney or enlarged spleen may preclude such an individual from participating in contact sports. The presence of CAD or asymmetric hypertrophic cardiomyopathy may preclude any sports participation until evaluation and therapy have been initiated. In determining an athlete's risk for sports participation, the physician must decide which types of activities may be appropriate for that individual.

Dynamic activity is highly aerobic and includes activities such as running, cross-country skiing, and swimming. These athletes must maintain an elevated cardiac output for an extended period of time, which leads to an increase in the thickness of the left ventricular wall and the volume of the left ventricle. Athletes who regularly engage in dynamic activity often have an increase in baseline vagal tone and may have resting pulses as low as 30 beats/minute.

Static or isometric exercise includes activities such as weight-lifting. This type of exercise involves a tremendous but brief increase in cardiac output against elevated peripheral resistance. Athletes who frequently engage in isometric exercise develop symmetric left ventricular thickening, in contrast to asymmetric thickening, which indicates possible pathology. Activities are then sorted by level of dynamic and static activities (e.g., billiards is low dynamic and low static; football is high dynamic and high static).

In addition, activities may also be categorized according to type of interaction with other athletes. For example, football, lacrosse, and rugby are examples of collision sports, whereas contact sports include soccer, basketball, wrestling, and others. Noncontact sports typically include tennis, track, golf, and swimming.

In adults over the age of 40 and in those with a family history of heart disease, CAD is the most common cause of sudden cardiac death. In association with physical exertion, individuals with CAD are vulnerable to MI or ischemia resulting from atherosclerotic plaque rupture. Hypertrophic cardiomyopathy is the most common cause of sudden death in athletes below 35 years of age, accounting for roughly 40% of cases. Hypertrophic cardiomyopathy is an autosomal dominant trait with variable expression; thus not everyone with the gene expresses the trait. Mutations of the beta cardiac heavy myosin chain results in asymmetric thickening of the left ventricular wall, which, with significant physical exertion, predisposes individuals to arrhythmias.

CLINICAL MANIFESTATIONS

HISTORY

The history can identify many athletes at risk for sudden cardiac death as well as those with medical conditions that might place them at an increased risk when participating in athletics. The patient's age, complete past medical history including previous surgeries and injuries, medications, heart murmurs, rheumatic fever, and previous athletic experience should be documented. Patients should be asked specifically about episodes of chest tightness, chest pain, palpitations, and shortness of breath with little or no exertion, light-headedness, head trauma, and syncope. Family history of sudden cardiac death before the age of 40, cardiomyopathy, Marfan syndrome, and prolonged QT syndrome should be assessed. In women, menstrual history is important. The use of illicit drugs such as cocaine and anabolic steroids should also be asked about.

PHYSICAL EXAMINATION

The patient's vital signs, height, and weight should be reviewed. General inspection should observe for body habitus consistent with Marfan syndrome (usually marked by greater than normal height, arm span greater than height, pectus excavatum, myopia, and displaced lenses). BP should be checked; if it is elevated, serial measurements should be taken to assess for HTN. Funduscopic examination is indicated in those with HTN. Cardiovascular assessment includes femoral and radial pulses to evaluate for coarctation of the aorta. Careful cardiac auscultation is important to detect murmurs, and, if present, note how they change with respiration and in the standing and sitting positions. Benign flow murmurs may increase with lying down or squatting but typically diminish or do not change with the Valsalva maneuver or upon standing. Murmurs associated with asymmetric hypertrophic cardiomyopathy will decrease in the supine or squatting positions and increase with Valsalva and standing. Any extra heart sounds or clicks should be documented. The abdominal examination should note surgical scars and the presence of hepato- or splenomegaly. The male genital examination should note developmental state and the presence of an inguinal hernia.

The musculoskeletal examination is another area of importance. Assessment of the neck, spine, shoulders, elbows, wrists, fingers, hips, knees, ankles, and feet for ROM and stability should be performed. Asymmetry should be noted and, if present, lead to a more focused examination. The spine should be examined for kyphoscoliosis. Upper extremity strength should be assessed by testing the different muscle groups; duck walking while squatting down can be performed to assess the lower extremities.

DIAGNOSTIC EVALUATION

The history and physical examination are sufficient evaluation for the vast majority of those who undergo sports PPEs. Routine screening ECGs and echocardiograms are not cost-effective interventions because of the low incidence of cardiac abnormalities in this group.

In patients with suspected hypertrophic cardiomyopathy, a chest x-ray, ECG, and echocardiogram are indicated. In patients with a history of syncope and no murmurs on physical examination, an event monitor or 24-hour Holter may be helpful in addition to the ECG and echocardiogram. A stress test is useful for older patients who complain of chest pain with exertion or those with significant risk factors for heart disease. Radiographs are not routinely indicated but may be indicated in patients with joint complaints or findings. Laboratory evaluation may be useful in patients with ongoing medical conditions such as hepatitis or diabetes but is seldom indicated otherwise.

TREATMENT

The vast majority of athletes who are seen in PPEs are cleared to play. In deciding not to allow an athlete to participate, the rationale for exclusion must be thoroughly discussed with the athlete, family, coaching staff, and other medical staff, with the emphasis on the activities in which the athlete *can* participate.

Athletes with active contagious infections should be excluded from all sports until their infections resolve. Participants with skin lesions such as tinea corporis, impetigo, or herpes simplex should not participate in contact sports. Individuals with joint injuries should rehabilitate the joint prior to returning to participation. Individuals with medical conditions such as recent concussion or splenomegaly should avoid sports that may involve collision contact. In athletes with an active medical illness such as uncontrolled diabetes or asthma, appropriate tests and treatment are recommended before allowing the athlete to participate. In patients with certain congenital or acquired conditions, referral to the appropriate specialist (e.g., nephrologist with solitary kidney, neurologist with seizure disorder) may assist in providing additional counseling regarding all the risks associated with participating in athletics. In patients with HTN, diet, lifestyle modification, and possibly medications to lower BP may be warranted before allowing the athlete to participate. Certain antihypertensive medications are banned by the National Collegiate Athletic Association (NCAA) and U.S. Olympic Committee, which is important to keep in mind for evaluating high-level athletes.

Finally, in those with a worrisome past medical history, significant family history, or an abnormality on cardiovascular examination or testing, cardiology consultation may be warranted to provide additional information regarding safe sports participation.

KEY POINTS

- The purpose of the PPE is to identify (a) medical conditions that may interfere with athletic performance and (b) possible life-threatening conditions that may prevent an athlete from participating in his or her sport safely.

- The history and physical examination are sufficient evaluation for the vast majority of those who undergo sports preparticipation evaluations.

- In patients with suspected hypertrophic cardiomyopathy, a chest x-ray, ECG, and echocardiogram are indicated.

- In deciding to not allow an athlete to participate, the rationale for exclusion must be thoroughly discussed with the athlete, family, coaching staff, and other medical staff; emphasis should be placed on the activities in which the athlete *can* participate.

Chapter

74

Preventive Care: 65 Years and Older

With increasing age, the effects of years of behaviors and accumulated medical disease result in different states of physiologic health for individuals of the same chronological age. Some individuals in their sixties and seventies are debilitated and reside in nursing facilities, while others in their eighties and nineties remain fully independent. The expected life span of a healthy individual at age 65 is approximately 15 years. However, the expected life span of patients with significant underlying medical conditions—such as severe COPD, cancer, or heart disease—may be considerably less. Preventive strategies should be tailored to an individual's health status and his or her personal preferences. For example, many patients in their eighties and nineties would no longer consider undergoing aggressive treatments, such as major abdominal or heart surgery, and may no longer wish to be screened for diseases that would require such treatment. Involving these patients and their families in decisions about the overall approach to the patient's care can help in deciding what is appropriate for each patient.

The most common causes of morbidity and mortality in the adult over age 65 are cardiovascular disease, cerebrovascular disease, cancers, and lung disease. Cardiovascular disease is the leading cause of death in the United States and is more prevalent with increasing age. Many types of cancer are also more prevalent in older populations. COPD is primarily a smoking-related disease with significant morbidity and mortality among the elderly. Pulmonary infections in older adults have a higher morbidity and mortality rate than in younger individuals.

CLINICAL CONSIDERATIONS

Most physicians recommend annual preventive care visits for older patients. In addition to preventive issues common to all age groups, the visits should focus on functional issues. For example, falls and

accidents are a significant cause of morbidity and mortality, and immobility a common cause of decline in function and loss of independence. Thus, issues surrounding fall prevention should be incorporated into preventive care discussions. Exercise is also important in preserving functional level, since inactive elders are at greater risk of becoming functionally dependent than are their more physically active counterparts.

A review of medications is important. Although the elderly comprise 12% of the population, they receive 32% of dispensed medications. Each year, an elderly individual takes an estimated 17 to 20 drugs. Age-related physiologic changes and drug interactions make the elderly adult more susceptible to an adverse reaction. Each visit affords an opportunity to review diagnoses and reassess the need for medications.

The driving ability of older adults, especially the frail elderly, needs review. Visual problems, hearing difficulty, and cognitive impairment occur more frequently in the geriatric population and may compromise driving ability. If there are concerns about driving safety, referral for testing may be warranted. Finally, soliciting the patient's wishes regarding future care and advance directives is important.

Blood pressure should be checked annually to screen for HTN. Treating HTN is of substantial benefit in the elderly and it reduces the incidence of strokes and other cardiovascular events such as congestive heart failure. Anticoagulation for patients with atrial fibrillation is also of value in reducing the risk of strokes in elderly patients. Despite concerns about the risk of falls and anticoagulation, the benefits of anticoagulation outweigh the risks for most patients with atrial fibrillation. Orthostatic blood pressure measurements should be checked when considering the use of antihypertensive medications and for those with gait instability. Cholesterol screening is recommended in men and women every 5 years, depending on the patient's functional status and expected life span. In patients with cardiovascular disease, treating hyperlipidemia is of benefit. One-time screening for abdominal aortic aneurysm is recommended for those men over age 65 who have ever smoked. Measurement of height, weight, and vital signs, along with a dietary history, can screen for obesity and malnutrition.

Counseling to promote a healthy diet—including appropriate amounts of calories, fat, vitamins, and fiber—is important. All patients with risk factors for osteoporosis should be counseled about the need for adequate calcium intake and weight-bearing exercise. The dietary calcium of many individuals is insufficient; they will therefore benefit from calcium and vitamin D supplementation. Some groups recommend routine osteoporosis screening for all postmenopausal women over age 65 and other high-risk groups younger than age 65 (Chapter 50). Those individuals with osteoporosis should be offered treatment to help reduce the risk of fracture. Diabetes screening is recommended, with a fasting glucose every 3 years. Many clinicians routinely screen for thyroid disease, although no formal recommendations support this at the present time. Routine dental care should be recommended.

Substance abuse is a common problem among geriatric patients and should not be overlooked. About 10% of patients over age 65 have problems with alcohol. Smoking is an important issue, since patients can benefit from smoking cessation even after years of smoking. If there are concerns about cognition or memory, additional history from family members and screening for dementia with a Mini-Mental Status Examination (MMSE) is indicated. Depression is common in the elderly population, and men over age 65 have the highest rate of completed suicide attempts. Screening for mental health and depression can be performed through the patient interview or with use of screening instruments such as the Yesavage Geriatric Depression Scale. If questions remain regarding a patient's mental functioning, referral for formal neuropsychiatric testing may be helpful.

CANCER SCREENING

Cancer screening continues to be a major focus of health screening in the geriatric population but is tempered to some degree by the presence of comorbid disease, the patient's past screening history, and the patient's wishes for continued screening. Cancer screening in women includes annual Pap smears and annual mammograms. Although women with significant comorbid disease may not benefit from continued breast cancer screening, healthy elderly women who desire mammography should be offered annual screening until their life expectancy falls below 5 to 10 years. Women over 65 who have had normal prior Pap smears and three consecutive normal results may be given the option of discontinuing cervical cancer screening. There are no recommendations to perform routine ovarian or uterine cancer screening. For men, annual prostate examination and PSA testing should be limited to those with a life expectancy of 10 years or more. Although there is no clear-cut age at which to discontinue colon cancer screening, most clinicians offer it to healthy individuals over age 65 until their life expectancy is less than 5 to 10 years. There is no evidence supporting routine screening for lung, skin, or oral cancers.

IMMUNIZATIONS

Tetanus immunization should be updated every 10 years. All patients over 65 years of age should receive pneumococcal and influenza vaccines. Influenza vaccines are administered annually. High-risk individuals are often given pneumococcal boosters every 5 to 7 years. Vaccination against herpes zoster is recommended as a one-time injection after age 60. TB screening is routinely recommended for all patients residing in long-term-care facilities and others at high risk. Patients at risk because of travel can be given hepatitis A or B vaccines.

SAFETY ASSESSMENT

Assessment of vision and hearing may be helpful in detecting a correctable deficit that may lead to improved function. Watching the patient walk down the hall may give clues to neurologic disease or need for assistive devices. Along with assessment of vision and gait, an environmental assessment and education of the family should be included to help with fall prevention. The walkways at home should be uncluttered, well lit, and free of throw rugs. Reinforcement of healthy behavioral measures should also be incorporated into the visit. These discussions can include topics such as seat belt use, bicycle helmet use, firearms and water safety, smoke detectors, and training in cardiopulmonary resuscitation (CPR) for household members. Exercise may be particularly beneficial in the elderly by decreasing the risk of falls, improving cardiovascular status and mood, and providing some protection against osteoporosis.

 KEY POINTS

- The most common causes of death in adults over age 65 are cardiovascular disease and cancer.

- In addition to recommendations common to all age groups, increasing focus in geriatric preventive care on functional issues and future care should be incorporated into the visits.

- Substance abuse and depression are common problems among geriatric patients.

- Along with assessment of vision and gait, an environmental assessment and education of the family should be included to help with the prevention of falls.

Chapter 75

Geriatric Assessment

Geriatric assessment is an interdisciplinary approach to the evaluation of an older individual's physical and psychosocial impairments and functional disabilities. This approach recognizes the complex medical and social problems facing many elderly individuals and requires sensitivity to their concerns and an awareness of the many unique aspects of their medical problems.

In the elderly, quality of life and maintaining function are critically important. Diseases should be diagnosed and assessed, but maintenance or restoration of function may be more important than curative treatment. Treatment of an illness always requires a detailed analysis of risk versus benefits.

FUNCTIONAL ASSESSMENT

Functional assessment measures an individual's ability to manage everyday life. Typically these assessments focus on an individual's ability to provide self-care, known as activities of daily living (ADLs); to perform higher-level functions, known as instrumental activities of daily living (IADLs); to maintain mobility; and to comprehend and communicate.

Geriatric assessment is important because of the high prevalence of disability among the elderly. In practice, comprehensive examination involves both assessment and the development of recommendations as well as plans for implementation. Measurement tools are often used as part of the assessment. Examples include depression scales, instruments that assess ADLs (toileting, eating, grooming, dressing, and transferring), and scales that measure IADLs (e.g., ability to shop or manage finances). Mobility is an important consideration, and observation of the patient provides the most insight. Observing whether the patient can get up easily from a chair, walk steadily, turn around, walk back, and sit down provides significant insight into his or her functional status. Checking an individual's balance with his or her eyes closed and hands at the sides is also important.

A geriatric assessment includes an evaluation of which ancillary support services and disciplines might be of benefit to the patient. For example, occupational therapy might make specific recommendations about environmental modifications that could

enhance safety and functional ability, and speech pathology might be helpful in someone with difficulty swallowing. Finally, the functional assessment should include a discussion of the patient's preferences and expectations, combined with the family's expectations and the willingness to provide care. It is of paramount importance that the patient's preferences receive the highest priority and to recognize that these may be in conflict with those of the family. Unrealistic expectations, inability to provide support, or reluctance of the family to help can doom any plan of care to failure.

HISTORY

Several common problems can make history taking more challenging in the elderly. Impaired hearing and vision are common and can interfere with effective communication. Eliminating extraneous noise, facing the patient, speaking slowly in deep tones, and providing good lighting can be helpful.

Many elderly patients ignore symptoms because of their cultural backgrounds or because they may feel that their symptoms are a normal concomitant of aging. Fear of illness may lead to denial and under-reporting of symptoms. Altered responses to illness are frequent and can lead to vague or absent symptoms (e.g., a painless MI). Impaired memory or cognitive function can also work against obtaining an accurate history.

At the other end of the spectrum are those elderly patients who have multiple complaints. Sorting through multiple symptoms and getting to know the patient may take time. By being alert to new or changing symptoms, the physician will be better able to detect potentially treatable conditions and avoid overlooking important issues.

The past medical history should include previous surgeries, major illnesses, and hospitalizations. As a general rule, surgeries or illnesses occurring within the previous 5 years are more relevant than remote events such as childhood illnesses. Immunization status and a review of past results of TB testing are frequently overlooked but also important.

Of paramount importance is reviewing all medications, both prescription and OTC. Elderly patients are more vulnerable to side effects, and OTC medications can cause significant side effects that may be overlooked unless specifically asked about. The "brown bag" technique, where the patient collects all his or her medications in a paper bag and brings them to the office, can be useful. It is also important to assess patients' knowledge of their medication regimes and their adherence to them.

PHYSICAL EXAMINATION

The complete physical examination is similar to that performed on younger individuals, with some special emphasis. Successful function requires that cognitive

skills be relatively intact and the Mini-Mental Status Examination is a useful screening tool for cognitive impairment. Formal cognitive testing may be helpful if there appears to be impairment despite a normal screening examination. The patient's general appearance and grooming can provide clues to functional problems, and poor hygiene may indicate a need for intervention.

Blood pressure should routinely be checked both sitting and standing, since elderly individuals often have significant orthostatic changes that contribute to falls. It is not uncommon for the elderly to have

■ TABLE 75-1 Commonly Abnormal Laboratory Values in Older Adults

Lab/Test	Finding
Albumin	Frequently low in the elderly but often a sign of poor nutrition.
Alkaline phosphatase	Mild asymptomatic elevations common. Liver or bone disease should be considered when values exceed 1.5 times normal.
Calcium	Unchanged in aging; abnormalities should prompt further evaluation. Need to correct for low albumin levels.
Chest x-ray	Mild interstitial changes or findings consistent with early COPD are common. A calcified aortic arch, old granuloma, and vertebral osteopenia are common age-related findings that are not a normal consequence of aging.
Creatinine	Low in the elderly due to decreases in lean body mass; high-normal and mildly elevated values may indicate significant renal impairment.
ECG	Nonspecific ST- and T-wave changes, PVCs, conduction abnormalities, and atrial arrhythmias are common in asymptomatic elderly and may not need further evaluation and treatment.
Electrolytes	Unchanged in aging; abnormalities should prompt further evaluation.
Fe/TIBC	Abnormal values are not due to aging and may indicate GI blood loss, poor nutrition, or chronic disease.
Glucose	Prevalence of glucose intolerance and type 2 diabetes increases with age.
Hemoglobin	Does not change with aging, but mild anemias due to chronic disease are often present. An acute drop or unexplained values under 12 g/dL generally merits investigation.
LFTs	Unchanged in aging; abnormalities should prompt further evaluation.
Platelet count	Unchanged in aging; abnormalities should prompt further evaluation.
PSA	Often elevated due to BPH, but marked elevations or increasing values suggest possible prostate cancer. Further evaluation of patients with possible prostate cancer should be undertaken only if the diagnosis would result in a change in management.
RA and ANA	Positivity in low titers often common and rarely indicative of disease.
Sedimentation rate	Mild elevations may be age-related. Levels >50 are more likely associated with disease.
TSH	Unchanged in aging; abnormalities should prompt further evaluation.
UA	Asymptomatic bacteriuria is common and does not merit treatment. Hematuria is never a normal finding and generally merits investigation.
WBC	Unchanged in aging; abnormalities should prompt further evaluation.

mild asymptomatic irregularities in their pulse; this finding seldom needs extensive workup or treatment. Sensory loss is common and hearing and vision screens are important for detecting impairment. Careful inspection of the oral cavity is part of the nutritional assessment, and palpation of the temporal arteries is important to screen for temporal arteritis. The abdominal examination may reveal a large aortic aneurysm. A careful rectal and genitourinary examination is important for helping to assess bowel and bladder function and detecting uterine prolapse, hernias, and testicular atrophy.

Assessing gait and station is particularly important, since the elderly are often at increased risk for falls and this examination may uncover correctable causes of unsteadiness. Careful assessment can identify physical evidence that a patient is at risk for abuse. Signs of abuse include trauma, burns, and weight loss. Poor nutrition is common, and a weight loss greater than 5 lb/month or losses in excess of 10 lb over 3 months merits investigation for underlying disease. Weight gain suggests edema or ascites.

DIAGNOSTIC EVALUATION

Most patients should have basic testing such as a CBC, chemistry profile, UA, and TSH if not recently available. Mammography and colon cancer screening utilizing fecal occult blood testing and/or endoscopy are recommended for patients until age 75, depending on patient preference and expected life span. Pap smear screening can be discontinued at age 65 if there has been regular testing and a normal Pap smear within the previous 3 years. Other tests should be ordered as clinically indicated.

Although abnormal laboratory findings occur regularly in an elderly population and are often attributed to aging, few are truly the result of advanced age. Misinterpretation can lead to either underdiagnosis or overtreatment. Table 75-1 lists some commonly abnormal laboratory tests in older adults.

ANCILLARY SPECIALISTS

There are many aspects of a comprehensive functional assessment that family physicians are not trained to complete. However, physicians should be familiar with these areas and orchestrate the assessment accordingly. The types of treatment often of value in an older population include physical therapy, occupational therapy, and speech therapy as well as the services of psychologists, case managers, dieticians, and nurses. The physician should be as detailed as possible in requesting ancillary services. Merely sending someone to physical therapy with an unspecified request is analogous to sending a patient to the pharmacy with a request for "drugs."

Social workers are invaluable in helping to manage a complex home situation. An experienced social worker or geriatric nurse making a home visit can assess the home environment and often suggest changes that might enhance an individual's ability to remain there. Examples include changes in the physical environment, such as entrance ramps and elevated toilet seats; special services, such as Meals On Wheels; increased social contact, such as a telephone checks; or increased participation in senior activities and arranging for the emergency provision of food or money.

KEY POINTS

- Geriatric assessment is an interdisciplinary approach to the evaluation of an older individual's physical and psychosocial impairments and functional disabilities.

- The functional assessment should include a discussion of the patient's preferences and expectations combined with the family's expectations and willingness to provide care.

- Most patients should have basic testing such as a CBC, chemistry profile, UA, and TSH if not recently available. Other tests should be ordered as clinically indicated.

- The types of treatments often of value in an older population include physical therapy, occupational therapy, speech therapy and the services of psychologists, case managers, dieticians, and nurses.

SENSORY IMPAIRMENT

HEARING LOSS

Hearing loss is the most common sensory impairment of old age; approximately 40% of elderly individuals have some type of hearing loss. Presbycusis or age-related hearing loss is a bilateral sensorineural impairment of the higher frequencies that may compromise speech comprehension. Other causes of hearing loss include ototoxicity, otosclerosis, Ménière disease, and cerumen impaction.

Hearing aids are usually worn in the ear and amplify sound. They are most effective in peripheral hearing loss and less helpful in those with a central auditory processing defect. Conduction loss from cerumen impaction may aggravate all forms of hearing loss and should be removed either manually or with ceruminolytic agents (e.g., Debrox).

VISION LOSS

Presbyopia is age-associated loss of the eye's ability to accommodate, and most individuals need glasses for reading by their fifties. The four most common ophthalmologic diseases encountered in the elderly are cataracts or lens opacification, macular degeneration, open-angle glaucoma, and diabetic retinopathy. Risk factors for cataracts include sun exposure, smoking, steroid use, and diabetes mellitus. Treatment consists of surgical removal of the lens and is indicated if the visual acuity is 20/50 or worse and/or there is significant functional impairment from the cataract.

Macular degeneration is the atrophy of cells in the central macula. It is the most common cause of visual impairment in Caucasian elderly, while glaucoma is the most common in African Americans. There are two types of macular degeneration, wet and dry. Lasar photocoagulation or newer intravitreal antiangiogenic antibody injections may be helpful for individuals with the wet type. Patients with macular degeneration should be monitored daily for visual changes with an Amsler grid. Antioxidant therapy (e.g., Ocuvite) is useful for reducing the risk of progression.

Glaucoma is characterized by an elevated intraocular pressure and an increased optic cup-to-disc ratio. If untreated, glaucoma can lead to the loss of peripheral vision and eventually blindness. Treatment is indicated when pressures are elevated (>25 mmHg) or in the presence of optic nerve atrophy or visual field loss. Pharmacologic treatment with drops that either decrease aqueous production (e.g., beta blockers, adrenergic agents) or increase aqueous drainage (e.g., miotics) can lower pressure. Surgery is indicated when pressures are poorly controlled by topical agents or visual loss progresses.

COMMON DISORDERS

WEIGHT LOSS

Involuntary weight loss in the elderly is a serious problem, and a 1-year documented unintentional weight loss of more than 4% is the best single predictor of death within 2 years. The causes of weight loss in older patients are similar to those in middle-age adults. The most common causes are depression and cancer, especially GI and lung malignancies. Cardiopulmonary disorders such as CHF or COPD can cause weight loss in later stages. Renal failure may present with anorexia and weight loss as an early symptom. Infection, especially TB, and endocrine disorders such as diabetes or hyperthyroidism are associated with weight loss. Medications may cause decreased appetite, altered taste and smell, or nausea, all of which can result in weight loss.

Elderly patients may also have reduced dietary intake from oral problems such as poorly fitted dentures, from functional impairments due to stroke or arthritis, or from difficulty swallowing. Access issues such as having insufficient resources to purchase food or the inability to shop or prepare meals may also limit adequate nutrition. In about 25% of cases no cause for an involuntary weight loss is identified.

If a complete history and physical examination fail to suggest the diagnosis, laboratory testing including CBC, ESR, comprehensive chemistry panel, UA, TSH, chest x-ray, PSA, and HIV testing in those with risk factors is sufficient to screen for organic disease. Treatment depends on the underlying cause. Collaboration with a social worker may be needed to identify services that address access needs or to provide meal assistance.

PARKINSON DISEASE AND PARKINSONISM

Parkinsonism is a clinical syndrome consisting of tremor at rest, rigidity, bradykinesia, and gait disturbance; it affects approximately 1% of individuals over age 60. Some 80% to 90% of patients will have idiopathic parkinsonism or Parkinson disease (PD). PD is clinically diagnosed after other less common disorders have been excluded. Box 76-1 lists criteria for the diagnosis of PD. Diagnosis requires three or more of these criteria to be met.

PD is a degenerative disorder of the substantia nigra and ventral tegmental area of the brain resulting in a depletion of striatal dopamine. On autopsy, individuals with PD have Lewy bodies (LBs), which are intracytoplasmic inclusion bodies in the nigral neurons. LBs are also found in the cerebral cortex, which may explain why about one-third of PD patients develop dementia later in the course of the disease.

PD may be confused with essential tremor (ET), another idiopathic movement disorder that is familial and increases with age. However, unlike the parkinsonian resting tremor, the tremor of ET is increased by movement and decreased by rest. Stroke is sometimes confused with PD. However, in PD, other features such as cogwheel rigidity and bradykinesia are present, while stroke-related defects such as weakness, decreased sensation, and abnormal reflexes are absent. Multiple small strokes can also mimic PD, but a MRI showing multiple small strokes in the basal ganglia and a poor response to levodopa usually distinguish the two.

Bradykinesia is probably the most disabling feature of PD, affecting almost all voluntary and many involuntary actions. As a result, many PD patients have difficulty initiating movements. PD patients often experience symptoms of autonomic dysfunction, including hypohidrosis, orthostatic hypotension, impotence, blurred vision, constipation, and incontinence. Phenothiazine drugs such as haloperidol and metoclopropamide can induce a reversible form of parkinsonism.

No cure is available for PD, but symptomatic pharmacologic treatment is helpful when symptoms begin to interfere with the patient's occupational and social functioning. Drugs for PD are listed in Table 76-1. Box 76-2 lists general prescribing guidelines.

Levodopa remains the mainstay of therapy. Combinations of levodopa and carbidopa are the most effective ways to get dopamine into the brain. Dopamine is ineffective because it does not cross the blood–brain barrier; however, levodopa is able to cross, and once in the brain is converted to dopamine through decarboxylization. Carbidopa inhibits only the peripheral decarboxylation of levodopa and lessens side effects by enhancing the central availability of levodopa and making it possible to reduce the therapeutic dose. Levodopa/carbidopa is commercially marketed as Sinemet and is available in a wide range of formulations, so that dosing can be titrated to an individual's needs. Levodopa is usually most effective for bradykinesia and rigidity and less so for tremors. If patients with suspected PD fail to respond at all to levodopa, one of the atypical PD states such as Wilson disease or a hereditary condition should be considered.

For younger patients with mild symptoms, anticholinergic or dopamine agonist medications may be adequate therapy. Anticholinergics are more effective for tremor than for rigidity or bradykinesia. Dopamine agonists act directly on the presynaptic and postsynaptic receptors and can allow for sparing the use of levodopa. The effectiveness of levodopa diminishes and the incidence of adverse effects increases over time with use of levodopa. For patients that require higher doses of levodopa, dopamine agonists can be added as adjunctive therapy.

Management of secondary parkinsonism depends on the cause. In arthrosclerotic parkinsonism and many other degenerative disorders, treatment is similar to that of PD. However, the response in these conditions is less marked than that in PD.

SKIN DISORDERS

XEROSIS

Xerosis (dry skin) is related to a decrease in sebum production and an increase in water vapor permeability. Treatment includes the frequent use of emollients and moisturizers, up to four times a day.

Pruritis, which is often due to xerosis, is most common in the winter and may be exacerbated by excessive bathing and harsh soaps or medications. Other causes include stress and systemic diseases such as renal insufficiency, hypothyroidism, hepatitis, anemia, diabetes, and malignancy. Therapy should be directed at the underlying cause. Symptomatic treatment includes emollients, nonmedicated soaps, limitation of soap usage to the axillae and genital areas, and the use of topical steroids and systemic antihistamines.

■ BOX 76-1 Criteria for Diagnosis of Parkinson Disease

Unilateral onset and persistent asymmetry
Resting tremor (typically pill rolling)
Progressive disability
Cogwheel rigidity
Bradykinesia
Excellent response to levodopa

■ TABLE 76-1 Pharmacologic Therapies for Parkinson Disease

Drugs	Comment	Side Effect
Dopamine precursors Levodopa/carbidopa	Mainstay of PD therapy	GI, dizziness, confusion, common dyskinesia.
Anticholinergics Trihexyphenidyl (Artane) Benztropine (Cogentin)	Effective for tremor/drool.	Confusion, constipation, urinary retention, dry mouth. Side effects more common in elderly.
Dopamine agonists Amantadine Bromocriptine (Parlodel) Pergolide mesylate (Permax) Pramipexole (Mirapex) Ropinirole (Requip)	Expensive, may be effective as single agent in early PD. Not as effective as Sinemet. Also used as adjunct in later stages. Effect of amantadine disappears in few months.	Nausea, dizziness.
Monoamine oxidase type B inhibitor Selegiline	Symptomatic benefit limited. Controversial but may have protective effect in early PD. Expensive.	
Catechol-O-methyltranferase transverse inhibitors Tolcapone (Tasmar) Entacapone (Comtan)	Enhance levodopa therapy.	Dizziness, diarrhea, dyskinesia. Use of tolcapone requires monitoring of liver function tests.

SCABIES

Scabies, caused by the scabies mite, produces an intensely pruritic rash that sometimes occurs in epidemics among nursing home residents. Itching usually begins 2 weeks after an infestation and typically worsens at night. Skin findings are variable and can range from a few to hundreds of small red papules. Many are covered with scaly crusts. The diagnosis of scabies can be confirmed by microscopic examination of skin scrapings. A specimen is placed on a glass slide with mineral oil and examined at low power to identify mites or their feces. Effective treatment of scabies may be accomplished by one of several scabicides including 1% gamma-benzene hexachloride lotion (Lindane), crotamiton (Eurax), or 5% permethrin cream (Elimite).

SEBORRHEIC KERATOSES

Seborrheic keratoses (SKs), a form of benign skin tumor, are quite common in older patients. They typically vary in color from tan to dark brown and range in size from lesions that are barely visible to several centimeters. They often have the appearance of being stuck on the skin. Removal of SKs may be indicated when they cause discomfort because of their location or if they cause cosmetic concerns. They may be removed using cryotherapy or by scraping them with a sharp dermal curette.

ACTINIC KERATOSES

Actinic keratoses (AKs) are precancerous lesions that are primarily seen in the middle-aged and elderly population. These lesions are induced by UV light and are

■ BOX 76-2 General Prescribing Guidelines for Parkinson Disease

Start treatment with one drug.
Start with lowest practical dose and increase gradually.
Make one change at a time unless patient is in crisis.
Eventually multiple drugs may be needed.

more common in fair-skinned individuals. Untreated, AKs have about a 1% per year risk of developing into squamous cell carcinomas. AKs are asymptomatic, red, rough, scaly lesions on sun-exposed sites such as the face, hands, and arms. Treatment consists of local destruction by one of several methods including cryotherapy or curetting. Extensive lesions may be treated with a topical agent such as 5-fluorouracil.

BASAL CELL CARCINOMA

Basal cell carcinoma (BCC) is the most common human malignancy. Risk factors include fair skin, history of sunburn, family history of skin cancer, and outdoor occupation. Approximately 80% of these lesions occur on sun-exposed areas of the head and neck. The typical appearance is that of a pink nodule that has a translucent or pearly quality with overlying telangiectatic vessels. BCC rarely metastasizes but can become locally invasive and destructive over the course of years. The diagnosis relies on clinical suspicion followed by biopsy of the lesion. The most common forms of therapy are surgical excision or curettage and electrodesiccation.

MALIGNANT MELANOMA

Malignant melanoma is a neoplasm that is especially important to diagnose because it is one of the few potentially fatal skin diseases. Patients at greater risk include those with fair complexions and light hair and eyes and those with excessive skin exposure. The diagnosis of malignant melanoma requires biopsy of clinically suspicious lesions. Management should be individualized for each patient, especially for the elderly individual. Survival is most closely related to the depth of tumor invasion.

KEY POINTS

- Hearing loss is the most common sensory impairment of old age; approximately 40% of elderly individuals have some type of hearing loss.

- The four most common ophthalmologic diseases encountered in the elderly are cataracts or lens opacification, macular degeneration, open-angle glaucoma, and diabetic retinopathy.

- Involuntary weight loss in the elderly is a serious problem; a 1-year documented weight loss of more than 4% is the best single predictor of death within 2 years.

- Parkinsonism affects approximately 1% of individuals over age 60. Some 80% to 90% of these patients will have idiopathic parkinsonism or PD.

77 Dementia

Dementia is a progressive decline in memory accompanied by a loss of intellectual capabilities severe enough to interfere with social or occupational function. In addition to memory loss, cognitive impairment can affect language, judgment, cognition, visuospatial skills, and personality.

The prevalence of dementia increases significantly with age, with roughly 1% of the population affected by age 60 and almost 50% after age 85. By the year 2030, nearly 20% of the population will be over age 65, and the societal burden of dementia will become an even greater health care concern. Although the majority of cases of dementia are irreversible, family physicians must be aware of the reversible causes, methods of diagnosing the various causes of dementia, and treatment options for both the patients and their families.

PATHOGENESIS

Alzheimer disease (AD) is the most common cause of dementia and accounts for over half of all cases. Postmortem analysis of patients with AD demonstrates brain atrophy, enlarged ventricles, and minimal evidence of vascular disease. Histologic findings usually located in the frontotemporal lobes include intracellular neurofibrillary tangles comprising tau proteins and extracellular plaques consisting of beta-amyloid protein. These lead to neuronal loss and subsequent disturbances in the cholinergic system, which accounts for the progressive cognitive decline. Although there is a rare autosomal dominant form of the disease involving the gene for the amyloid protein, most cases are sporadic. Risk factors for AD include advanced age, female gender, and a family history of the disease. The apolipoprotein APO-E4 on chromosome 19 is associated with an increased risk for AD. However, testing for APO-E4 is neither sensitive nor specific enough to justify its use as a screening test.

Vascular dementia is the second most common cause of dementia and results from tissue damage due to cerebral ischemia and hypoxia. Patients with HTN, diabetes, a history of smoking, and known arterial disease are at risk. Multi-infarct dementia due to a series of small-vessel infarctions known as lacunar strokes is one type of vascular dementia. The multiple infarcts typically cause patients to experience discrete episodes of worsening cognition that occur in a stepwise manner. In older patients, AD and vascular dementia may occur together.

Severely depressed patients may present with cognitive slowing and poor memory, a condition termed pseudodementia, which mimics dementia. These individuals usually improve once treatment is initiated. Depression is also common in patients with an underlying dementia, particularly early in the course of the disease.

Lewy body (LB) dementia is characterized by the presence of LBs, or intracytoplasmic inclusions, and by decreased neuronal density in the hippocampus, amygdala, cortex, and other portions of the brain. Patients with LB dementia have a rapid clinical decline, visual hallucinations, episodic delirium, and extrapyramidal motor signs.

Space-occupying lesions such as subdural hematoma and tumor, infections such as syphilis and HIV, and other neurologic disorders such as MS, PD, and Huntington disease may disrupt neural pathways involved with cognition and memory. Normal-pressure hydrocephalus is characterized by ataxia, incontinence, and dementia and occurs due to diminished absorption of CSF, resulting in compression of the affected neural pathways. Medical disorders such as hypothyroidism, hypercalcemia, vitamin B_{12} or folate deficiency, and acute intoxication can lead to memory impairment. Medications such as sedatives, opiates, antihypertensives, and neuroleptics may cause or exacerbate some of the mental status changes associated with dementia.

CLINICAL MANIFESTATIONS

HISTORY

Because most patients with dementia lack objective insight into their condition, the history is often best obtained through family members, friends, and caregivers. Dementia may also be suspected during a routine evaluation if a patient has difficulty recalling medications, recent events, and medical history. Questions should be asked about patient orientation, episodes of forgetfulness, ADLs, and job duties. Examples include instances of patients getting lost; forgetting words, names, or recipes; neglecting personal hygiene; and not knowing common facts such as their own address and current events. Episodes of social withdrawal, frustration with emotional outbursts, and difficulty driving are common in patients with dementia and should be ascertained. The time course of symptoms (e.g., abrupt vs. gradual), duration, and course (e.g., continuous, fluctuating, or stepwise) are helpful in determining the type of dementia.

Past surgical and medical history should focus on episodes of head trauma, previous vascular surgery, meningitis, and other neurologic diseases. Having a family history of a first-degree relative with dementia and being female increase the risk for dementia.

All medications must be reviewed and alcohol intake and nutrition assessed. Sexual history determines risk for HIV and syphilis. Review of systems should focus on signs of depression, thyroid disorder, and other neurologic disorders.

PHYSICAL EXAMINATION

The physical examination should include mental status evaluation, neurologic examination, and a general examination aimed at identifying illness that may be contributing to the patient's cognitive decline. A general assessment also provides information about hygiene, nutritional status, and attentiveness. The physical examination can also identify problems such as hearing or vision loss and orthopedic problems that may be interfering with ADLs.

The MMSE is a standardized test that is useful in determining the presence of dementia. Specifically, the MMSE provides insight into patient orientation, recall, attention, language ability, visuospatial ability, and executive functioning. The score can be corrected for the level of education and followed over time.

A complete neurologic examination can detect abnormalities suggesting prior stroke, a mass, or evidence of PD. Abstract reasoning can be assessed by asking the meaning of phrases such as "People in glass houses shouldn't throw stones." Psychiatric assessment determines the presence of depression and other psychiatric disorders. Neuropsychiatric testing can also be done to differentiate the type of dementia as well as its extent.

DIFFERENTIAL DIAGNOSIS

Box 77-1 lists the causes of dementia. AD accounts for about 50% of cases, and about 15% have a vascular dementia. Other patients may have a mixed dementia, which is caused by a combination of AD and vascular disease, LB dementia (10% to 15%), and frontotemporal dementia (5% to 10%). Dementia

■ BOX 77-1 Differential Diagnosis for Dementia

Alzheimer disease
Multi-infarct dementia
Lewy body dementia
Depression (pseudodementia)
Normal-pressure hydrocephalus
Thyroid disorder
B_{12} deficiency
Folate deficiency
Syphilis with CNS involvement
HIV with CNS involvement Subdural hematoma
Medications:
Opiates
Neuroleptics
Antidepressants
Anticholinergics
Multiple sclerosis
Parkinson disease
Huntington disease
Down syndrome
Intoxication

must also be distinguished from other causes of mental confusion, such as depression and delirium.

Delirium, referred to as an acute confusional state, affects memory and cognition. Delirium typically occurs suddenly over hours to days and is associated with a clouding of consciousness and disruption of the sleep cycle. It is often reversible. Patients with dementia are at increased risk for developing delirium. Acute changes in mental status merit ruling out a toxic reaction to medicine as well as physical illnesses such as infection, dehydration, hypoxia, electrolyte imbalance, anemia, and hepatic failure. Depression may mimic dementia. Typically symptoms of depression precede memory loss and depressed patients appear apathetic.

DIAGNOSTIC EVALUATION

There are no definitive tests for diagnosing most of the disorders that cause dementia, including AD. The diagnostic evaluation should focus on recognizing potentially treatable causes of dementia and identifying treatable coexisting illnesses that may be contributing to impaired cognition. History, physical

■ **BOX 77-2** Indications for Neuroimaging

Recent onset dementia
Rapid progression
History of head trauma
Younger age
Urinary incontinence and gait disorders
Focal abnormalities on neurologic examination

■ **BOX 77-3** Managing Patients With Dementia

Optimize Function
Treat medical conditions that impair function
Optimize hearing and vision
Avoid medications that impair cognition
Encourage physical and social activity
Assess nutrition
Identify and Manage Behavioral Complications
Psychosis
Agitation and aggression
Depression
Wandering
Caregiver Education and Support
Discuss prognosis and progression of disease
Discuss advance directives
Discuss community resources
Recommend legal and financial counseling
Review ethical issues
Offer opportunities for new treatments

examination, and laboratory testing are indicated to rule out conditions that mimic dementia. Appropriate tests include a CBC, ESR, serum electrolytes, calcium, albumin, BUN, creatinine, LFTs, TSH, vitamin B_{12} and folate levels, and UA. Hearing and vision screening are often useful. A chest x-ray and ECG are commonly recommended, and if the patient has risk factors, HIV testing is indicated.

There is controversy about whether all patients with dementia should have some type of neuroimaging procedure such as a CT or MRI. Some authorities recommend testing all patients to rule out conditions such as a subdural hematoma, normal-pressure hydrocephalus, a mass lesion, or vascular dementia. Since the yield for finding conditions that change management is small, others advocate limiting imaging to those with atypical presentations or focal neurologic findings. Box 77-2 lists some indications for imaging. A lumbar puncture is useful in evaluating for vasculitis, CNS infection, and MS; it may improve symptoms in those with normal-pressure hydrocephalus. Formal neuropsychological testing determines more precisely the extent of cognitive impairment and may be useful in patients with atypical deficits or only a mild cognitive decline.

TREATMENT

Patients found to have reversible causes of dementia should receive prompt and appropriate treatment. For example, those with depression should be started on antidepressants and re-evaluated for cognitive improvement. However, because dementia is most often irreversible, the focus is to maintain quality of life and maximize function. Patients and their caregivers should be educated about creating a safe, familiar, and nurturing environment for the patient; managing behavioral problems; and treating comorbid conditions that may exacerbate cognitive decline. Box 77-3 summarizes the management of patients with dementia.

If disruptive behavior persists after optimizing function and using behavioral strategies, the atypical antipsychotics such as quetiapine (Seroquel) are the preferred agents to help control behavior that presents a risk to the patients or others. Phenothiazines (e.g., haloperidol, risperidone) and anticonvulsants are occasionally needed to control disruptive behavior. Since cognitive impairment may be exacerbated by the use of psychoactive medications such as tranquilizers, sleeping pills, anxiolytics, and drugs with anticholinergic activity, they should be used cautiously with careful dosage titration and periodic reassessment of both their indication and dosage. Side effects also include an increased incidence of falls, increased sedation, and—in the case of the phenothiazines—tardive dyskinesia. The dosage and continued use of psychoactive medications should be monitored.

Patients with multi-infarct dementia should have optimal control of HTN, diabetes, and hyperlipidemia; if they are smokers, they should be told to stop. If not contraindicated, they should receive an antiplatelet medication such as aspirin or Plavix. Serial lumbar punctures or the placement of a ventricular shunt may provide benefit for patients with normal-pressure hydrocephalus. Medications thought to be contributing to or exacerbating the dementia should be changed or discontinued.

Patients with suspected AD may benefit from the use of reversible acetylcholinesterase inhibitors such as tacrine (Cognex), donepezil (Aricept), rivastigmine (Exelon), or galantamine (Reminyl). These all appear to slow the progression of AD and typically result in a small improvement in symptoms followed by a gradual decline to a level below baseline, a pattern that on average correlates to a 2- to 7-month delay in loss of cognition. A newer medication for moderate to severe AD is memantine (Namenda). It is an *N*-methyl-D-aspartate (NMDA) receptor antagonist and can be used along with the acetylcholinesterase inhibitors. Caregivers of those with AD must be educated regarding home safety, long-term-care options, and the importance of a living will. Since they are at high risk for burnout, caregivers may also benefit from joining support groups, which can help them to cope with the task of taking care of their loved ones.

KEY POINTS

- Dementia is a progressive decline in memory and a loss of intellectual capabilities severe enough to interfere with social or occupational function.
- Multi-infarct dementia due to a series of small-vessel infarctions causes patients to experience discrete episodes of worsening cognition, which occur in a stepwise manner.
- Patients with dementia are diagnosed by history, physical examination, and laboratory testing to rule out conditions that mimic dementia.
- Patients with suspected AD may benefit from the use of reversible acetylcholinesterase inhibitors and NMDA receptor antagonists.

Urinary Incontinence

Urinary incontinence (UI) is defined as the involuntary loss of urine severe enough to cause social and hygiene problems. It is a significant cause of disability and dependency and can lead to social isolation, depression, skin breakdown, UTI, and falls; it also incurs significant economic cost. UI is so common in the elderly population that it is considered a classic geriatric syndrome. Approximately one-third of community-dwelling women and one-fourth of elderly men experience some degree of incontinence, and the prevalence increases with age. About one-half of patients who are homebound or live in long-term-care facilities suffer from incontinence. Despite this prevalence, 50% of incontinent patients have never discussed it with their physicians. Many patients feel that incontinence is part of the aging process and are embarrassed to discuss it or believe that there is no treatment for it.

PATHOGENESIS

Normal urination is a complex process; knowledge of the pathophysiology is needed to understand the causes of UI.

The lower tract consists of the bladder and urethra. The urethra has two sphincters, an internal one, consisting of smooth muscle, and an external one, with both smooth and striated muscle. The bladder is made up of a smooth muscle called the detrusor muscle, which is innervated primarily by cholinergic neurons from the parasympathetic system. When these neurons are stimulated, bladder contraction occurs. The sympathetic system innervates both the bladder and the internal sphincter. The beta-adrenergic system in the bladder produces relaxation and the alpha-adrenergic receptors cause sphincter contraction. The striated muscle of the external sphincter allows voluntary interruption of voiding. Additional voluntary control comes from the CNS, which inhibits the autonomic processes described above through the pontine micturition center. Normal pelvic geometry is important for adequate sphincter function, since it allows intra-abdominal pressure to be distributed equally, preventing urine leakage from activities such as coughing, sneezing, laughing, or straining. All of these are associated with increased intra-abdominal pressure.

Three basic mechanisms cause urinary incontinence. These are overactivity of the bladder detrusor muscle (urge incontinence), malfunction of the urinary sphincters (stress incontinence), and overflow from the bladder (urinary retention). **Urge incontinence** occurs when uninhibited bladder contractions are sufficient to overcome urethral resistance. **Stress incontinence** is involuntary loss of urine during coughing, sneezing, standing, or exercising. In **overflow incontinence,** either obstruction of urine outflow or ineffective bladder contractions cause urinary retention. As the bladder distention reaches maximum capacity, there is a point at which urethral sphincter pressure is exceeded and overflow leakage from the bladder occurs.

CLINICAL MANIFESTATIONS

HISTORY

Since at least one-half of patients with UI can be helped with relatively simple measures, it is important to identify patients with UI. Questions such as "Do you have trouble holding your urine?" are an effective way to open a discussion about UI and should be part of the initial evaluation.

Patients with incontinence need a complete history, including an obstetric and surgical history, especially about previous abdominal or pelvic surgery. The medical history should identify problems such as diabetes, CHF, stroke, Parkinson disease (PD), and UTI. Review of medications should include both prescription and over-the-counter meds. Classes of drugs associated with UI include sedatives, pain medications, diuretics, anticholinergics, and calcium channel blockers. There is often a temporal connection between these drugs and the onset or worsening of incontinence. History can also provide important clues to the type of precipitating factors of urinary incontinence. Box 78-1 lists important aspects of the history.

PHYSICAL EXAMINATION

The goals of the physical examination are to identify precipitating factors and establish the pathophysiology. In addition to a general examination, the focus should be on the abdominal, genitourinary, and neurologic

■ **BOX 78-1** History Taking for Urinary Incontinence

Duration of symptoms
Characteristics of UI—for example, timing and amount of incontinent episodes
Fluid intake
Caffeine and alcohol intake
Other urinary symptoms—for example, nocturia, frequency, hematuria, dysuria
Associated events—for example, surgery
Alteration of bowel function
Use of pads or protective devices

■ **BOX 78-2** Drip Mnemonic

D:	delirium, drugs
R:	restricted mobility, retention
I:	infection, inflammation, impaction
P:	polyuria

examinations. Important findings include a distended bladder, enlarged prostate, uterine prolapse, cystocele, or rectocele. Examining patients for sphincter tone, perineal sensation, and fecal impaction, and for the presence of a rectal mass is important. The neurologic examination should detect evidence of cognitive impairment, spinal cord disease, and CVA.

DIFFERENTIAL DIAGNOSIS

The initial classification can be divided into acute reversible forms and persistent UI. Persistent incontinence occurs over time and is unrelated to an acute event. It can usually be classified by pathophysiology—that is, into stress, urge, or overflow incontinence. Stress incontinence, or the involuntary loss of urine when intra-abdominal pressure increases, is most frequently caused by relaxation of the pelvic musculature. It is more common in women who have had vaginal deliveries of children but also occurs in men whose sphincters may have been damaged by transurethral surgery or radiation therapy. Urge incontinence is usually associated with involuntary detrusor activity. Many neurologic problems such as stroke, dementia, PD, and spinal cord injury are associated with this problem. If no neurologic disease is present, the condition is called detrusor instability. Patients often complain of having the sudden urge to go and being unable to get to the bathroom in time. Occasionally, individuals who have bladder instability can have impaired contractions, creating a combination of urge incontinence and urinary retention. Overflow incontinence, caused by overdistention of the bladder, can be caused by anatomic obstruction (e.g., prostate disease), urethral stricture, or neurologic factors such as diabetes or MS that result in an underactive bladder. Medications such as sympathomimetics, anticholinergics, or narcotics may also cause retention. Functional incontinence is the loss of urine from factors outside the urinary tract. In this situation,

the urinary system is normal but the patient cannot reach the toilet because of reasons such as decreased awareness, as seen in dementia, poor mobility, or inadequate access to bathroom facilities. Often UI is a mixture of causes, as in the case of someone with urge incontinence whose impaired mobility may cause the loss of urine.

Acute reversible UI usually has a sudden onset and is associated with an illness. Acute factors may contribute to worsening of chronic UI. A useful mnemonic to evaluate incontinence, DRIP, is outlined in Box 78-2. Acute infection is a common cause of UI, along with fecal impaction and inflammatory conditions such as cystitis or urethritis. Any cause that precipitates polyuria, such as uncontrolled diabetes, alcohol ingestion, diuretics, and CHF can cause incontinence, as can the introduction or alteration of medications.

DIAGNOSTIC EVALUATION

Goals of the initial evaluation are to identify correctable causes, determine who needs further evaluation, and assess which patients can be treated without extensive testing. Generally this can be accomplished with a clinical assessment and a few simple tests. All patients should have a UA, which can detect infection (a common cause of reversible incontinence), uncontrolled diabetes, and hematuria, which suggests the need for further workup.

Postvoid residual (PVR) can be assessed by either US or bladder catheterization. Catheterization is commonly used in women, while US is often preferred in men because catheterization may be more difficult or traumatic. PVRs of less than 75 mL are considered normal and levels of 75 to 200 mL borderline. Any PVR of more than 200 mL requires further investigation.

If no recent laboratory work is available, baseline values—including serum electrolytes, BUN, creatinine, glucose, and calcium—should be assessed to determine renal function and identify conditions causing polyuria.

After the initial laboratory and clinical assessment, most potentially reversible causes of UI can be identified and the nature of the incontinence classified. Characteristics suggesting the need for further evaluation and testing include an unclear diagnosis, recent history of pelvic surgery, symptomatic pelvic prolapse, UI with recurrent symptomatic infection, hematuria without infection, PVR greater than 200 mL, prostate nodules, an abnormality suggesting neurologic disease, and failure to respond to adequate treatment. Commonly, when further evaluation and testing are indicated, the patient is referred to a urologist or gynecologist who may then elect to perform urodynamic testing and/or cystoscopy.

TREATMENT

Treatment of UI consists of behavioral, pharmaceutical, and surgical intervention. Generally the least invasive treatment should be used first. Often a combination of therapies is helpful. Behavioral techniques present little risk but often are not very effective. Bladder retraining involving progressive increases in the intervals between voiding may be helpful in patients with urge incontinence. Scheduled voiding, where patients are toileted on a regular basis, is most successful in patients with functional incontinence. Kegel exercises involving repetitive contraction of the pelvic floor muscles can strengthen the pelvic floor. These exercises are helpful for improving or controlling stress incontinence. In addition to behavioral techniques, assessing the environment and improving access to toileting or improving the call system for assistance may improve incontinence. Simple lifestyle changes may also be of help in mild incontinence. Restriction of fluids and decreased intake of alcohol and caffeine should be recommended.

Several medications may be helpful. These drugs should be started at a low dose and gradually titrated upward to maximize benefits and reduce side effects. Oxybutynin, imipramine, and tolterodine can help to control urge incontinence. Calcium channel blockers may be useful in patients with concomitant medical conditions, such as hypertension. Drugs such as pseudoephedrine, with alpha-adrenergic properties that stimulate the internal sphincter, may improve stress incontinence. Estrogen may be helpful in patients with atrophic vaginitis and can be used in combination with pseudoephedrine. Effective drugs for overflow incontinence work by stimulating bladder contractions or relaxing the sphincter. Cholinergic agents such as bethanechol stimulate the bladder and may be helpful in patients with an atonic bladder due to neurologic conditions such as diabetic neuropathy; however, medical treatment in overflow incontinence caused by bladder contractility problems is not very effective. Alpha-adrenergic blockers such as terazosin, prazosin, or tamulosin are often used in men

with BPH to relax the internal sphincter. Surgery should be considered in patients with severe stress incontinence. Options include periurethral bulking agents, transvaginal suspensions, slings, and sphincter prostheses. Patients with an obstructive disease (e.g., BPH or urethral stenosis) may also benefit from surgery.

In patients with intractable UI, a variety of absorbent pads, garments, and collection systems are available. The goal of these products is urine containment and prevention of skin breakdown. Pessaries should be tried in women with cystocele and uterine prolapse who will not consider surgery. Although urethral catheters should generally not be used, external collection devices (Texas catheters) are preferable to indwelling catheters in patients who have not been helped by other measures. However, external devices are not widely available for women. If internal catheterization is necessary, an intermittent or suprapubic method is recommended so as to decrease bacteriuria. Indwelling catheters should be reserved for comfort in terminally ill patients, to prevent worsening of pressure ulcers, and for patients with inoperable outflow obstruction.

KEY POINTS

- Approximately one-third of community-dwelling elderly women and one-fourth of elderly men experience some degree of UI; the prevalence increases with age.

- Three basic mechanisms cause UI. These are overactivity of the bladder detrusor muscle (urge incontinence), malfunction of the urinary sphincters (stress incontinence), and overflow from the bladder (urinary retention).

- All patients should have a UA, which can detect infection—a common cause of reversible incontinence, uncontrolled diabetes, and hematuria, which suggests the need for further workup.

- PVRs of less than 75 mL are considered normal and levels of 75 to 200 mL borderline; levels greater than 200 mL require further investigation.

- Treatment of UI consists of behavioral, pharmaceutical, and surgical intervention.

Nursing Home and End-of-Life Care

Nursing homes (NHs) or long-term-care facilities (LTCs) are institutions that offer around-the-clock nursing care as well as medical, social, and personal services to individuals unable to fully care for themselves or who are in need of rehabilitation to restore this capacity. About one-half of women and one-third of men in the United States will spend some time in an NH before they die. Admissions rise with age and NH admissions increase rapidly after age 85.

NH residents are nearly evenly divided between short-term (less than 6 months) and long-term (greater than 6 months) residents. Short-term residents are evenly divided by those admitted for rehabilitation and those admitted for terminal care. LTC residents typically have physical or cognitive impairments that make them unable to live in the community. Among LTC residents, the prevalence of mental disorders such as dementia, delirium, and mental illness approaches 90%.

COMMON MEDICAL PROBLEMS

Physicians caring for patients in NHs encounter several common problems repeatedly. Some degree of incontinence occurs in more than half of NH admissions and often precipitates admission. More than two-thirds of NH patients fall at least once a year, often with serious injury. Risk factors for falls include psychoactive drugs, overmedication, balance problems, weakness, poor functional status, and intermittent use of restraints. Physical therapy to increase strength and balance may reduce falls, and aggressive treatment of osteoporosis may reduce the risk of fractures resulting from falls.

Nutrition problems are also common among NH residents, and weight is an important parameter to follow. Loss of more 5 lb in 1 month or 10 lb in 6 months is considered significant. Underlying medical conditions common in LTC residents—such as poor dentition, cancer, movement disorders, and mechanical problems such as difficulty swallowing—can contribute to malnutrition. Poor nutrition impairs wound healing and the ability to mount an immune response, placing NH patients at greater risk for infection, pressure sores, and other significant problems.

Infections in particular are a serious issue, and up to 15% of NH residents suffer from infection at any given time. Frequently encountered infections include pneumonia, UTI, infected pressure sores, and cellulitis. In addition to fever, infections in the LTC setting present with nonspecific symptoms such as confusion, change in behavior, loss of appetite, and weight loss, weakness, or lethargy.

Medication can cause serious side effects. On average, LTC residents take more than eight medications. Medications should be monitored and periodically reviewed for their continued need. Reviewing the diagnosis, symptoms, and severity should be part of evaluating whether a medicine is appropriate, and dosages should be assessed and lowered whenever possible. Psychoactive and antipsychotic medications in particular should be evaluated on a regular basis. Relevant symptoms should be documented, along with evidence that the treatment helps. Attempts to reduce dosages or eliminate psychoactive medications should be considered and documented. As a general rule, NH patients benefit more from reducing the number of medications than adding additional ones.

MONITORING CARE

The goal of the NH is to provide a safe and supportive environment for chronically ill and dependent individuals. Quality of life should be maximized and chronic conditions stabilized, with management directed at delaying the progression of disease and improving function. Each visit merits asking the patient about any new complaints and asking the nurse if there are any changes of status.

A change in status should prompt an assessment for infections such as pneumonia or UTI, fecal impaction, or medication side effects. Symptoms relevant to existing conditions should be sought (e.g., edema and dyspnea in patients with CHF); if these are present, they should be addressed, along with special tests relevant to patients with chronic disease (e.g., blood sugars in patients with diabetes mellitus and electrolytes in patients with CHF). It is important to review nursing notes, to listen to patients even if they are cognitively impaired, and to make sure that patients are examined and touched.

The physical examination should include weight, vital signs, and a targeted examination to evaluate new complaints and follow active conditions. The assessment should address the stability of active chronic conditions and new complaints or changes in status. The plan should include a medication review, appropriate labs, testing, consultations, and other therapies that might benefit the patient. Yearly, a more detailed examination and functional assessment—including the MMSE as well as testing of vision and hearing—should be considered.

END OF LIFE

Many cognitively ill patients have lost the capacity for decision making. Advance directives made when the patient is competent allow the patient's wishes to be honored and followed in the event that the patient should no longer be able to communicate these wishes. Despite the recent emphasis on advance directives, only about 15% of the general adult population has completed a directive of this type.

ADVANCE DIRECTIVES

In discussing advance directives, it is important to assure patients that their clinical care will be consistent with their preferences. Shared decision making among the patient, his or her proxy, and the physician gives the proxy an opportunity to voice his or her concerns and to be aware of the patient's preferences.

Two common types of advance directives are a living will and health care power of attorney. A living will contains information about the patient's wishes if the patient were to become incapable of communicating those wishes. The health care power of attorney appoints an individual or surrogate to act as the patient's medical decision maker if the patient should become incapable of making such decisions. Since conflict may develop between family members or the physician about what is in the patient's best interests, discussion in advance about resuscitation, invasive interventions, and enteral nutrition can decrease the stress of making a decision at a time of crisis.

HOSPICE

Hospice care is a type of care provided to patients whose life expectancy is 6 months or less. Hospice care may be provided in the home or in an institutional setting such as an NH. Although traditionally associated with cancer care, hospice is appropriate for end-stage patents with conditions such as CHF, COPD, dementia, and chronic renal failure.

Hospice care shifts the emphasis toward palliation, emphasizing symptomatic treatment and comfort measures. The management of pain and relief of symptoms is the primary concern. Special attention is paid to the patient's physical, emotional, and spiritual needs rather than trying to cure his or her illness or prolong life.

KEY POINTS

- About one-half of women and one-third of men in the United States will spend some time in an NH before they die. NH admissions increase rapidly after age 85.

- Up to 15% of NH residents suffer from infection. Frequently encountered infections include pneumonia, UTI, infected pressure sores, and cellulitis.

- The goal of the NH is to provide a safe and supportive environment for chronically ill and dependent individuals.

- A change in status merits looking for infections such as pneumonia or UTI, fecal impaction, or medication side effects.

- A living will contains information about the patient's wishes if the patient were to become incapable of communicating those wishes; the health care power of attorney appoints an individual or surrogate to act as the patient's medical decision maker if the patient should become incapable of making such decisions.

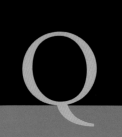

Questions

1. A 7-year-old child moved to the United States 6 months ago. His past medical history and physical examination are unremarkable. You review his immunization records and note that he has missed a few immunizations. When providing "catch-up" shots, which of the following immunizations can you safely omit at this age?
   a. Mumps, measles, rubella (MMR)
   b. Influenza
   c. Hemophilus influenzae
   d. Pertussis
   e. Hepatitis B

2. A 23-year-old female presents for a colposcopy and cervical biopsy. Which of the following is a true statement about obtaining informed consent on this patient?
   a. Informed consent is not needed
   b. Informed consent is implied by the patient allowing the procedure to be performed
   c. Risks and benefits of the procedures must be included in the discussion
   d. Alternative forms of treatment do not need to be reviewed
   e. Patient can be told that there are possible side effects, but specific side effects do not need to be reviewed

3. Mr. Jones presents to your office with a desire to quit smoking. He would like to set a date to quit but first wants get nicotine replacement or other therapy to help with his attempt. You determine that he is in which of the "stages of readiness" to quit smoking.
   a. Precontemplation
   b. Contemplation
   c. Preparation
   d. Action

4. Which of the following is important in deciding that a test is appropriate for screening?
   a. A low prevalence of disease being tested
   b. Lack of effective therapies for the disease
   c. High specificity of the test
   d. High sensitivity of the test
   e. Both c and d

5. A 40-year-old male presents for an annual physical examination. He has no significant family history and a normal physical examination. Which of the following tests will you recommend for screening this patient?
   a. Cholesterol
   b. PSA
   c. Colonoscopy
   d. Stress treadmill
   e. Glucose

6. A 2-month old presents for a well-child exam and is noted to have bruising on the torso and extremities. The mother seems unconcerned and states that she thinks he fell. An appropriate course of action would now include:
   a. Observation
   b. Notification of child protective services
   c. Referral for hematology consultation
   d. Supplementation with vitamin with iron
   e. Psychiatric evaluation of the mother

7. An 86-year-old male presents with the following skin lesion. Treatment options for this would include:
   a. Topical clindamycin
   b. Salicylic acid topically
   c. Retinoic acid topically
   d. No therapy
   e. Surgical excision

8. A 74-year-old female presents with a flat affect, poor eye contact, and limited interaction during the interview. Upon physical examination, there is no rigidity, bradykinesia, or tremors noted and the neurologic examination appears to be normal. During the Mini-Mental Status Examination (MMSE) questions she responds to many of the questions with "I don't know." A likely diagnosis in this patient is:
   a. Parkinson disease
   b. Dementia
   c. Delirium
   d. Stroke
   e. Depression

9. An 85-year-old male presents with his daughter who notes that he has had a gradually progressive loss of function resulting in forgetfulness and inability to live alone because of loss of IADLs. He scores a 22/30 on his MMSE and otherwise has a nonfocal neurologic examination. Which of the following is the most likely cause for his findings?
   a. Multi-infarct dementia
   b. Lewy body dementia

c. Parkinson disease

d. Alzheimer disease

e. Huntington disease

10. When assessing a patient to distinguish dementia from delirium, which of the following is true?
    a. Both have a gradual onset and are progressive
    b. Delirium is only associated with alcohol withdrawal
    c. Sleep is unaffected by delirium
    d. Patients with dementia rarely develop delirium
    e. Medication reactions and infections commonly cause delirium

11. A 70-year-old male presents with a rhythmic tremor in his right hand while sitting and talking with you. Upon testing his neurologic function in that hand, the tremor disappears. Although the man moves about very slowly, his exam is otherwise normal. Which of the following are true regarding his diagnosis and treatment?
    a. He has an essential tremor and needs no treatment
    b. Urgent therapy is needed utilizing levodopa
    c. Parkinson disease is unlikely since it is asymmetric
    d. He has suffered a stroke and requires hospitalization
    e. Metoclopramide (Reglan) may induce or aggravate his condition

12. A 75-year-old female presents with history of urinary incontinence. She notes that she cannot get to the bathroom in time when she feels the sensation to urinate. She has no pain or fever. She takes sertraline for anxiety but otherwise is healthy. Initial steps in management of this patient include:
    a. Discontinuing the sertraline
    b. Urinalysis and culture
    c. Cystoscopy
    d. Use of anticholinergic medication such as oxybutynin
    e. Advising her to curtail her liquid intake

13. When performing a geriatric assessment, which of the following tests should be considered routine?
    a. PSA
    b. Rheumatoid factor
    c. Gait evaluation
    d. Liver function tests
    e. Serum iron

14. When considering involuntary weight loss in the geriatric population, which of the following is true?
    a. More than 4% loss is predictive of death within 2 years
    b. Only about 5% have no identifiable cause
    c. Hyperthyroidism is the most common cause
    d. Functional impairments rarely cause weight loss

15. The family of an 85-year-old patient with advance dementia approach you and are inquiring about hospice care. When counseling this family, which of the following considerations will be important to advise?
    a. Hospice care can only be provided in a hospital setting
    b. Hospice is not appropriate for dementia patients
    c. Over 90% of patients enrolled in hospice have cancer as their diagnosis
    d. Patients enrolled in hospice should not be told because it will demoralize them
    e. An important criteria for hospice is life expectancy less than 6 months

16. A 75-year-old male presents with increasing difficulty reading and has loss of central vision. He reports no additional problems related to bright lights. You make a referral for him to see an ophthalmologist because you are concerned about which of the following?
    a. Presbyopia
    b. Glaucoma
    c. Cataracts
    d. Macular degeneration
    e. Strabismus
    f. Psych

17. You are seeing a patient in your office with elevated liver enzymes on recent blood testing and suspect alcohol abuse as a potential cause. You administer the "CAGE" questionnaire. When utilizing this test, which of the following must you consider?
    a. Results provide a conclusive diagnosis
    b. Sensitivity of the test is greater than 95%
    c. Specificity of the test is around 90%
    d. The test requires referral for accurate interpretation
    e. Over half of adults meet criteria for substance abuse

18. Somatization is characterized by which of the following?
    a. Onset after age 50 years
    b. More common in men
    c. Extreme loyalty to one physician
    d. Symptoms in an isolated organ/system
    e. Exaggeration of patient complaints

19. You are seeing a 14-month-old male for a well-child visit. Which of the following are recommended at this age as screening or preventive care measures?
    a. Blood lead level
    b. Serum glucose
    c. Serum bilirubin
    d. Human papillomavirus vaccine
    e. Serum cholesterol

20. Which of the following medical conditions may present as an anxiety disorder?
    a. Posttraumatic syndrome
    b. Obsessive–compulsive disorder
    c. Postconcussion syndrome
    d. Panic disorder
    e. Phobias

21. You are implementing a smoking cessation program within your office and in setting up the program will be providing education to the staff. Important considerations to emphasize include:
    a. You should wait for patients to show interest in quitting before discussing smoking with them
    b. Older patients will derive no health benefit from quitting
    c. Teenagers are a low-risk subgroup for smoking
    d. Lung cancer risk is never reduced by quitting
    e. Risk of a second heart attack drops by 50% in 1 to 2 years

22. An 65 year-old male presents with his wife who notes that he is getting up every 2 hours to urinate. He denies any pain or fever. Physical examination is unremarkable other than a slightly enlarged prostate with a firm nodule. Urinalysis by dipstick in the office is negative. His PSA value is 8 ng/mL. To evaluate this patient further, which of the following is indicated?
    a. CT scan of the abdomen and pelvic
    b. Ultrasound of the renal system
    c. No further testing
    d. Serum glucose
    e. Needle biopsy of the prostate

23. A 50-year-old male presents with a painful red eye and notes that in the affected eye, he sees halos around lights. Upon eliciting the history and performing the examination, which of the following confirms the need for urgent referral?
    a. Unilateral involvement
    b. Purulent discharge
    c. Severe itching
    d. Dilation of the pupil
    e. A nodular lesion on the lid margin

24. You are seeing a 45-year-old male who noted onset of back pain 1 week ago after working in his yard and doing heavy lifting. When considering the causes for his back pain, which of the following would be most common?
    a. Muscle strain
    b. Malignancy
    c. Infection
    d. Herniated disc
    e. Nephrolithiasis

25. A 40-year-old female presents with asymptomatic hematuria with eight RBCs/HPF. This is confirmed by a repeat urine examination on another occasion. At this point, which of the following would you recommend?
    a. Renal biopsy
    b. MRI
    c. Antinuclear antibody test
    d. Urine culture
    e. Cystoscopy

26. You are seeing a 76-year-old male with constant leaking of urine and a postvoid residual of 210 cc of urine. Appropriate initial treatment of this patient would include which of the following?
    a. Pseudoephedrine
    b. Oxybutynin
    c. Urecholine
    d. Foley catheterization
    e. Finasteride

27. Which of the following represents age-related hearing loss?
    a. Meniere disease
    b. Otosclerosis
    c. Acoustic neuroma
    d. Presbycusis
    e. Labyrinthitis

28. A 21-year-old female presents with a history of a breast lump on her right side. She initially noted the lump about 18 months ago. It is not painful. She believed it had begun after getting hit in the chest during a basketball game. It initially grew for 2 to 3 months but has been stable in size since. The presentation of this mass is most consistent with which of the following?
    a. Breast cancer
    b. Fibroadenoma
    c. Fibrocystic breast disease
    d. Mastitis
    e. Intraductal papilloma

29. A 42-year-old male has painful joints in the hands, especially the metacarpophalangeal joints. On exam there is soft tissue swelling about the joints and x-ray reveals bony erosion in the periarticular bone. Which of the following would be the most likely cause for these joint pains?
    a. Systemic lupus erythematosis
    b. Wegener granulomatosis
    c. Osteoarthritis
    d. Rheumatoid arthritis
    e. Scleroderma

30. A 65-year-old male presents for follow-up on his congestive heart failure and hypertension. His last echocardiogram revealed an ejection fraction of 65% with diastolic dysfunction. He has been very stable on his current medical regimen that includes aspirin, carvedilol, lisinopril, furosemide, and digoxin. He has not been hospitalized or symptomatic in over 3 years and his current exam reveals clear lungs, regular heart rate and rhythm with an S4 but no murmurs and no edema. He would like to discontinue some of his medications. Which of the following medications should be discontinued initially?
    a. Carvedilol
    b. Lisinopril
    c. Digoxin
    d. Furosemide
    e. Aspirin

31. A mother brings in her 12-year-old daughter with concerns about weight. The daughter is obese with a BMI of 31. The mother wants an evaluation to find out why she is overweight and you proceed to educate the mother with the following information:
    a. Secondary causes are common and treatable
    b. Therapy for obesity in children involves taking a daily diet pill
    c. The causes for obesity are multifactorial
    d. Thyroid replacement cures most cases
    e. To lose one pound of fat, the patient must have a 2000 calorie deficit

32. A phlebotomist in your office is drawing blood from a patient who is HIV-positive. She accidentally is stuck by the needle after drawing his blood. She comes to see you immediately and you advise which of the following:
    a. Check HIV titers in 2 weeks
    b. Wait and see if she becomes ill, then draw labs and consider treatment
    c. Since no blood was injected into her, she is not at risk
    d. Begin pneumocystis, toxoplasmosis, and mycobacteria prophylaxis now
    e. Begin antiviral prophylactic therapy for HIV now

33. You are evaluating an 18-year-old male for a preparticipation sports exam. He was noted to have proteinuria and a 24-hour sample was collected with separate daytime and nighttime samples. He has daytime proteinuria but virtually no protein is excreted into the urine at night. Further evaluation or counseling of the patient should include:
    a. He may not participate in sports until the proteinuria resolves
    b. Strict bedrest with re-evaluation of his urine in 2 weeks
    c. Referral for renal biopsy
    d. Reassurance that his condition is benign and not needing treatment
    e. Four weeks of a steroid burst and re-evaluation of his urine

34. A 35-year-old female has been treated for *Helicobacter pylori* and now has recurrence of epigastric discomfort. Her diagnosis was initially made by testing for serum *H. pylori* antibodies. In order to determine whether her exposure to *H. pylori* currently represents an active disease state, which of the following would you recommend?
    a. Repeat serology
    b. Barium swallow
    c. Ambulatory esophageal pH monitoring
    d. Abdominal CT scan
    e. Stool for *H. pylori* fecal antigen

35. A 46-year-old patient presents for follow-up care for his hypertension, elevated lipids, and diabetes. His current medications include glipizide, simvastatin, enalapril, and verapamil. He notes increasing problems with constipation since his last visit. Appropriate management of his symptoms would include which of the following?
    a. Referral for colonoscopy
    b. Initiation of laxative therapy
    c. Metoclopropamide 10 mg orally four times daily
    d. Changing his verapamil to alternative therapy
    e. Recommending a low fat diet

36. You are evaluating a 60-year-old male for new onset of jaundice. He is experiencing no pain and minimal symptoms. His skin has a yellowish hue and his sclera are icteric. You plan to order labs and perform additional testing to determine the etiology. Match the following labs with the disease that it can assist with diagnosis:
    1. Antismooth muscle antibodies   a. Hemochromatosis
    2. Ferritin   b. Hemolytic anemia
    3. Ceruloplasmin   c. Autoimmune hepatitis
    4. Antimitochondrial   d. Wilson disease
    5. Haptoglobin   e. Primary biliary cirrhosis

37. A 32-year-old male presents with an enlargement in his axilla that he believes has been there and unchanged for the past 2 weeks. There has been no injury, pain, or drainage from the lesion. He notes no other arm problems or injuries. On exam, you note a 2 cm enlarged, soft, mobile lymph node in the patient's left axilla. There is no redness and the remainder of the upper extremity exam is normal. There are no other areas of lymphadenopathy noted. Which of the following would you recommend for your patient at this time?
    a. Observation for 4 weeks
    b. Surgical removal
    c. Fine needle aspiration
    d. Empiric cephalexin for 10 days
    e. PET scan imaging

38. A 58-year-old male presents with complaints of vomiting less than 1 hour after eating and often, nearly immediately after eating. This has been present for the past 4 months and he believes he has lost some weight as a result. After vomiting, he feels fine until this recurs the next time he eats. It occurs nearly every time he eats and is not associated with nausea, fever, diarrhea, or other abdominal symptoms. He has tried over-the-counter antiemetics, such as Dramamine, with no change in symptoms. He takes no other medications, does not drink, occasionally smokes, and is physically very active. In addition to ordering labs tests, which of the following would you recommend?
    a. Colonoscopy
    b. Abdominal ultrasound
    c. Barium esophogram
    d. Abdominal CT scan
    e. Chest x-ray

39. A 10-year-old male presents with a red, warm patch on his left arm that you believe is consistent with cellulitis. In prescribing an antibiotic for this patient, which of the following organisms should be included in the coverage?
a. *Pseudomonas aeruginosa*
b. *Staphylococcus aureus*
c. *Hemophilus influenzae*
d. *Clostridium difficile*
e. *Streptococcus pneumoniae*

40. A 5-month-old girl presents with fever to 103.8°F. Besides a slight increase in crying and a slight decrease in appetite, there are no other obvious symptoms. Specifically, there is no cough, congestion, emesis, diarrhea, or rash. On exam, the ears, mouth, lungs, and skin are all clear and the child has a soft fontanelle and normal neurologic exam for age. Labs include a WBC count of 16,000 and urinalysis with 5 to 10 WBCs per hpf. Appropriate management would include which of the following?
a. Admit and obtain urine and blood cultures along with empiric antibiotic coverage
b. Counsel about medications for fever and follow-up with phone call the next day
c. Start oral amoxicillin for a 10-day course
d. Obtain chest x-ray
e. Reassure the parents and follow-up prn

41. A 2-year-old male presents with an upper respiratory infection and his mother is concerned about his breathing. He has laryngitis and a harsh barking cough along with some obvious dyspnea. On auscultation, he has good air entry, minimal inspiratory, and expiratory stridor but no retractions or cyanosis. His oxygen saturation is 99% on room air. Appropriate management of this patient would include which of the following?
a. Albuterol by nebulizer every 4 hours as needed
b. Albuterol syrup orally three times per day
c. Prednisone 1 mg/kg daily for 7 days
d. Inhaled racemic epinephrine
e. Oral dexamethasone for one dose

42. A 4-year-old male presents after a seizure described as generalized and lasting 5 minutes. He is currently somnolent but without any focal deficits. His temperature is 102°F. He has nasal congestion and an erythematous pharynx. Management of this patient should include which of the following?
a. Lumbar puncture
b. CT scan of the brain
c. Initiate therapy with phenytoin
d. Administer antipyretic medications
e. Empiric therapy with IV ceftriaxone

43. An 18-year-old female presents for physical examination before heading off to college. She has had regular care throughout childhood. She currently has no complaints. She has no significant past medical history. Her parents and siblings are healthy. She has been sexually active for 1 year. She has a boyfriend and is currently on contraception and states she regularly uses condoms. In providing her preventive health care, which of the following are recommended at this time?
a. Pap smear screening
b. Cholesterol screen
c. STD screening
d. Urinalysis
e. Electrocardiogram

44. A mother brings in her 7-year-old male for evaluation for possible Attention Deficit Disorder. His teacher has noted inattentiveness, impulsivity, and that he forgets to take home or bring back necessary books or assignments. He has a calm demeanor and does not seem fidgety in the office. He is quiet during your exam, which is otherwise normal. To diagnose Attention Deficit Disorder, which of the following is true?
a. CT scan of the brain is part of the evaluation
b. Ages and Stages questionnaire can accurately diagnose ADHD
c. TSH should be obtained in all patients
d. ADHD is a clinical diagnosis
e. Hyperactivity is a universal element of this disorder

45. A 14-year-old girl presents for evaluation of amenorrhea. She has never had a menstrual period and is of normal weight and body build. Upon physical examination, you note that she is lacking both breast development and pubic hair but otherwise appears to have normal genital anatomy. Next steps in the evaluation and management of this patient should include:
a. Karyotype
b. MRI of brain
c. Serum gonadotropin levels
d. Medroxyprogesterone challenge test
e. Serum testosterone

46. A 35-year-old female presents at her 6-week postpartum visit with complaints of feeling down. She notes frequent crying spells and that she is very fatigued. Most days she is so tired that she does not shower or change out of her pajamas until her husband gets home from work in the evening. She denies any suicidal or homicidal thoughts. She has a past medical history of depression for which she took medication. Her husband has returned to work but is extremely supportive and helps with all childcare and housework. Her family is out of town but call frequently and offer support. Which of the following are important considerations in caring for this patient?
a. Depression is unlikely after a happy event such as childbirth
b. Her prior history of depression puts her at increased risk for postpartum depression

c. Her supportive family puts her at low risk for postpartum depression

d. She cannot take antidepressant medication during the postpartum period

e. This degree of fatigue and "postpartum blues" is normal in the postpartum period

47. A 35-year-old female presents for contraceptive care and advice. She has four children and is currently married in a monogamous relationship. They are still unsure if they want additional children. Her last two children were conceived unintentionally in association with first condoms and then oral contraceptive use. The patient admits to having an irregular schedule and to not being reliable with use of these contraceptive choices. Which form of contraception would be most appropriate in meeting her current needs?
a. Intrauterine device
b. Hormonal contraceptive patch
c. Postcoital contraception
d. Female condoms
e. Tubal ligation

48. A 24-year-old female with a history of one lifetime sexual partner undergoes an annual gynecologic examination and is found to have atypical cells of undetermined significance on her Pap smear. Reflex testing for HPV is negative. Follow-up for this patient should include which of the following?
a. Loop electroexcision procedure (LEEP)
b. Repeat Pap smear in 4 months
c. Repeat Pap smear in 12 months
d. Colposcopy
e. Conization

49. You are caring for a 21-year-old G1P0 who on initial screen is found to have a positive urine culture for *Escherichia coli*. The *E. coli* is sensitive to all antibiotics tested. She is afebrile, asymptomatic and has no allergies. Appropriate follow-up care for this patient would include which of the following?
a. Repeat culture to confirm true infection
b. Treatment with amoxicillin
c. Treatment with ciprofloxacin
d. Ultrasound of her kidneys
e. No treatment is necessary

50. A 25-year-old G2P1 female presents for routine glucose testing during her pregnancy. When counseling her about gestational diabetes and its treatment, which of the following is true?
a. Intrauterine growth retardation occurs with inadequate treatment
b. Goals of therapy are to prevent maternal retinopathy and neuropathy
c. Dietary treatment is the only option during pregnancy
d. The maternal risks associated with diabetes resolve upon delivery
e. Oral diabetic medications are now a common part of treatment

51. A 20-year-old waitress complains of cough and a low-grade fever. She feels tired and has shortness of breath on exertion. She denies any pleuritic pain or night sweats. Her temperature is 100.6°F (41.1°C), heart rate 100, and respiratory rate 22. Examination of the ears, nose, and throat is normal. Auscultation of the lungs reveals a few fine crackles at the right lung base. The heart rate is regular with no murmurs. The next step in the management of this patient is:
a. Treat with antibiotics for sinusitis
b. Treat with a cough suppressant for postviral syndrome
c. Order a chest x-ray for suspected pneumonia
d. Obtain sputum for Gram stain and culture
e. Initiate incentive spirometry to treat atelectasis

52. A 25-year-old woman complains of vaginal itching and burning. The pH of the vaginal discharge is 4. The most likely diagnosis is:
a. Atrophic vaginitis
b. Candidal vaginitis
c. Trichomoniasis
d. Bacterial vaginosis
e. Human papillomavirus

53. A 52-year-old man presents with a complaint of dyspnea, which has troubled him for the preceding 8 months. He has had minimal prior medical care, notes no prior medical problems, and denies any medication use. He admits to having smoked a pack of cigarettes daily for the past 30 years. He is currently stable and his physical examination is remarkable for a prolonged expiratory phase and diminished breath sounds bilaterally. In evaluating this patient, which of the following is the most likely cause for his chronic dyspnea?
a. Pulmonary embolus
b. Chronic obstructive pulmonary disease
c. Diabetes mellitus
d. Myocardial infarction
e. Pneumonia

54. An asymptomatic 15-year-old youth presents for a preparticipation sports examination and is found to have a systolic ejection murmur at the left sternal border that decreases with squatting and increases on standing. With regard to hypertrophic cardiomyopathy, which of the following is true?
a. Most patients with hypertrophic cardiomyopathy have symptoms
b. It is the most common cause of sudden cardiac death in those over the age of 50
c. It is an autosomal recessive trait
d. Diagnosis is made via echocardiogram
e. Squatting decreases venous return and thus decreases the intensity of the murmur

55. A 40-year-old man presents with a painful, swollen right knee and a low-grade temperature. The most useful test for this individual is:
a. CBC
b. Uric acid level

c. ESR
d. Rheumatoid factor
e. Joint fluid analysis

56. A previously healthy 26-year-old man presents with abdominal cramping and fever that has lasted for 2 days. He has had 10 stools in the last 24 hours. A stool specimen reveals the presence of blood and WBCs. The most likely diagnosis is:
   a. Staphylococcal food poisoning
   b. Rotavirus
   c. Crohn disease
   d. Shigellosis
   e. Irritable bowel syndrome

57. A 22-year-old woman complains of a severe unilateral throbbing headache accompanied by emesis and photophobia. She has a history of "bad headaches" and states that her mother and sister also have "headache problems." The patient takes no medications, is afebrile, and other than being moderately uncomfortable, has a normal physical examination. The most likely diagnosis is:
   a. Tension headache
   b. Sinusitis
   c. Meningitis
   d. Temporal arteritis
   e. Migraine headache

58. A 30-year-old obese woman presents with right upper quadrant pain and low-grade fever. Her symptoms started 2 weeks earlier with myalgias, fatigue, and anorexia. They are worsening progressively; now she also has nausea and vomiting. Her physical examination reveals mild jaundice and right upper quadrant pain. The CBC shows mild elevation of the WBC count. Hemoglobin, hematocrit, and platelet levels are within normal limits. The liver function test shows elevated AST, ALT, and total bilirubin with a high conjugated fraction. Which of the following is the best management option?
   a. Since the patient has abdominal pain with nausea and vomiting, admit her for possible appendicitis
   b. Since she has three risk factors for gallstone disease as well as right upper quadrant pain, she needs a cholecystectomy
   c. Her jaundice is secondary to hemolysis and should be evaluated and treated accordingly
   d. Advise the patient to continue oral fluids and bed rest and order a hepatitis profile to determine the type of hepatitis
   e. Endoscopic retrograde cholangiopancreatography should be performed to assess for a pancreatic mass

59. A 21-year-old sexually active woman comes in with complaints of pain in the genital area, mild vaginal discharge, and painful urination. On examination, painful vesicles and ulcers are noted on the cervix. You tell the patient the most likely diagnosis is:

a. Syphilis
b. Urinary tract infection
c. Yeast vaginitis
d. Herpes simplex
e. Cervicitis

60. A 41-year-old obese woman presents with an acute onset of sharp intermittent right upper quadrant pain associated with eating. She denies any fever or chills. On examination, there is no abdominal mass or tenderness. The CBC is normal. Liver function tests show elevated total and conjugated bilirubin levels as well as alkaline phosphatase. The next step in management is:
   a. Ultrasound of the right upper quadrant
   b. Magnetic resonance imaging of the abdomen
   c. Esophagogastroduodenoscopy (EGD)
   d. Empiric proton pump inhibitor therapy
   e. Liver biopsy

61. A 76-year-old man complains of progressively worsening fatigue over the preceding 6 months. He has difficulty walking two blocks because of this. He also has a poor appetite and has lost 15 pounds. Physical examination reveals pale conjunctivae. The lungs are clear to auscultation bilaterally. The heart rhythm is regular and the rate is 96 beats per minute. There are no heart murmurs. The CBC shows hemoglobin of 7 with decreased mean corpuscular volume (MCV). The total iron-binding capacity is increased and the ferritin level is low. This patient's anemia is most likely secondary to:
   a. Thalassemia
   b. Anemia of chronic disease
   c. Folate deficiency
   d. B_{12} deficiency
   e. Iron deficiency anemia

62. A 15-year-old white adolescent girl complains of "bad skin." On examination, the patient is noted to have whiteheads and blackheads as well as some papules and pustules on her face and upper back. Treatment options are many for this patient. The medication reserved for severe acne is:
   a. Tretinoin (Retin A)
   b. Sulfur preparations
   c. Isotretinoin (Accutane)
   d. Topical clindamycin
   e. Benzoyl peroxide

63. A 55-year-old black man complains of pain and some swelling in his right great toe. He has also noticed some "bumps" in his skin. On examination, his toe is swollen, red, and very painful. There are scattered tophi on his skin. Many causes of arthritis have systemic manifestations. A common association is:
   a. Nail pitting and psoriatic arthritis
   b. Tophi and rheumatoid arthritis
   c. Malar rash and scleroderma
   d. Fingertip atrophy and telangiectasias with SLE
   e. Erythema migrans and dermatomyositis

64. A 60-year-old woman presents with complaints of fatigue for the past 6 months. Her condition has been worsening progressively. Now she is beginning to notice weakness and unsteadiness in her gait. Physical examination shows pale conjunctivae. Her lung and heart examinations are unremarkable, but the neurologic examination shows a decreased vibration sense. The hemoglobin level is 8 and the MCV is high. The most common cause of her condition is:
   a. Iron deficiency anemia
   b. Folate deficiency
   c. Pernicious anemia
   d. Anemia of chronic disease
   e. Thalassemia

65. A 32-year-old gravida 3, para 2–0–0–2 presents for her prenatal visit. Based on her last menstrual period, the current gestational age is 10 weeks and 4 days. The patient states that she is sure of her dates. She denies any problems. Her BP is 125/80. On physical examination, the uterus is barely palpable above the pubis. Fetal heart sounds are heard at a rate of 140 beats per minute. Management of this patient should include:
   a. Laboratory evaluation for preeclampsia
   b. Routine care with follow-up in 4 weeks
   c. Ultrasound to confirm gestational age
   d. Amniocentesis to evaluate chromosomes
   e. Abdominal x-ray to rule out any pelvic masses

66. A 32-year-old woman presents with palpitations, tachycardia, and exophthalmos. You are concerned she may have Graves disease. With regard to that disease, which of the following statements is true?
   a. Serum TSH is decreased whereas free T4 is elevated
   b. Thyroid scan shows a "hot" nodule
   c. Tests for thyroid antibodies are negative
   d. Both serum TSH and free T4 are elevated
   e. Fine-needle aspiration is required for diagnosis

67. A 20-year-old man with no past medical problems complains of a runny nose, which he has had for several months. The nasal discharge is watery and clear. He also has a nonproductive chronic cough for which he has tried several over-the-counter medications, with no relief. His symptoms are worse at night. On physical examination, the patient has a pale nasal mucosa. The bridge of the nose also has a nasal crease. The most likely diagnosis is:
   a. Vasomotor rhinitis
   b. Allergic rhinitis
   c. Sinusitis
   d. Rhinitis medicamentosa
   e. Nasal foreign body

68. A 40-year-old man with no past medical problems complains of left-sided chest pain with no radiation. He denies any nausea or diaphoresis. His pain is located at midclavicular line at the fourth intercostal space. The pain becomes worse with inspiration. His vital signs are stable. Physical examination shows a tender spot at the fourth intercostal space. The remainder of the physical examination is unremarkable. The ECG shows a normal sinus rhythm at 70 beats per minute. The most likely diagnosis is:
   a. Myocardial infarction
   b. Pneumonia
   c. Costochondritis
   d. Esophageal spasm
   e. Pericarditis

69. A 55-year-old man with history of hemorrhoids complains of weakness and dizziness. Over the last 2 days, he has had two episodes of painless rectal bleeding. He denies any fever or chills. Vital signs are BP 100/60, temperature 98.4°F (36.8°C), respiratory rate 22, and heart rate 98. The conjunctiva is pale. His lungs and heart exam are unremarkable. The abdomen is not distended. The bowel sounds are active. There is no abdominal tenderness. Rectal examination shows bright red blood per rectum (BRBPR). His hemoglobin level is 7 with microcytic and hypochromic RBCs, and the WBC count is 8000. Which of the following is the most likely diagnosis with this presentation?
   a. Diverticulosis
   b. Colon cancer
   c. Ulcerative colitis
   d. Irritable bowel syndrome
   e. *Clostridium difficile* colitis

70. A 30-year-old woman, gravida 1, para 0, comes in for her second trimester prenatal visit at 16 weeks' gestation. She has had prenatal care since her pregnancy diagnosis at 8 weeks' gestation and has had all routine prenatal testing performed according to schedule. In continuing to provide routine care, which one of the following tests should now be offered?
   a. A CBC to rule out anemia
   b. Atypical antibody screen
   c. Hepatitis B surface antigen
   d. Triple marker screen
   e. Glucose screening for diabetes

71. A 68-year-old white woman comes in to discuss the results of her dual-energy x-ray absorptiometry (DEXA) scan. Her T score is –2.7. You explain that she has osteoporosis and requires treatment. Management of osteoporosis includes:
   a. Daily intake of 500 mg of calcium
   b. Avoidance of weight-bearing exercise
   c. Taking bisphosphonates on a full stomach
   d. Smoking cessation
   e. Estrogen replacement therapy

72. A 60-year-old man complains of left-lower-quadrant abdominal pain, fever, and chills, which he has had for the past 2 days. His appetite is poor and he feels nauseous. Vital signs are as follows: blood pressure 140/90, temperature 101°F (38.3°C), respiratory rate

22, and heart rate 90. The patient looks sick and appears to be in pain. The lung and heart examinations are unremarkable. His abdomen is distended, with decreased bowel sounds. The left lower quadrant is tender to palpation. The rectal examination is normal. The CBC shows leukocytosis of 15,000 and hemoglobin of 12. The test of choice to diagnose this patient's condition is:

a. Ultrasound
b. Computed tomography of the abdomen
c. Barium enema
d. Bleeding scan
e. Colonoscopy

73. A 20-year-old man with no prior medical problems complains of a dry cough, which he has had for the past month. He denies any fever, chills, or night sweats. The cough started with a runny nose and low-grade fever. All the other symptoms resolved within a week but the cough has been persistent. His vital signs are stable, and the physical examination is unremarkable. The most likely diagnosis is:

a. Sinusitis
b. Postviral syndrome
c. Pneumonia
d. Psychogenic cough
e. Asthma

74. A 9-month-old Native American boy is brought in by his mother; he has had a fever of 101°F (38.3°C) since the day before. She denies any diarrhea, nausea, or vomiting. Lately he has been pulling on his right ear. All his symptoms started after a cold, which began a couple of days ago. He has had four other similar episodes in the past 6 months. The mother is very concerned and states that antibiotics usually take care of the problem. His vital signs show a temperature of 100°F (37.7°C). The child is irritable but consolable. Examination of the ear shows an erythematous tympanic membrane with decreased mobility. The remainder of the physical examination is unremarkable. The best management option for this child should include:

a. Observation; this is most likely a viral URI
b. Treatment for acute otitis media with antibiotics
c. Antibiotics for acute otitis and then prophylaxis for 6 months
d. Antibiotics for acute otitis and then daily oral decongestants
e. Referral to ENT specialist for myringotomy and tympanostomy tube placement

75. A 62-year-old black man complains of fever, cough, and chest pain. On examination, the patient has a temperature is 102°F (39.8°C) obvious chills and rales at the left lung base. The patient should be admitted if he has:

a. Pulse greater than 120
b. O_2 saturation less than 95%
c. Age greater than 50

d. Systolic BP less than 110
e. Pleural effusion

76. A 60-year-old woman presents with chronic dyspnea and a long history of smoking. Based on the history and physical examination, you diagnose chronic obstructive pulmonary disease and initiate treatment to relieve the patient's symptoms. In addition to this therapy, additional recommendations should include:

a. Spiral computed tomography scan of the chest
b. Exercise avoidance
c. Smoking cessation
d. *Haemophilus influenzae* b vaccination
e. Referral for bronchoscopy

77. A 40-year-old woman complains of intermittent palpitations, which began 3 weeks earlier and occur daily. The symptoms are not associated with any medication use, activity, or other symptoms. The physical examination, including heart rate, is within normal limits. CBC, FSH, and TSH testing is within normal limits and event monitor testing shows sinus rhythm during the occurrence of symptoms. Which of the following is most likely in this patient?

a. Menopause
b. Cardiac arrhythmias
c. Anemia
d. Panic attacks
e. Hyperthyroidism

78. A 70-year-old man has been treated for a gastric ulcer—positive for *Helicobacter pylori*—diagnosed 6 weeks earlier. He presents for follow-up and is asymptomatic. Current recommendations should include which of the following?

a. Lifetime use of a proton pump inhibitor
b. Rotating antibiotic use every 6 weeks
c. Esophagogastroduodenoscopy (EGD)
d. Observation for recurrence of symptoms
e. *H. pylori* antibody testing

79. A 23-year-old woman complains of dizziness. On questioning, she says that she sometimes feels the room spinning. She has no significant past medical history, is on no medications, and has not been ill recently. On physical examination, she is noted to have vertical nystagmus unaffected by position. Her physical examination, including vital signs and orthostatic BP and pulse readings, are normal. A hearing evaluation is performed and is within normal limits. Which of the following diagnoses should be considered in the further evaluation of this patient?

a. Multiple sclerosis
b. Ménière disease
c. Benign positional vertigo
d. Vestibular neuronitis
e. Psychiatric disease

80. A 65-year-old man presents for preoperative medical evaluation for a vascular procedure to treat symptoms of claudication. He has a past medical history of hyper-

tension that has been well controlled the past 2 years with angiotensin converting enzyme (ACE) inhibitors. He is on no other medications except for one aspirin per day. He has had two prior uncomplicated surgeries for an inguinal hernia and a herniated lumbar disk. He quit smoking 10 years ago. Other than decreased peripheral pulses, his physical examination is within normal limits. The surgeon has requested that the patient have a CBC, basic metabolic profile, ECG, and chest x-ray performed. What other testing is indicated in this patient before proceeding with surgery?

a. Prothrombin time
b. Cardiac stress test
c. Pulmonary function tests
d. Echocardiogram
e. Venous duplex scan

81. The parents of a 4-year-old and a newborn child present for wellness care and are seeking counseling with regard to vaccinations for their children. Which of the following is a true statement that may be part of the counseling you provide to encourage appropriate vaccination?

a. Hepatitis A vaccine is recommended for all children
b. Inactivated poliovirus vaccine (IPV) has been associated with vaccine-related polio infection
c. Pneumococcal vaccine is recommended only for high-risk adults
d. Chronic hepatitis B infection develops in 90% of infected teens and adults
e. Children receiving aspirin therapy should not receive influenza or varicella vaccines

82. A mother brings in her 12-year-old son for a routine health care visit. She expresses concern about their family's history of elevated cholesterol and heart disease. She would like her son to have his cholesterol evaluated. A true statement regarding cholesterol and cholesterol screening in children is:

a. Normal cholesterol in children is ≤240 mg/dL
b. Childhood cholesterol levels are predictive of adult levels
c. Screening is recommended for children with a parental history of hypercholesterolemia
d. Cholesterol values in children are unaffected by diet and physical activity
e. Screening is recommended for children beginning at 12 months of age

83. A 35-year-old man presents for an initial physical examination. He has had no significant past medical history and reports that both of his parents are alive and well, as are his siblings. He does not smoke or drink and exercises regularly. He received his last tetanus shot 5 years ago. His physical examination, including vital signs and weight, is normal. You now recommend which of the following:

a. Electrocardiogram
b. Chest x-ray
c. Lipid profile

d. Exercise stress test
e. Occult blood testing of stool

84. You are seeing a 15-month-old boy for follow-up on a pruritic skin rash that you have diagnosed as atopic dermatitis. The child has erythema, scaling, and lichenification of the flexural creases of the arms and legs. There is a family history of eczema and allergies. No identifiable triggers have been identified for the child's atopic dermatitis, and he is otherwise well. The mother is concerned about the long-term implications of this condition. You advise her that:

a. Atopic dermatitis is a rare condition
b. Resolution of the atopic dermatitis by age 2 is common
c. Affected children rarely develop allergic rhinitis or asthma
d. Most cases are diagnosed after age 2
e. In teenagers, the face and cheeks are most commonly affected

85. A 15-year-old adolescent girl presents with recurrent episodes of wheezing, which she experiences three or four times per year in association with upper respiratory infections. During the episodes, medical evaluation has documented a peak expiratory flow of 70% predicted. She has no nocturnal symptoms and no other significant past medical history. You diagnose asthma and now recommend which of the following therapies:

a. Oral steroids daily
b. Short-acting beta agonists as needed
c. Inhaled steroids daily
d. Inhaled nedocromil daily
e. Antibiotics to be used with exacerbations

86. A 40-year-old overweight Hispanic woman complains that she has feelings of hopelessness, insomnia, recent weight gain, constipation, and no energy. On examination, the patient cries, makes little eye contact, has a somber affect, and shows psychomotor retardation. Depression is diagnosed. Possible treatment strategies would include:

a. Use of buproprion because of the insomnia
b. Use of antidepressants for 6 to 12 months for the first episode of depression
c. Use of a selective serotonin reuptake inhibitor (SSRI) if agitation is a complaint
d. Use of mirtazapine because of weight gain
e. Use of trycyclic antidepressants to relieve constipation

87. A 30-year-old white woman complains of fatigue, sore throat, and low-grade fever. On examination her throat is mildly erythematous and there are shotty cervical nodes. The heterophile test is negative. The most common cause of a heterophile-negative, mononucleosis-like syndrome is:

a. Cytomegalovirus
b. Toxoplasmosis

c. Rubella
d. HIV
e. Hepatitis A

88. A 10-year-old male presents for evaluation of his asthma. He reports daily symptoms and wakes from sleep about once a week because of symptoms. He is currently using albuterol as needed for his symptoms. Current therapeutic recommendations should include:
    a. Oral steroids daily
    b. Antibiotics for 10 days
    c. Nedocromil daily
    d. Inhaled steroids and long-acting beta agonists
    e. No change in therapy

89. A 45-year-old previously healthy male presents for a physical examination. His last physical was performed 10 years earlier and was normal. He has no significant past medical history and is on no medications. He does not smoke and consumes two to three alcoholic drinks weekly. His family history is significant for hypertension in his mother. He denies any physical complaints. His physical examination is normal with the exception of a BP of 148/98. You recommend a recheck on his BP in 1 month; the repeat measurement is then found to be 150/100. Further evaluation of this patient should include which of the following:
    a. Serum and urine catecholamines
    b. Cardiac stress testing
    c. Electrocardiogram
    d. No testing
    e. Renal scan

90. An 18-year-old man presents for a preparticipation sports examination. He has no significant past medical or family history and a normal physical examination. His mother asks whether he should have any cardiac screening performed. Which of the following statements are true and helpful in addressing her concerns?
    a. Routine screening with an ECG or echocardiogram has been shown to be cost-effective
    b. History taking is used to identify those at risk for sudden cardiac death
    c. In those below age 40, coronary artery disease is the most common cause of sudden cardiac death
    d. Aortic stenosis is the most common cause of sudden death in those over age 40
    e. Stress testing is recommended routinely for preparticipation sports examinations

91. A 20-year-old woman presents with concerns that her thyroid gland is overactive, because her mother had a similar condition and she has not been feeling well. In the evaluation of this patient, which of the following would be a symptom of hyperthyroidism?
    a. Palpitations
    b. Weight gain

c. Constipation
d. Depression
e. Fatigue

92. A 30-year-old woman complains of fatigue, cold intolerance, and dry skin. She has no other medical problems and takes birth control pills. Her physical examination is normal. Laboratory evaluation reveals TSH, at 8.9, to be elevated. The next step in evaluating her thyroid function would be:
    a. Arrange for a thyroid scan
    b. Start her on thyroxine and recheck her TSH in 3 months
    c. Administer TRH
    d. Order a thyroid ultrasound
    e. Test free T4

93. A 26-year-old man presents to the emergency department with complaints of the acute onset of the "worst headache of my life." Appropriate diagnostic evaluation/treatment would include which of the following?
    a. Sumatriptan 6 mg SC
    b. CT scan of the head which, if negative, should be followed by lumbar puncture
    c. CT scan of the head
    d. Ibuprofen 600 mg PO every 6 hours
    e. Erythrocyte sedimentation rate and, while awaiting results, corticosteroid therapy

94. A 56-year-old white man expresses concerns regarding diabetes. His mother has diabetes, which is controlled with glipizide, and his brother was just diagnosed with the disease, controlled by diet. Appropriate screening is guided by the following criteria:
    a. High-risk individuals should be screened with a hemoglobin A_{1C}
    b. All patients over 55 years of age should be screened with a fasting blood sugar every 4 years
    c. Random blood glucose greater than 200 with polyuria, polydipsia, and polyphagia establishes a diagnosis of diabetes
    d. A single fasting blood sugar greater than 126 signifies diabetes
    e. For patients over age 30 with diabetes, screening for microalbuminemia should be done every 6 months

95. An otherwise healthy 18-year-old, sexually active white man complains of a persistent watery discharge in both eyes. On examination, both conjunctivae are slightly erythematous with a watery discharge. The likely diagnosis for this patient's red eye is:
    a. Blepharitis
    b. Bacterial conjunctivitis
    c. Viral conjunctivitis
    d. Iritis
    e. Inclusion (chlamydial) conjunctivitis

96. A 39-year-old gravida 5, para 2 comes in for a prenatal visit. She is 20 weeks pregnant and at her last visit a maternal serum alpha-fetoprotein was ordered; it is decreased. The most probable cause is:
   a. Twin pregnancy
   b. Neural tube defects
   c. Pregnancy-induced hypertension
   d. Trisomy 21
   e. Trisomy 18

97. A 5-year-old child is brought in by her mother for follow-up. She was diagnosed with acute otitis media 2 weeks earlier and given an antibiotic. The child's fever and ear pain have resolved. On examination you note that the effusion behind the ear is still present. The tympanic membrane is normal. Management of this child should include:
   a. Antibiotics
   b. A tympanostomy tube
   c. Observation
   d. Referral to an ear–nose–throat (ENT) specialist
   e. Hearing evaluation

98. A 68-year-old man presents for routine physical examination. In addition to obtaining a complete history and examination, which of the following would you routinely recommend?
   a. Chest x-ray
   b. Hepatitis B vaccine
   c. DEXA scan
   d. Pneumococcal vaccine
   e. Electrocardiography

99. A 42-year-old woman returns from a business trip and notes the sudden onset of dyspnea along with a pleuritic right-sided chest pain. Her past medical history is unremarkable. She is currently on birth control pills. Her vital signs are BP 120/70, heart rate 100, regular respiratory rate 24, and temperature 98.6°F (37.0°C). Cardiac and lung examinations are unremarkable. There is no chest wall tenderness. Examination of her extremities reveals no cyanosis or clubbing, but there is pitting edema in her right leg. Testing should be done promptly to exclude the following:
   a. Fibromyalgia
   b. Costochondritis
   c. Pulmonary embolus
   d. Lymphedema
   e. Varicose veins

100. A 50-year-old man complains of recurrent chest pain that radiates down his left arm and has been occurring over the past 9 months. The pain is described as a retrosternal pressure. It is brought on by walking or other strenuous exercise and is relieved by 2 minutes of rest. His vital signs are stable and the physical examination is unremarkable. The most likely diagnosis is:
   a. Myocardial infarction
   b. Stable angina
   c. Unstable angina
   d. Pericarditis
   e. Pleurisy

QUESTIONS

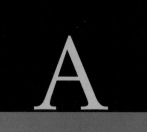

Answers

1. Correct Answer: C (Chapter 4 [Table 4-1])

is correct because H flu type B vaccine (Hib) is not administered after the age of 5 since children at this age generally achieve a natural immunity and are not significantly impacted by the disease. Hib should be administered at 2 months, 4 months, 6 months, and a fourth dose should be administered between 12 and 15 months of age. Not administering this vaccine to these young children could be devastating as H influenza B can lead to devastating illnesses such as meningitis and encephalitis.

A is incorrect because the first MMR vaccine is due when the child is 12 months old and the second MMR is due when the child is between 4 and 6 years old. Omitting these could lead to devastating consequences regardless of the age group. Mumps is associated with parotitis, orchitis, oophoritis, pancreatitis, myocarditis, and encephalitis. One to three out of 1000 inflicted with measles die as a result of neurologic and respiratory complications. Rubella is one of the TORCH infections and is associated with ophthalmologic, cardiac, and neurologic defects, including mental retardation in those children born to mothers with this infection during the pregnant state.

B is incorrect because the influenza vaccine is recommended for all children above 6 months of age. The influenza intramuscular vaccine is recommended for children 6 months of age or older with risk factors including but not limited to asthma, HIV, cardiac disease, sickle cell disease, and diabetes, health care workers, and other household members in close contact with high-risk groups. The recommendation for universal vaccination for children over 6 months of age replaces previous recommendations restricting vaccine use under 24 months to high-risk children. This is due to this age range being at highest risk for hospitalizations secondary to influenza. Healthy people ages 5 to 49 years are recommended to receive the intranasal live attenuated influenza vaccine. Due to the vaccine's live attenuated virus, viral shedding can occur for up to 7 days, so it is not recommended for health care workers, asthmatics, immunocompromised individuals, or those within close contact to them.

D is incorrect because pertussis, along with diphtheria and tetanus (TdaP), should be administered in four doses at 2 months, 4 months, 6 months, and then anywhere from 15 to 18 months. The fifth and final dose of the series should be given at age 4 to 6 years. Furthermore, TdaP should be given at age 11 and 12 years

if at least 5 years have elapsed since the last dose of tetanus and diphtheria toxoid-containing vaccine. Subsequent routine Td boosters are recommended every 10 years thereafter provided that one booster of pertussis has been given during the teen years. In individuals with potentially contaminated wounds with more than a 5-year lapse since their last dose, a booster should be given. In individuals with high-risk wounds, passive immunization with tetanus immunoglobulin (TIg) in addition to starting the primary series is indicated at initial presentation for wound care.

E is incorrect because the hepatitis B vaccine should be given at birth, before hospital discharge, or at least before 2 months of age. The second dose should be given between 1 and 4 months of age (at least 4 weeks after the first dose). The third dose should be given between 6 and 18 months of age (at least 16 weeks after the first dose and 8 weeks after the second) and this dose should not be given before 24 weeks of age. Infants born to hepatitis B surface antigen (HbsAg) positive mothers should receive HepB and 0.5 ml of HepB immunoglobulin (HBIG) at separate sites within 12 hours of birth. The second dose is recommended at age 1 and 2 months. The final dose of the immunization series should not be administered before 24 weeks of age (same as above). HBsAg and anti-HBs antibody testing should be performed on these infants between 9 and 15 months of age.

2. Correct Answer: C (Chapter 2).

Informed consent must be granted for patients undergoing surgical or other invasive procedures. Describing the nature of the patient's condition and its consequences, including whether it is disabling or life-threatening must be included as elements of informed consent. Recommended treatment and alternatives should also be reviewed, including benefits, risks, costs, discomfort, and specific side effects.

3. Correct Answer: C (Chapter 2 [Table 2-1]).

The patient is ready to make a change by setting a specific quit date; at this stage nicotine replacement and further therapy should be offered to help the patient achieve this goal.

A is incorrect because in the precontemplation stage the patient is not considering quitting, may not believe they are able to quit, and/or may not believe they are susceptible to severe illness due to their habit. At this stage, it is appropriate to ask the patient about their knowledge of the health consequences of smoking.

B is incorrect because at the contemplation stage the patient is merely considering cessation. They also recognize the dangers of smoking and may still be upset by previous failed attempts. At this stage, it is appropriate to encourage the patient to quit and provide educational materials.

D is incorrect because the patient is not in the process of cessation. At this point, support and positive reinforcement are most appropriate, as well as discussing strategies if relapse were to occur. Maintenance is when a patient has successfully quit smoking and is continuing to live tobacco-free. Continuing support of this and aiding if relapse occurs are most appropriate at this stage.

4. Correct Answer: E (Chapter 3).
High sensitivity and specificity are both desirable characteristics of a screening test. Sensitivity is the measure of percentage of cases that a test may detect. Specificity is a measure of the percentage of patients who test negative. A low prevalence of disease being tested (**A**) would increase the cost/benefit ratio of the disease being screened in a population. A lack of effective therapies for the disease (**B**) would not warrant a screening test as it would not decrease the morbidity or morality associated with early detection of a disease. As a review, positive predictive value is the likelihood percentage that a person with a positive test has the disease. A negative predictive value is the likelihood percentage that a person who tests negative for the disease does

	Disease Present	Disease Absent
Positive test	A	B
Negative test	C	D
Sensitivity	A/(A+C)	
Specificity	B/(B+D)	
Positive predictive value	A/(A+B)	
Negative predictive value	D/(B+D)	

	Disease Present	Disease Absent
Positive test	80	40
Negative test	20	60
Sensitivity	[80/(80+20)]×100%=80%	
Specificity	[60/(40+60)]×100%=60%	
Positive predictive value	[80/(80+40)]×100%=66%	
Negative predictive value	[60/(20+60)]×100%=75%	

not indeed have it. Below are examples of how to calculate each of the quantities in variable as well as numerical forms.

5. Correct Answer: A (Chapter 5).
A cholesterol screening is warranted for this patient, as he is over the age of 35. Routine cholesterol screening is recommended every 5 years starting at age 35.

B is incorrect. Yearly prostate cancer screening, including a PSA, as well as digital rectal exam is recommended for men above the age of 50, unless the male is African American or has a family history of prostate cancer. In the latter two cases, PSA and DRE should be performed annually starting at the age of 40.

C is incorrect. The patient is below the age of 50 and has no risk factors for colon cancer or prostate cancer based on his family history and medical history; therefore he is not at increased risk for the above-mentioned cancers. A colonoscopy is recommended by the United States Preventative Services Task Force for all patients at and above the age of 50 years and is required every 10 years. This may be substituted by annual occult blood testing along with flexible sigmoidoscopy every 5 years for colon cancer screening given a negative medical and family history of colon cancer before the age of 50. However, if risk factors such as anemia, weight loss, heme-positive stools, or other malignancy suspecting situations occur, a full colonoscopy is warranted in this age group.

D is incorrect. Stress testing is warranted if one suspects cardiac disease such as angina. This is not the case in this man.

E is incorrect. Glucose testing in the form of fasting glucose and subsequent glucose tolerance testing is only warranted earlier than age 45 if family history or personal history causes suspicion for diabetes mellitus. Beginning at age 45 diabetes screen including fasting blood glucose checks should be obtained every 3 years.

Additional tests in this age group for women include mammography every 1 to 2 years (by ACS differs from USPTFS) starting at age 40 and continuation of pap smears every 3 years in low risk women.

6. Correct Answer: B (Chapter 7).
In any case of suspected child abuse or neglect, local child protective service agencies must be contacted. The story given for why the child is bruised seems to be vague, and more importantly the lack of concern for the child's injuries suggests abuse or at the very minimum neglect. Observing (**A**) the situation may expose the child to further neglect or abuse. Referral for a hematology consultation (**C**) might be considered if no obvious causes are detected and in situations where there is appropriate parental concern for the child's welfare, may be considered earlier. Supplementation with iron (**D**) is appropriate therapy for given iron deficiency anemia; however, there is currently no evidence to suggest the child has this condition. A psychiatric evaluation (**E**) may be appropriate in the future, but the

immediate concern is for the safety and well-being of the child.

7. Correct Answer: E (Chapter 76).

The pink nodular, pearly white translucent appearance with inverted edges and telangiectatic vessels are typical of basal cell carcinoma. Biopsy is diagnostic and the most common therapies include surgical excision or curettage and electrodesiccation. This malignancy rarely metastasizes but can become locally invasive and destructive over the course of years. This lesion occurs on sun-exposed areas (80% on the head and neck) and other risk factors include fair skin, family history of skin cancer, history of sunburns, and outdoor occupations. Squamous cell carcinoma is another common skin malignancy that more readily metastasizes and can have a prior premalignant lesion called actinic keratoses. These premalignant lesions are primarily seen in older individuals, are induced by UV light, are common in fair skinned individuals, and appear as asymptomatic, rough, scaly lesions on sun-exposed sights. Actinic keratoses have a 1% yearly risk of developing into squamous cell carcinoma. Actinic keratoses can be treated by cryotherapy or curettage. Extensive lesions can be treated with a topical agent such as 5-fluorouracil. Malignant melanoma is one of the few potentially fatal skin diseases. It readily metastasizes, and risk factors include fair complexion, light hair and eyes, and those with excessive skin exposure. Biopsy is required of suspicious lesions. Survival is most closely related to depth of tumor invasion.

8. Correct Answer: E (Chapter 42).

This patient is demonstrating lack of interest in the interviewer's questions and possibly poor concentration. She also is demonstrating a lack of emotions through her flat affect. Depression presents as a 2-week or greater history of depressed mood and/or disinterest with an impairment of function accompanied by at least four of the following: weight changes, sleep disturbance, loss of energy, feelings of worthlessness or guilt, poor concentration, psychomotor retardation or agitation, thoughts of death, or recurrent suicidal ideations.

The patient does not have Parkinson disease (**A**) due to her lack of cogwheel rigidity, bradykinesia, and tremors. Dementia (**B**) would be suspected if the patient had difficulty recalling objects or recent events, had marked forgetfulness, had a history of getting lost, neglecting personal hygiene, was socially withdrawn, had frustrating emotional outbursts, or difficulty driving. Delirium (**C**) is referred to as an acute state of confusion, which affects memory and cognition. It usually occurs suddenly over hours to days and is associated with a clouding of consciousness and disruption of the sleep cycle. None of these appear to be the case with this patient. Stroke (**D**) could present as an acute confused state, as a sudden loss in motor function or loss of vision. No acute events such as these are depicted in this scenario.

9. Correct Answer: D (Chapter 77).

Progressive memory loss accompanied by loss of instrumental activities of daily living is consistent with a diagnosis of Alzheimer disease. These activities routinely include driving and emotional outburst control. Patients with Alzheimer also usually will develop social withdrawal. It is the most common cause of dementia and accounts for over half of the cases of dementia. Histologic findings include intracellular neurofibrillary tangles comprising tau proteins and extracellular plaques consisting of beta-amyloid proteins. These lead to neuronal loss and subsequent disturbance in cholinergic system, which results in cognitive decline. Most cases are sporadic, but an autosomal dominant form involving the amyloid protein has been described. Risk factors include advanced age, female gender, family history of the disease. APO-E4 apolipoprotein on chromosome 19 is associated with increased risk for AD.

A is incorrect. Multi-infarct dementia is a type of vascular dementia. It presents in discrete episodes of stepwise worsening cognition. Multi-infarct dementia is due to a series of lacunar strokes (due to small vessel hyaline arteriolosclerosis). Risk factors for all types of vascular dementias include HTN, diabetes, history of smoking, and known arterial disease.

B is incorrect. Lewy body dementia patients have a rapid clinical decline, visual hallucinations, episodic delirium, and extrapyramidal motor signs. This patient does not have these signs. Lewy body dementia is characterized by the presence of Lewy bodies (intracytoplasmic inclusions) and by decreased neuronal density in the amygdala, hippocampus, cortex, and other portions of the brain.

C is incorrect. Parkinson disease is characterized by bradykinesia (slowing of voluntary muscle movements), a resting tremor, described as "pill-rolling," micrographia, blunting of affect, a shuffling gait, and cogwheel rigidity. Dementia occurs in some cases, but it is not a consistent or diagnostic finding. The pathophysiology of Parkinson disease is degeneration of dopaminergic neurons in the substantia nigra. This patient lacks the motor symptoms mentioned above.

E is incorrect. Huntington chorea is an autosomal dominant disease that may interrupt the pathways involved in memory and cognition; however, chorea (spasmodic movements of body and limbs), muscle rigidity, and dementia. The pathophysiology involves atrophy/loss of neurons of the globus pallidus, putamen, and caudate. This patient again does not possess these motor symptoms.

10. Correct Answer: E (Chapter 76).

Delirium, or an acute confusional state that affects memory and cognition, typically occurs over hours to days (**A** is incorrect) and is commonly caused by medications, infection, dehydration, hypoxia, electrolyte imbalance, anemia, and hepatic failure (not just alcohol withdrawal, **B** is incorrect). It is associated with a clouding of consciousness and disruption of the sleep cycle (**C** is incorrect), and commonly occurs in patients with dementia (**D** is incorrect).

Dementia is a progressive decline in memory and intellectual capabilities severe enough to cause interference in social or occupational functioning. This includes impairment in language, judgment, cognition, visuospatial skills, and personality. This typically is a decline over years. One per cent of the population is affected by age 60 and almost 50% by age 85. Dementia is usually subcategorized into either the Lewy body type, Alzheimer, Parkinson disease, Huntington chorea, or multi-infarct dementia. For further explanations of the above types of dementia please see the answer to question 9.

11. Correct Answer: E (Chapter 76).
This patient has Parkinson disease. Metoclopramide (Reglan), which stimulates GI tract motility, does so by blocking the gastric dopamine receptor. This can cause dystonic reactions, restlessness, drowsiness, parkinsonism, and will exacerbate parkinsonian symptoms in patients with the disease.

B is incorrect. The treatment of choice for Parkinson disease is levodopa with carbidopa. Levodopa is a dopamine precursor that can cross the blood–brain barrier and helps to replenish the dopaminergic loss in the substantia nigra typically associated with Parkinson. Administration of carbidopa, a peripheral dopa decarboxylase inhibitor, increases the bioavailability of levodopa in the brain and inhibits its peripheral conversion to dopamine, thus limiting peripheral side effects. This also helps to decrease the daily requirements of levodopa by approximately 75%.

A is incorrect because an essential tremor is a tremor associated with voluntary movements, not a resting tremor as in Parkinson disease.

C is incorrect because parkinsonian tremor usually begins as a "pill-rolling tremor" (as though a pill were being rolled between the thumb and fingers with mild external and internal rotation of the wrist) unilaterally, but usually progresses to include both hands. Tremor may also include the chin, lips, legs, and trunk and may be exacerbated by stress. The important thing here is that it typically has a unilateral onset.

D is incorrect because the patient has no history significant for a stroke, such as a focal or hemi deficit. This patient has the bradykinesia and resting tremor associated with Parkinson disease.

12. Correct Answer: D (Chapter 78).
This patient has detrusor instability. Her symptoms of urgency and incontinence point toward urge incontinence due to contractions of the bladder with filling. It is idiopathic in most cases but can be neurogenic. Cystometry (electronic measure of pressure changes as water fills and is expelled from the bladder), not cystoscopy (**C**) is diagnostic. It shows bladder contraction on filling. Anticholinergic medications such as oxybu-

tynin (Ditropan), tolterodine tartrate (Detrol LA), propantheline bromide (Pro-banthine), or imipramine (Tofranil) are the medications of choice to treat detrusor instability. Additionally behavior modification such as timed voiding, not inhibiting liquid intake (**E**) can also be beneficial.

A is incorrect as sertraline, a selective serotonin reuptake inhibitor, does not cause urinary symptoms, but may cause GI upset, insomnia, somnolence, sexual dysfunction (anorgasmia), dry mouth, weight loss, and exacerbation of Mania.

B is incorrect as a urinalysis and culture are appropriate in the workup for urinary tract infection, which would typically present with dysuria or can sometimes be asymptomatic. It does not present with such urgency associated with incontinence.

13. Correct Answer: C (Chapter 75).
Gait evaluation is particularly important since geriatric patients are at increased risk for falls and this exam may uncover correctable gait disturbances such as peripheral neuropathy secondary to vitamin B12 deficiency, or may uncover other disturbances as the bradykinesia and shuffling gait associated with Parkinson disease.

A is incorrect as prostate specific antigen (PSA) is often elevated due to benign prostatic hypertrophy, but marked elevations or increasing values are suggestive of prostate cancer. Further evaluation of patients with possible prostate cancer should be undertaken only if the diagnosis would result in a change in management.

B is incorrect. Rheumatoid factor and antinuclear antibody (ANA) tests are both commonly positive in low titers and rarely indicate disease in the elderly.

D is incorrect as liver function tests (LFTs) are unchanged with aging and may indicate necessity for further evaluation for hepatitis, cirrhosis, or hepatocellular carcinoma.

E is incorrect as serum iron is important in the evaluation of microcytic anemia, as in iron deficiency anemia, which may be secondary to oncologic causes, such as cancers of the GI tract.

14. Correct Answer: A (Chapter 76).
Unintended weight loss of 4% over 1 year is the single best predictor of death within 2 years in the geriatric population. The causes of weight loss in the geriatric population are similar to those in middle-age adults. The most common causes are depression, cancer, especially gastrointestinal and pulmonary malignancies (not hyperthyroidism, **C** is incorrect). Congestive heart failure and chronic obstructive pulmonary disease can both cause weight loss in later stages. Other causes of weight loss in this population include renal failure (anorexia and weight loss as early symptoms), infection (such as tuberculosis), endocrine disorders such as diabetes and medication induced decrease in appetite. Alteration in taste and nausea is also associated with weight loss in this population. **D** is incorrect. Functional impairments such as from poorly fitted

dentures, secondary to stroke or arthritis, or from difficulty swallowing can also cause weight loss in this population. **B** is incorrect. In about 25% (not 5%) of cases weight loss remains unexplained and no identified cause is found.

15. Correct Answer: E (Chapter 79).

Hospice care is a type of palliative care provided to patients whose life expectancy is 6 months or less. Hospice care emphasizes symptomatic treatment and comfort measures. The management of pain and relief of symptoms is the primary concern. Special attention is paid to the patient's physical, emotional, and spiritual needs rather than trying to cure his or her illness or prolong life. It is important for the patient to be cognizant of their enrollment in hospice care as it will help them to fulfill the needs mentioned above.

D is incorrect. As this is not always possible, due to dementia and severe prolonged bouts of delirium, an attempt is made as hospice care also provides a way for the patient to take control of how they are affected by their disease as their life comes to an end.

A is incorrect. Hospice care can be provided at the patient's place of residence (home, nursing home).

B is incorrect. Hospice care is appropriate for end-stage patients with conditions such as cancer, congestive heart failure, chronic obstructive pulmonary disease, chronic renal failure as well as dementia.

C is incorrect. Although traditionally associated with cancer care, these other end-stage diseases make up far more than 10% of enrolled patients in hospice care (only 41.3% had cancer as a primary diagnosis, not 90%). National Hospice and Palliative Care Organization reported in October of 2008 that the previous year's noncancer-related admissions were at 58.7%.

16. Correct Answer: D (Chapter 76).

Macular degeneration is atrophy of the cells in the central macula. It is associated with a loss of central vision and blurring of vision. It is the most common cause of visual impairment in Caucasian elderly. There are two types of macular degeneration. Wet macular degeneration involves formation of new, abnormally weak blood vessels under the macula. These break and leak blood and fluid and can lead to central vision loss. Photocoagulation can be helpful in this type of macular degeneration. Dry macular degeneration involves formation of deposits, drusen, under the retina. This can lead to wet macular degeneration as well. This type can lead to wet macular degeneration. Patients with macular degeneration should be monitored for visual changes with an Amsler grid (grid with black dot in middle used to monitor changes in central vision. Antioxidant therapy (including using Ocuvite) helps to reduce progression.

A is incorrect. Presbyopia is an age-associated loss of the ability of the eye to accommodate. It is not associated with a loss of central vision. Most of these individuals need glasses for reading by their fifties.

B is incorrect. Glaucoma, left untreated, leads to a loss of peripheral vision (not central) and eventual blindness. Glaucoma is characterized by an elevated intraocular pressure (measured by tonometry) and increased optic cup-to-disc ratio. There is an increase in pressure of the aqueous humor (produced by ciliary bodies) as it flows from the posterior chamber to the anterior chamber of the eye past the trabecular meshwork into the canal of Schlemm. Open angle glaucoma is a slower progressing blockage of outflow of aqueous humor, while closed angle glaucoma (acute blockage of the canal of Schlemm by the Iris) can present as an acute crisis. Treatment is indicated if intraocular pressures exceed 25 mmHg or in the presence of optic nerve atrophy or visual field loss. Pharmacologic treatment includes drops that either decrease the aqueous production (beta blockers, adrenergic agents) or increase aqueous drainage (mitotic) and thus lower the pressure. Surgical intervention is only indicated when pressures are poorly controlled by topical agents or when visual loss progresses. Glaucoma is the most common cause of blindness in African Americans.

C is incorrect. Cataract is a loss of transparency of the crystalline lens (cloudy appearance). Risk factors for cataracts include sun exposure, smoking, steroid use, and diabetes mellitus. Treatment consists of surgical removal of the lens and is indicated if the visual acuity is 20/50 or worse and/or if there is functional impairment from the cataract. It is a generalized clouding of vision and does not begin as a loss of central vision specifically.

E is incorrect. Strabismus is a misalignment of one of both eyes. It involves inability of the eyes to coordinate focus on an object. It is thought to be a problem with the muscles of the eyes. It generally presents in childhood. When a child is found to have unilateral strabismus, the eye without the defect is covered for a significant amount of time to allow the defected eye's muscles to strengthen. There are different types of strabismus including esotropia (crossed eyes) and exotropia ("wall-eyes," or eyes directed laterally). This is not a defect in central vision of the eyes (like macular degeneration).

17. Correct Answer: C (Chapter 35).

The specificity ranges between 85% and 95%. The CAGE questionnaire is not diagnostic as many factors go into diagnosing substance abuse. The CAGE questionnaire is used when abuse is suspected:

Have you ever felt the need to "*C*ut down" on your drinking?

Are you "*A*nnoyed" by people criticizing your drinking?

Have you ever felt "*G*uilty" about your drinking?

Do you ever need a drink in the morning to steady your nerves or hangover? ("*E*ye-opener")

A is incorrect. The test is a screening test and does not diagnose substance abuse, but is a useful tool, as the diagnosis depends on a constellation of medical, social, and psychological clues.

B is incorrect. When using the CAGE test and given 2 "yes" answers, the sensitivity ranges from 70% to 85% and the specificity ranges from 85% to 95%.
D is incorrect since interpretation of the CAGE questionnaire is straightforward. However, the CAGE questionnaire is a screening test and is not diagnostic; therefore, further questioning, testing, or referral would be indicated to arrive at a diagnosis of substance abuse in those instances of a positive screen.
E is incorrect. 13% of the adult population meets the diagnostic criteria for substance abuse and 20% of U.S. adults are at risk for substance abuse.

18. Correct Answer: E (Chapter 31).
Somatization is defined as emotional or psychological distress that is experienced and expressed as physical complaints. Somatization disorder is the most common type of somatiform disorder. It is characterized by multiple, unexplained symptoms in multiple organs (D is incorrect) before the age of 30 (A is incorrect). Most patients with somatiform disorder will "doctor shop" (search for the answers to their health disparity from multiple doctors) (C is incorrect). Women who have this somatization disorder outnumber men by 6:1 (B is incorrect). *Diagnostic and Statistical Manual of Mental Disorders*, fourth edition (DSM-IV) criteria require the presence of four pain symptoms, two GI symptoms, one sexual symptom, and one pseudoneurological symptom (headaches, ataxia, etc.) in order to diagnose somatization disorder. Other somatiform disorders include hypochondriasis and conversion disorders.

19. Correct Answer: A (Chapter 66).
Blood lead and hemoglobin levels are generally obtained between 9 and 15 months of age. Serum glucose and bilirubin levels are obtained shortly after birth (B and C are incorrect). Patients born to diabetic mothers may have hypoglycemia due to increased insulin, due to the mother's elevated blood sugar. Bilirubin levels can be high in the immediate neonatal period due to immaturity of the newborns hepatobiliary system. This may result in clinical jaundice that may require therapy.
D is incorrect. The human papilloma virus vaccine has been developed as a preventive tool for prevention of cervical cancer. It is active against the strains of virus most commonly associated with cervical cancer. It is recommended for girls beginning at 11 years of age. Pap smears are recommended within the first 3 years of a woman's sexual activity. Repeat smears are recommended every year and can be spaced out every 2 to 3 years if a woman is in a monogamous relationship (or not sexually active) and has had three normal Pap smears. Human papilloma virus DNA testing is recommended for sexually active females with abnormal PAP smears.
E is incorrect. Annual serum cholesterol measurements are recommended for men age 35 and older and women age 45 without significant risk factors for cardiac disease. For men and women with an increased risk for CHD, however, screening should begin at age 20. In children with a family history of CHD at a young age, cholesterol screening is recommended beginning at age 2 years.

20. Correct Answer: C (Chapter 37).
Posttraumatic stress disorder, obsessive–compulsive disorder, panic disorder, and phobias are all different forms of anxiety disorders. Postconcussion syndrome refers to a state of nervous instability following mild or moderate head injury. The main features are dizziness, headache, fatigue, and difficulty in concentration. An uneasy or anxious feeling is also a common symptom that is reported.
A is incorrect. Posttraumatic stress disorder is a psychiatric disease that is a form of anxiety disorder. Anxiety symptoms lasting at least 1 month develop after an individual experiences a distressing event outside the normal human response. There may be delayed onset and the patient may experience flashbacks.
B is incorrect. Obsessive–compulsive disorder also is a psychiatric disease and a variety of anxiety disorder. This condition involves intrusive, unwanted thoughts and repetitive behaviors performed in a ritualistic manner.
D is incorrect. Panic disorder is a specific form of anxiety disorder that involves episodic of intense fear or apprehension accompanied by at least four somatic complaints: for example, diaphoresis, dyspnea, dizziness, or flushing, accompanied by behavior changes because of unrealistic and persistent worry.
E is incorrect. Phobias are anxiety disorders characterized by persistent or irrational fear of a specific object, activity, or situation.

21. Correct Answer: E (Chapter 54).
Smoking reduces the risk of a second myocardial infarction by 50% within 1 to 2 years of smoking cessation. Even older individuals benefit from stopping tobacco use after years of smoking or after quitting subsequent to a smoking-related illness (B is incorrect). Lung cancer risk drops significantly 10 years after a smoker quits (D is incorrect). Adolescent smoking has fallen very little since its peak in the 1970s, and in teenage girls it has increased in recent years (C is incorrect). This is despite the fact that smoking in the United States has declined to about 25%.
A is incorrect. The National Cancer Institution lists four "A's" for office-based intervention.

1. *Ask* about smoking at every opportunity possible. Ask those who smoke whether they are interested in cessation.
2. *Advise* every smoker with a clear, unambiguous direct message. Tailor the advice to the patient's individual situation.
3. *Assist* patients in their efforts to stop. If a smoker is ready to quit, ask him or her to set a date. Offer

self-help material and pharmacologic therapy, such as nicotine replacement. Consider a referral to a formal smoking cessation program. If the individual is ready to quit, discuss the benefits and barriers to smoking cessation. Make the information as relevant to the individual as possible. Advise the smoker to avoid exposing family members to secondhand smoke. Indicate a willingness to help in the future, when the smoker is ready, and continue to ask about quitting in follow-up visits.

4. *Arrange* and negotiate a follow-up appointment generally within 1 to 2 weeks after the quit date. Make sure to congratulate those who have successfully quit and reinforce the benefits of giving up smoking. Discuss high-risk situations for relapse and review coping mechanisms. For those who fail to quit, provide positive reinforcement for taking the first step towards quitting. Ask about what obstacles the patient encountered and discuss strategies to overcome these in the future. Encourage the patient to set another quit date.

22. Correct Answer: E (Chapter 51).

Any firm nodule in the prostate should be biopsied. Ultrasound guided biopsy with anywhere from 6 to 12 biopsies is the usual procedure. The patient's PSA is in an abnormal range, but in a range often due to benign conditions. Values under 4 are considered normal, while those above 10 are considered suspicious for carcinoma. For the above value of 8 (between 4 and 10) additional PSA measures such as the percent of free PSA or the ratio of free PSA: total PSA can help determine the need for biopsy. Using a cutoff of 25% free PSA in patients with values of 4 to 10 may eliminate many unnecessary biopsies without significant loss in sensitivity. Urinalysis helps to rule out transitional cell carcinoma of the bladder (blood in urine) as well as other less malignant diseases such as cystitis or renal lithiasis.

A is incorrect. CT scan of the abdomen and pelvis is not indicated for patients with prostatic symptoms or physical findings. CT scan does not show the prostate well. In patients with suspected metastases, CT scan can be beneficial in assessing for spread to the solid organs.

B is incorrect. Renal ultrasound is the visualization method of choice for urinary obstruction, renal tumors, renal vein thrombosis, and is part of the evaluation for renal failure. Renal ultrasound would not be helpful for assessing a prostate nodule or elevated PSA.

C is incorrect. Evaluation of prostate cancer, though usually lower mortality rate than most other cancers, can cause significant morbidity in a symptomatic patient. In elderly males with significant comorbidities, one possible choice may be to manage symptoms and not pursue invasive procedures. Screening PSA testing is generally not recommended for geriatric patients with a life expectancy of less than 10 years.

D is incorrect. Generally, glucose testing would be indicated to evaluate polyuria such as is present in this patient. However, this patient has an advanced age, no glucosuria, and an enlarged prostate with a suspicious nodule. Glucose testing could be performed to be thorough but is not the test of choice for evaluating this patient's findings.

23. Correct Answer: D (Chapter 76).

The patient is suffering from closed angle glaucoma. It typically presents with blurred vision, halos around lights, pain, redness in the eye, and a moderately dilated pupil that does not respond to light. Dilation of the pupil helps to distinguish closed angle glaucoma from other causes of a painful red eye (e.g., iritis). Emergent treatment is needed to prevent permanent loss of vision.

Review question 16, as the following information is given. Glaucoma left untreated leads to a loss of peripheral vision (not central) and eventual blindness. Glaucoma is characterized by an elevated intraocular pressure (measured by tonometry) and increased optic cup-to-disc ratio. There is an increase in pressure of the aqueous humor (produced by ciliary bodies) as it flows from the posterior chamber to the anterior chamber of the eye past the trabecular meshwork into the canal of Schlemm. Open angle glaucoma is a slower progressing blockage of outflow of aqueous humor, while closed angle glaucoma (acute blockage of the canal of Schlemm by the Iris) can present as an acute crisis. Treatment is indicated if intraocular pressures exceed 25 mmHg or in the presence of optic nerve atrophy or visual field loss. Pharmacologic treatment includes drops that either decrease the aqueous production (beta blockers, adrenergic agents) or increase aqueous drainage (mitotic) and thus lower the pressure. Surgical intervention is only indicated when pressures are poorly controlled by topical agents or when visual loss progresses. Glaucoma is the most common cause of blindness in African Americans. **A** is incorrect. Many diseases (such as those mentioned below) can present with unilateral involvement. Unilateral involvement does not indicate a need for emergent treatment.

B is incorrect since purulent discharge would suggest an infectious etiology such as conjuncitivits or dacrocystitis, neither of which should affect vision. These infections are usually due to *Staphylococcus aureus* or beta hemolytic *Streptococci*. They are usually unilateral conditions, but can be bilateral.

C is incorrect. Itching of the eye is not typical of acute angle glaucoma. It is more consistent with allergic conjunctivitis.

E is incorrect. A nodular lesion can be either a chalazion, which presents with discomfort of the eye lid (a chronic granulomatous lesion of the melbomian gland, which is hard and painless) or a hordeolum, which is an abscess over the upper or lower eye lid. An external hordeolum is known as a stye while an internal one is abscess of the melbomian gland. Neither of these eye nodules present with halos around lights.

24. Correct Answer: A (Chapter 9).
The onset of pain following heavy lifting in an adult under 50 years of age suggests a muscular cause for this patient's pain.

B and C are incorrect as tumor, infection, or inflammation can cause nighttime awakenings due to pain that does not improve with rest.

D is incorrect as disc herniations usually occur after a very trivial stress (may even just be a cough or sneeze). The most common levels for these to occur are L5–S1 (nerve root for S1) and L4–L5 (nerve root for L5). Recall nerve root L5 includes motor function for extension of the great toe, as well as sensory for the dorsum of the foot/base of the first great toe. The nerve root for S1 includes the ankle jerk reflex, plantar flexion (motor), and sensory for the buttock, posterior thigh, calf, lateral ankle, and foot.

E is incorrect. Although nephrolithiasis can cause back pain, the pain usually radiates to the groin unilaterally. If this were the case, a UA would be necessary and if the lithiasis were less than 4 mm, the patient would probably be able to pass it with adequate hydration within 1 to 2 weeks. The urine must be strained during this time, and an F/U KUB in 1 to 2 weeks should be recommended. If the stone is not passed in 2 weeks or if the nephrolithiasis were larger than 4 mm then extracorporal shockwave lithotripsy or surgical intervention would be necessary.

25. Correct Answer: D (Chapter 18).
In asymptomatic individuals the initial test for evaluation of hematuria is a urine culture. An entirely normal repeat study after treatment of an infection in healthy individuals below 35 to 40 years of age usually requires no further evaluation other than a follow-up urine analysis in 1 to 2 months. If just one UA is positive for blood (greater than 1 RBC/high power field), then a repeat UA is performed before having the patient evaluated further. Although there are many causes of hematuria, including systemic lupus erythematous (+ANA), henoch–schonlein purpura (presents with purpura on lower extremities and buttock), various other forms of nephritis, renal vein/artery embolus, tuberculosis, polycystic kidney disease, bladder carcinoma (if suspected diagnostic modality of choice is cystoscopy), medullary sponge kidney, renal cell carcinoma (warrants CT scan or MRI) exercise, trauma, renal stones, foley placement, prostatitis, BPH, and so on the key to this question is making sure to rule out more benign and easily treatable causes such as infection before putting the patient through unnecessary treatments or diagnostic imaging studies.

A, B, C, and E are incorrect due to the answers given above.

26. Correct Answer: E (Chapter 78).
This 76-year-old man is most likely suffering from overflow incontinence secondary to benign prostatic hypertrophy. Finasteride is a 5-alpha-reductase blocker that is used to reduce BPH and therefore help alleviate obstruction to voiding. Overflow incontinence usually presents with constant leakage of urine with a postvoid residual greater than 200 ml. It can be caused by anatomic obstruction (prostate disease, urethral stricture) or neurologic factors such as diabetes or multiple sclerosis, or can be caused by medications such as narcotics, anticholinergics (disinhibits beta relaxation of bladder), or sympathomimetics (increases beta relaxation).

B is incorrect. Oxybutynin is an anticholinergic used to control urge incontinence; this would worsen overflow incontinence, which is usually due to detrusor muscle instability, or may be secondary to stroke, dementia, Parkinson disease, or spinal cord injury. Patients often complain of having the sudden urge to go to the bathroom but are unable to get to the bathroom before micturition occurs.

C is incorrect. Urecholine is a cholinergic that is used to stimulate bladder contraction in conditions such as atony due to diabetes mellitus. It is not hydrolyzed by cholinesterase and therefore has a longer duration of action than similar parasympathomimetics like bethanechol, which is also used in overflow incontinence in diabetics. However, in general medical treatments of overflow incontinence due to bladder contractility problems are generally not very efficacious.

D is incorrect, as catheterization usually predisposes the patient to bacteria not native to their urethra, bladder, or kidneys. If necessary a suprapubic catheter is inserted or intermittent catheterization is recommended. Indwelling catheters should be reserved for comfort in terminally ill patients, to prevent worsening of pressure ulcers, or for patients with inoperable outflow obstruction.

27. Correct Answer: D (Chapter 76).
Presbycusis is a bilateral loss of hearing related to aging. It is a sensorineural hearing loss, which particularly affects hearing at higher frequencies. It is associated with age-related degeneration of the hair cells of the cochlea and giant stereocilia and is thought to result from cumulative noise-induced damage over time.

Meniere disease is an acquired condition, not age-related, that affects the inner ear and can affect balance and hearing. It is characterized by episodes of tinnitus and progressive hearing loss. The hearing loss associated with Meniere disease is low-pitched in nature as is any associated tinnitus. It is usually unilateral and caused by endolymphatic hydrops, resulting in increased pressure within the semicircular canals and damage to the sensory hair cells. Hyperacusis and nystagmus may also be present. It usually develops when a person is between 30 and 60 years of age and has an undetermined etiology, and chronic therapy includes diuretics (acetazolamide or hydrochlorothiazide) and salt restriction.

Otosclerosis is a hereditary disorder in which ossification of the labyrinth of the inner ear occurs, which results in tinnitus and eventual conductive hearing loss. The ossification can lead to fusion of the ossicles that causes the conductive hearing loss. Treatment is generally surgical through referral to an otolaryngologist. This is not an age-related phenomenon. An acoustic neuroma is a schwannoma of the eighth cranial nerve that gradually grows to compress the eighth cranial nerve and eventually the brainstem. This can occur sporadically or can be found in neurofibromatosis type 2 (MISME syndrome, multiple inherited schwannomas, meningiomas, and ependymomas). Acoustic neuromas are treated surgically.

Labyrinthitis is an inflammation of the labyrinth and often follows an upper respiratory tract infection. It is usually caused by a viral infection and causes vomiting and severe vertigo. Recovery is generally within 1 to 6 weeks. Meclizine, dimenhydrinate, antiemetics, and benzodiazepines are used in the treatment of labyrinthitis. Long-term sequelae can include dysequilibrium and dizziness, which can last for months to years.

28. Correct Answer: B (Chapter 60).

Fibroadenomas commonly present in younger women as discrete, painless rubbery masses. After an initial several month period of growth, fibroadenomas generally stabilize in size, remain mobile, and do not spread to adjacent lymph nodes. They can be observed but are often surgically removed because of the associated anxiety and discomfort.

Breast cancer typically presents in a postmenopausal woman as an isolated painless mass discovered on self-examination or as part of routine screening. The mass usually does not have discrete borders, but may be mobile or fixed. Over time cancerous masses will enlarge, become fixed, and may be associated with palpable lymph nodes. Other signs of breast cancer include skin dimpling, nipple inversion, nipple discharge in a nonlactating woman (especially bloody discharge), and skin edema or inflammation. Although this woman's mass is painless, the age and stability in growth over 18 months make a diagnosis of breast cancer highly unlikely in this woman.

Fibrocystic breast disease usually presents as diffusely lumpy tender breasts. Fibrocystic changes will vary with the menstrual cycle and are most commonly found in young women. Cysts that persist through the menstrual cycle fail to resolve with aspiration or those with bloody aspirate may be malignant. This woman's mass is not painful, is discrete, and does not vary with her menstrual cycle. Fibrocystic change is not likely the cause for the mass in this case.

Mastitis usually presents in a lactating woman and appears as an erythematous, painful area on the breast. Purulent discharge may be present. *Staphylococcus aureus* is usually the implicated pathogen. It is recommended to continue breast feeding or pumping of the affected breast. Antibiotics with appropriate methicillin-resistant *S. aureus* coverage should be used for 2 to 4 weeks duration, and heat or ice packs may be used for 24 hours for symptom relief. If an abscess is present and can be percutaneously drained with complete resolution, the patient may be monitored conservatively. If the patient is not lactating, inflammatory carcinoma must be ruled out, and referral for possible biopsy would be warranted. Intraductal papillomas usually present with nipple discharge (bloody or serous). Grossly they appear as pink to tan, friable, lesions within the duct and are attached to the involved duct by a stalk. They are generally not palpable on clinical breast exam. They are rarely malignant, but if multiple lesions are present (usually in younger women), they may undergo malignant transformation.

29. Correct Answer: D (Chapter 23).

Rheumatoid arthritis usually presents in the MCP joints. It is a chronic multisystem disease of unknown cause. The characteristic feature of established RA is persistent inflammatory synovitis of the peripheral joints, including MCP, wrist, knee, and joints of the feet, in a symmetric distribution. Two-thirds of patients present with an insidious onset of fatigue, anorexia, generalized weakness, and vague musculoskeletal symptoms until appearance of synovitis. Stiffness is frequent following periods of inactivity. Morning stiffness is common, as in many inflammatory joint diseases. X-rays show bony erosions in the periarticular bone of the wrists or hands. The earliest changes, however, occur in the wrists or feet and consist of soft tissue swelling and juxta-articular demineralization. Treatment may include NSAIDs or COX-2 inhibitors, but disease-modifying antirheumatic drugs (DMARDs), such as methotrexate, should be started as soon as the diagnosis is certain to prevent long-term disfigurement and preserve function. Systemic lupus erythematous may present with arthritis of the hands and wrist, but x-rays do not show bony erosions. Diagnosis is based on at least four of the following at any point in the patient's history: malar rash, discoid rash, photosensitivity, oral ulcers, arthritis, serositis, renal disease, seizures or psychosis with no other known cause, hemolytic anemia or leukopenia, anti-double-stranded DNA, anti-Smith antigen or antiphospholipids, and antinuclear antibodies. Severe systemic illness requiring glucocorticoid therapy can occur with fever, anemia, prostration, and weight loss.

Wegener granulomatosis is a small vessel vasculitis which affects both the upper and lower respiratory tracts as well as presents with glomerulonephritis. Presenting symptoms include upper respiratory symptoms (nasal congestion, sinusitis, otitis media, mastoiditis, inflammation of the gums, or stridor) but can also include migratory oligoarthritis specifically in the large joints, ocular disease, dysesthesia secondary to neuropathy, purpura, fever, and weight loss. Three-fourths of patients have renal involvement, which may be subclinical until renal insufficiency is advanced. Induction treatment includes prednisone and cyclophosphamide (or prednisone and methotrexate).

Osteoarthritis usually presents in the cervical, or lower lumbar vertebrae, first metacarpal phalangeal, hip, knee, and first metatarsal phalangeal, and distal and proximal interphalangeal joints. There is usually joint space narrowing on x-ray along with osteophytes, but erosions do not occur. Osteoarthritis is uncommon in adults under age 40 and highly prevalent in those aver age 60. Scleroderma is a multisystem disease that frequently presents with Raynaud phenomenon, gastroesophageal reflux disease with or without dysmotility, skin changes, swollen fingers, and arthralgias. The American College of Rheumatology diagnostic criteria include thickened skin changes proximal to the metacarpophalangeal joints or at least two of the following: sclerodactyly, digital pitting (loss of tissue on finger pads secondary to ischemia), and bibasilar pulmonary fibrosis. A diagnosis can also be made if the patient has three out of five features of CREST syndrome (calcinosis, Raynaud phenomenon, esophageal dysmotility, sclerodactyly, and telangiectasias). A positive ANA is usually present in patients with scleroderma. This patient does not satisfy either criterion for a diagnosis of scleroderma.

30. Correct Answer: C (Chapter 41).

Digoxin can improve left ventricular contractility in patients with systolic congestive heart failure and can help to control heart rate in patients with atrial fibrillation. There is no data to suggest benefit of patients in sinus rhythm with diastolic congestive heart failure. Initial management could include discontinuing the digoxin. Patients with diastolic heart failure generally benefit from reduction in heart rate and increased left ventricular relaxation and filling time. Beta blockers, such as carvedilol, are useful therapeutic agents in achieving these goals and thus are a cornerstone of therapy for diastolic heart failure. In addition, carvedilol was associated with significant (65%) reduction in all-cause mortality, during the U.S. Carvedilol trial. This effect was independent of sex, age, etiology of heart failure, or ejection fraction.

Lisinopril should be maintained to provide afterload reduction and adequate blood pressure control. ACE inhibitors are beneficial in heart failure, particularly in those with diabetes mellitus, hypertension, or additional cardiovascular risk factors.

Acutely, patients with diastolic congestive heart failure will benefit from aggressive diuresis. Once fluid retention is no longer a concern, the diuretic dose may be reduced to the minimal level necessary to maintain euvolemia. In many cases, diuretics may ultimately be discontinued. In this patient, discontinuing furosemide

may be a logical next step after he is off the digoxin.

Aspirin continues to be recommended as a preventive medication for myocardial infarction and ischemia in those patients with cardiovascular disease or risk factors.

31. Correct Answer: C (Chapter 49).

The exact causes for obesity are still being researched and are yet to be precisely determined, but appear to be multifactorial. Important factors most likely include not only genetic disposition but also psychosocial factors such as socioeconomic status.

Many patients present wanting to find an underlying medical condition that would account for their being overweight or obese. Secondary causes for obesity are unusual and the medical examination and laboratory workup for obesity generally does not uncover a cause. Very often patients want to take a pill to fix their condition. The current state of knowledge and treatment for obesity do not lend itself to this approach. Even in the cases where hypothyroidism is incidentally discovered, treatment of the hypothyroidism results in a euthyroid overweight or obese patient. Hypothyroidism may cause symptoms but it is generally not the cause for obesity. Treatment efforts focus on diet and exercise with the goal of increasing caloric expenditure and limiting intake to healthy less-calorie dense choices. Expenditure of 3500 more calories than are taken in can result in weight loss of one pound.

32. Correct Answer: E (Chapter 45).

Antiviral prophylaxis with AZT should be instituted as soon as possible after a health care provider is exposed to HIV-infected material. Early chemoprophylaxis may destroy the virus and prevent infection. Waiting to check titers or to see if she becomes ill puts her at unnecessary risk of developing infection that may then become a long-term health problem. Even though she did not "inject" blood into herself, the accidental stick with a needle that contained blood from an HIV-positive patient potentially exposes her to the HIV virus from any residual blood on or in the needle. Prophylaxis for pneumocystis, toxoplasmosis, or mycobacteria would not be appropriate until active HIV infection is established. Initiating such therapies is determined based on the patient's CD4 counts. Pneumocystis prophylaxis with trimethoprim-sulfamethoxazole begins with a CD4 count of 200. Toxoplasmosis begins with a CD4 count of less than 100. Mycobacterium avium complex prophylaxis with clarithromycin begins with a CD4 count of 50.

33. Correct Answer: D (Chapter 26).

Orthostatic proteinuria is a benign condition of unknown etiology. Proteinuria is often discovered incidentally during a school or sports examination. Causes for proteinuria can include a variety of causes including intrinsic renal diseases such as minimal change disease, glomerulosclerosis, polycystic kidney disease, or Alport syndrome. Other conditions associated with proteinuria include diabetes, immunologic or connective tissue diseases, medications, and cancers such as multiple myeloma. These conditions are associated with a continuous proteinuria that is not dependent on the upright or supine position. Orthostatic proteinuria is associated with protein leakage into the urine in significant quantities only upon assuming the upright posture and diminishing in the supine position. The exact cause for this condition is unknown but patients have been studied for years and uniformly follow a benign course with no additional follow-up or treatment being required. Thus, no additional workup or restrictions are needed for this patient.

34. Correct Answer: E (Chapter 17).

Testing the stool for *Helicobacter pylori* antigen would determine if the infection is active. Other means to test for active disease would include the CLO test performed on samples obtained via endoscopy, pathologic examination of biopsy specimens, and urea breath testing. Use of the fecal antigen testing is a good means to detect disease activity because it is more readily available than urea breath testing and it is not invasive.

Serologic testing is highly sensitive and specific and would be more convenient than fecal antigen testing. Unfortunately, this test remains positive indefinitely in patients who have had a history of *H. pylori* infection, even post-treatment. Barium swallow is a useful test for detecting anatomic abnormalities such as esophageal cancers, achalasia, or esophageal pouches but is not sensitive for detecting the surface inflammatory changes associated with the *H. pylori* gastritis. Ambulatory pH monitoring is useful in correlating heartburn symptoms with gastroesophageal reflux in patients with symptoms but no visible changes detected on esophagogastroduodenoscopy. This test would not be helpful in detecting *H. pylori*–related disease. Abdominal CT would play no role in diagnosing heartburn-related symptoms. CT scans are obtained in many cases of acute and chronic abdominal pain to help define the anatomy and any associated abnormalities that may be the cause for pain. CT scans are very helpful in acute abdominal pain where diseases such as nephrolithiasis, pancreatitis, appendicitis, or diverticulitis are suspected. CT scans are also obtained in cases of bowel obstruction to help identify the level of the obstruction and the possible etiology.

35. Correct Answer: D (Chapter 11).

Verapamil, a calcium channel blocker, can cause constipation. Changing Verapamil to an alternative medication may relieve this patient's symptoms. Other medications that may cause constipation include opiates, anticholinergics, tricyclic antidepressants, diuretics, antacids, clonidine, levodopa, and laxative abuse.

Other causes of constipation include insufficient dietary fiber, inactivity, hypokalemia, hypercalcemia, hypothyroidism, scleroderma, amyloidosis, pregnancy, neurological disorders such as Parkinson disease, paraplegia, prior pelvic surgery, diabetes mellitus, irritable bowel syndrome, colonic mass, Hirschsprung disease, perianal pathology such as fissure/es, hemorrhoids, rectoceoles, rectal prolapse, and diverticular disease. If the patient had no other potential causes for his change in bowel habits, then consideration should be given to the possibility of a lesion such as colon cancer. Since there is an identifiable potential cause for his symptoms, these should be addressed first. If his symptoms resolve with a change in medication, then he should undergo routine colonoscopy at age 50 or age 40 in those with a first-degree relative with colon cancer.

Laxative medication or preferably an increase in activity level and fiber and fluid intake are measures that can be taken to try to relieve symptoms of constipation. Dietary and behavioral measures should be undertaken before additional medications are prescribed. In addition, continual use of motility agents, although not proven, has been thought to cause damage to the myenteric nerves, thus negatively impacting GI motility. Metoclopramide is a promotility agent used in treatment of nausea and vomiting and has its primary effect on the esophagus and gastroesophageal sphincter. Metoclopropamide would not have a role in treating constipation.

Recommending a low-fat, high-fiber diet is part of constipation management, and may be beneficial in long term in those who are prone to constipation. This step could be taken along with modification of the patient's medication regimen. Other important steps in evaluation of constipation include treating underlying disorders causing constipation, such as hypothyroidism, bowel obstruction, or anal fissure (or any of the above-mentioned causes). For functional constipation, increasing fluid and fiber intake is the first step to be taken. Patients should drink eight 8-oz glasses of water per day and consume large amounts of bran, fresh fruit, vegetables, beans, and whole grains. Other means to increase dietary fiber in those who are having difficulty ingesting sufficient quantities include over-the-counter products, such as bulk-forming agents, which increase stool volume by absorbing water such as psyllium (Metamucil), methylcellulose (Citrucel), polycarbophil (FiberCon). Patients may also benefit from bowel retraining, which involves devoting 10 to 15 minutes each day to a quiet and unhurried time on the commode. This should take place at the same time each day and occur following a meal, to take advantage of the gastrocolic reflex. Bowel retraining often requires 2 to 3 weeks before becoming effective. Other medications include osmotic laxatives such as lactulose, magnesium salts, and sorbitol, which are nonabsorbable solutes that draw water fluid into the intestinal lumen by creating an osmotic gradient. Stimulant agents such as phenolphthalein (Ex-Lax) and bisacodyl (Dulcolax) alter mucosal permeability and stimulate intestinal smooth muscle activity. Stool softeners like docusate sodium (Colace), which is used for hard stools that are difficult to pass, decrease surface tension, and allow water and fat to mix in the stool. Stool softeners must be taken with plenty of water to work optimally. Enemas and suppositories work by distension and stimulation of the rectum, which leads to evacuation, and is especially useful in bedridden patients and those with stool impaction.

36. (Chapter 19).

1. **Correct Answer: C.** Antismooth muscle antibodies can be found in type 1 and type 2 autoimmune hepatitis. Antinuclear antibodies (ANAs) are usually also elevated in autoimmune hepatitis.
2. **Correct Answer: A.** Ferritin is used to help in the diagnosis of hemochromatosis. Elevated ferritin, decreased transferrin, and increased transferrin saturation are indicative of hemochromatosis, which is a iron storage disease affecting many organs including the liver.
3. **Correct Answer: D.** Decreased ceruloplasmin is found in 90% of Wilson disease patients; however, 20% of carriers also have reduced rates of serum ceruloplasmin. Kayser–Fleischer rings are present in 99% of patients with the neurologic form of the disease; however, only 30% to 50% of patients present with the purely hepatic or presymptomatic states of Wilson disease. These rings are diagnosed definitively using an ophthalmologist's slit-lamp exam. Definitive diagnosis of the disease is made by liver biopsy and with quantitative copper assays. Wilson disease involves abnormal excretion of copper with subsequent buildup in the liver, the iris, and the brain causing parkinsonism. Trientine is the chelator being used more often in treatment, as it is less toxic than penicillamine.
4. **Correct Answer: E.** Antimitochondrial antibodies are used to screen for primary biliary cirrhosis. Primary biliary cirrhosis is a disease with insidious onset characterized by autoimmune destruction of the intrahepatic bile ducts and cholestasis.
5. **Correct Answer: B.** Haptoglobin is a glycoprotein synthesized in the liver that binds free hemoglobin. It is increased in obstructive liver disease or diseases associated with increased erythrocyte sedimentation rate (ESR). It is decreased in any type of hemolysis, liver disease, anemia, mildly with oral contraceptives, or in childhood and infancy.

37. Correct Answer: A (Chapter 21).

Deciding when to aggressively work up a patient with lymphadenopathy can be difficult. Important considerations include assessing for inciting causes and associated symptoms that may indicate increased risk for serious causes such as metastatic cancer or lymphoma. Fever, weight loss, and generalized lymphadenopathy are examples of symptoms that suggest infection or malignancy as potential etiology. Frequently, localized adenopathy can be the result of a viral infection or local inflammatory condition (e.g., tinea pedis, onychomycosis) or injury that may not be apparent at the time of the lymph node evaluation. When there are worrisome signs or symptoms, then observation is one option. It is recommended to observe for up to 4 weeks. Nodes that are unchanged or larger after 4 weeks should be biopsied. Nodes that have not resolved in 12 weeks should also be evaluated for possible biopsy.

Fine needle aspiration is one method for obtaining tissue to evaluate the etiology of the lymphadenopathy. However, fine needle aspirates often obtain inadequate samples and for this reason surgical excision is generally the preferred method for evaluating undiagnosed lymphadenopathy.

If there were signs of infection, such as redness, tenderness, fever, or an identified lesion, then empiric cephalexin would be reasonable during the observation period for resolution of the node. PET scanning has no role in evaluating this type of patient and is generally reserved for evaluating patients with known malignancies for metastastes.

38. Correct Answer: C (Chapter 22).

The symptoms this patient is experiencing are suggestive of an esophageal obstruction. Lesions that could cause obstruction of this nature include cancer, stricture, and achalasia. A barium esophogram and upper endoscopy are tests that would be helpful in identifying these types of lesions that may cause obstruction with the swallowing process. A colonoscopy may be warranted as a routine screening tool in patients this age but would not be warranted as part of the evaluation for these symptoms. Other indications for colonoscopy would include change in bowel habits and melena or hematochezia.

Abdominal ultrasound is not a useful tool for examining the esophagus, the stomach, or the intestines. The only exception to this is that ultrasound has been used to assess for appendicitis, particularly in children. Ultrasound is useful in examining the organs both intra-abdominally and in the pelvis. This would include the liver, kidneys, pancreas, uterus, and ovaries.

Abdominal CT is useful for assessing the organs and for inflammatory conditions such as pancreatitis, diverticulitis, and appendicitis. CT, like ultrasound, is not as useful for evaluating the esophagus, stomach, or intestines except for more advanced disease where there may be significant wall thickening or mass effect. Chest x-ray would not be expected to show any significant findings. Without contrast material, the esophagus is generally not apparent on chest x-rays, although on occasion, lesions such as a hiatal hernia are apparent due to the associated "gas bubble" that can be seen.

ANSWERS

39. Correct Answer: B (Chapter 53).

Staphylococcus aureus is the most common cause of cellulitis. *Streptococcus pyogenes* is also a common offending agent. With *S. pyogenes* a golden crust is often present. Oral or intravenous B-lactams, including dicloxacillin, cefazolin, and cephalaxin are commonly used for treatment.

Pseudomonas aeruginosa is a common respiratory pathogen in patients with cystic fibrosis or those that are immunocompromised. Pseudomonas is also associated with osteomyelitis in sickle cell patients and is a cause of foot infections since it has been found to grow well in tennis shoes.

Hemophilus influenza type B is a common cause of epiglottitis. Nontypeable H. flu is the second most common cause of otitis media infections and sinusitus, and it is implicated in many acute pneumonias in COPD patients.

Clostridium difficile is the cause of pseudomembranous collitis. These infections can occur after eradication of normal gut flora that then leads to an overgrowth of enteric *C. difficile*. The change in gut flora is generally associated with use of antibiotics that kill off the normal flora but not *C. difficile*.

Streptococcus pneumoniae is the most common cause of otitis media, sinusitis, and a common cause of pneumonia, as well as of bronchitis, bacteremia, meningitis, and other infectious processes.

40. Correct Answer: A (Chapter 71).

Children between the age of 3 months and 3 years, with a temperature over 102 degrees Fahrenheit, are at increased risk of occult bacteremia and an underlying bacterial infection. One approach to these children is to first obtain a CBC. Those with WBCs greater than 15,000 should be admitted and urine and blood cultures should be ordered. A chest x-ray in these children is indicated if respiratory symptoms are apparent. Children in whom cultures are obtained should generally receive empiric antibiotic coverage until culture results are available. Admitting the patient and starting antibiotics would be reasonable. The risk of bacteremia is higher in younger children, is increased in those with a temperature over 102 degrees, and is higher in those with WBCs over 15,000. For these reasons, empiric treatment with antipyretics or antibiotics or observation would not be recommended. Children, in this age category, with temperatures above 102 who are not admitted should have follow-up the next day.

For neonates (birth to 1 month of age) and ill-appearing infants (age 1 to 3 months), the workup involves a full septic workup that entails a CBC, blood cultures, chest x-ray, urinalysis, urine culture, and lumbar puncture. Hospitalization and empiric antibiotic coverage is indicated to cover the most common pathogens until culture results are available. Infants 1 to 3 months of age who appear well have normal laboratory studies, and a WBC between 5000 and 15,000 may be discharged with a follow-up in 24 hours. Empiric coverage (such as ceftriaxone IM) is usually provided pending follow-up and culture results. In children older than age 3, occult bacteremia is less common and clinical evaluation by history and physical exam can usually distinguish the source of fever. Laboratory evaluation in these older children is dictated by clinical findings.

41. Correct Answer: E (Chapter 69).

This patient has mild croup and no signs of respiratory distress. Dexamethasone as a single dose has been shown to lessen the need for re-evaluation and hospitalization in children with croup. Croup is a respiratory infection or laryngotracheobronchitis generally caused by the parainfluenza virus. Children may appear nontoxic and with crying or activity may experience respiratory distress. Since lungs are not affected, oxygen saturation is generally within normal limits, except in very severe cases. Anterior–posterior soft tissue neck x-ray will demonstrate steeple sign of upper tracheal narrowing; this helps to confirm the diagnosis.

Inhaled racemic epinephrine is used in patients with moderate-to-severe croup. Following therapy with racemic epinephrine, the child should be observed for 2 to 3 hours to assure that rebound symptoms do not occur. This may entail an extended emergency room stay or often the child is admitted. Dexamethasone is generally also prescribed along with any racemic epinephrine treatments. Nebulized or oral albuterol (beta-2 agonist) is indicated for treatment of asthma or COPD. Albuterol is not indicated in treatment of croup.

Oral prednisone at a dose of 1 to 2 mg/kg is given as treatment for asthma for 3 to 10 days or until peak expiratory flow returns to above 80%. This is used during acute exacerbations or when initiating therapy. This is not indicated in the treatment of croup.

42. Correct Answer: D (Chapter 69).

Febrile seizure occurs with fever and rate of rise of temperature as the predominate. With this in mind, treatment attempts should be made to control or reduce the fever with antipyretics. Therapy with antiepileptics is not indicated for simple febrile seizures. After this is accomplished, the second step should be to assess and treat the underlying cause of the fever. Lumbar puncture or CT scan would only be indicated if based on the history or physical exam; postictally, there were signs or symptoms suggesting meningitis, encephalitis, or other CNS lesions might be present. Presence of a febrile seizure, particularly when there is an identifiable cause for the fever, is not an indication for these tests. Likewise, antibiotics are not routinely recommended because of the seizure, but must have an indication based on the evaluation of the source of the fever.

43. Correct Answer: C (Chapter 52).

Sexually transmitted diseases (infections) should be tested for at this time, as the patient is sexually active and is in a high-risk age group for sexually transmitted infections.

A Pap smear should begin within 3 years of a patient's first sexual intercourse to check for dysplasia.

B is incorrect. Cholesterol screens are indicated in male patients beginning at 35 years of age and female patients at 45 years of age.

Routine urinalysis testing, although done in childhood, is not routinely indicated as part of adolescent care. Electrocardiograms are indicated in specific disease conditions, such as hypertension and heart disease, but are not a part of routine health screening at this age.

44. Correct Answer: D (Chapter 70).
ADHD is a clinical diagnosis based on the following DSM-IV criteria for ADHD: I: Either A or B or combined type. A: Six or more of the following symptoms of inattention have been present for at least 6 months to a point that is disruptive and inappropriate for developmental level. Inattention: (1) Often does not give close attention to details or makes careless mistakes in schoolwork, work, or other activities. (2) Often has trouble keeping attention on tasks or play activities. (3) Often does not seem to listen when spoken to directly. (4) Often does not follow instructions and fails to finish schoolwork, chores, or duties in the workplace (not due to oppositional behavior or failure to understand instructions). (5) Often has trouble organizing activities. (6) Often avoids, dislikes, or does not want to do things that take a lot of mental effort for a long period of time (such as schoolwork or homework). (7) Often loses things needed for tasks and activities (e.g., toys, school assignments, pencils, books, or tools). (8) Is often easily distracted. (9) Is often forgetful in daily activities. B: Six or more of the following symptoms of hyperactivity–impulsivity have been present for at least 6 months to an extent that is disruptive and inappropriate for developmental level. Hyperactivity: (1) Often fidgets with hands or feet or squirms in seat. (2) Often gets up from seat when remaining in seat is expected. (3) Often runs about or climbs when and where it is not appropriate (adolescents or adults may feel very restless). (4) Often has trouble playing or enjoying leisure activities quietly. (5) Is often "on the go" or often acts as if "driven by a motor." (6) Often talks excessively. Impulsivity: (1) Often blurts out answers before questions have been finished. (2) Often has trouble waiting one's turn. (3) Often interrupts or intrudes on others (e.g., butts into conversations or games). II: Some symptoms that cause impairment were present before age 7 years. III: Some impairment from the symptoms is present in two or more settings (e.g., at school/work and at home). IV: There must be clear evidence of significant impairment in social, school, or work functioning. V: The symptoms do not happen only during the course of a pervasive developmental disorder, schizophrenia, or other psychotic disorder. The symptoms are not better accounted for by another mental disorder.

CT scanning and TSH testing are not indicated as part of the evaluation. The Ages and Stages questionnaire is an evaluation used to screen for developmental problems in children in four domains: cognitive, motor, self-help, and language. It is used for ages 3 months to 5 years.

45. Correct Answer: C (Chapter 59).
This patient has primary amenorrhea and because she is also lacking secondary sex characteristics, her hypothalamic/pituitary function needs to be determined. If the FSH and LH are within normal limits, then an ultrasound should be performed to determine presence or absence of a uterus and ovaries. If the FSH and LH are abnormally elevated or if on ultrasound there is no evidence of a uterus or ovaries, then genetic testing will determine the karyotype. If the FSH and LH are abnormally low, then the patient should be evaluated for hypogonadotropic hypogonadism including assessment for medical illnesses and an MRI of the brain. The medroxyprogesterone challenge test would be performed if there were evidence of both a uterus and presence of estrogen (e.g., breast development). This test evaluates the presence of estrogenic action on the uterus and the presence of an intact outflow tract. Testosterone would be useful if there were virilization or clitoral hypertrophy.

46. Correct Answer: B (Chapter 65).
History of major depression puts this patient at increased risk for developing postpartum depression. Postpartum depression is relatively common after events such as childbirth. Although this patient has a supportive family, the strongest predictors of postpartum depression include prior psychopathology (such as depression), low levels of social support, stressful life events, and poor marital status. This patient, despite having strong family support, is still at significant risk due to her personal history of previous depression. Postpartum depression should be treated immediately to minimize impairment to caregiving mothers. Selective serotonin reuptake inhibitors are usually first-line agents, although breast-feeding mothers should take caution. Cognitive-behavioral therapy and group therapy can also be helpful. Postpartum blues has an onset of 2 to 14 days after childbirth and has a duration of less than 2 weeks. It is a heightened emotional reactivity that can develop in 50% of women. The key thing here is both duration and severity of symptoms.

47. Correct Answer: A (Chapter 61).
An intrauterine device is an ideal choice for a woman in a monogomous relationship, who may still want to have children in the future. Furthermore, the patient's irregular schedule would not be of concern if using an intrauterine device. Intrauterine devices such as Progestasert have theoretical and actual failure rates of 2.0. This device works by interfering with sperm mobility and fertilization. IUDs are highly effective, inexpensive, and reversible. Complications include pregnancy,

undiagnosed vaginal bleeding, and pelvic inflammatory disease. Relative contraindications include nulliparity, prior ectopic pregnancy, history of multiple partners, as well as history of STIDs or abnormal Pap smear. Complications include PID, ectopic pregnancy, spontaneous abortions, increased menstrual flow and pain, and uterine perforation during insertion.

Hormonal contraceptive patches still require weekly changes and may not be ideal for this woman with such an irregular schedule and failure of prior hormonal contraception. Postcoital contraception requires taking the equivalent of two oral contraceptive pills within 72 hours of coitus as well as 12 hours later. Levonorgestrel 0.75 mg may be given in two doses 12 hours apart or taking both together. An alternate form of postcoital contraception utilizes Ethinyl estradiol 50 mcg with 0.5 mg norgestrel that is given in a regimen of two tabs initially followed by two tabs 12 hours later. Both of these methods have nausea as potential adverse effects. Emergency postcoital contraception prevents at least three of four pregnancies that would have occurred. These methods should not be relied upon as a means of contraception.

Female condoms have an actual failure rate of 21.0 to 26.0 (although theoretical failure rate of 6%), and also requires use every time coitus occurs. This patient's history suggests poor use of such contraception.
This patient is not sure if she desires more children. A tubal ligation should be considered permanent and would be inappropriate in this case.

48. Correct Answer: C (Chapter 57).
The patient has ASCUS, but has no history of previous abnormal Paps and most importantly, a negative HPV test. This patient should have a repeat Pap smear in 12 months. A subsequent abnormal Pap smear is indication for colposcopy. If the patient is at risk for not adhering to this regimen, then immediate colposcopy should be scheduled.

Higher grade lesions, positive endocervical curettage, or an inadequate colposcopy may require conization or loop electroexcision procedure (LEEP). Lower grade lesions may be treated with observation, laser, cryotherapy, or by LEEP, depending on size and location of the lesion.

49. Correct Answer: B (Chapter 64).
The patient should be treated with amoxicillin, nitrofurantoin, or cephalexin for 7 to 10 days. All pregnant women should be screened and, if positive, treated for asymptomatic bacteriuria. Acute pyelonephritis of pregnancy requires hospitalization and parenteral antibiotic therapy. After treatment a culture to document clearing of infection is indicated, and cultures should be repeated monthly thereafter until delivery. If infections are recurrent, continuous low-dose prophylaxis with nitrofurantoin is indicated. All asymptomatic bacteriuria in pregnancy should be treated so as to avoid complications of pyelonephritis, given the mild physiologic hydronephrosis of pregnancy (predisposes to development of pyelonephritis).

Ciprofloxacin, other fluoroquinolones, and tetracyclines should be avoided in pregnancy for risk of teratogenicity in the fetus.

Ultrasound of the kidneys of a pregnant woman is likely to show mild hydronephrosis that is physiologic of pregnancy not secondary to a disease process. Ultrasound would be useful in cases of pyelonephritis to evaluate for obstruction.

Although most patients are not treated for asymptomatic bacteriuria, pregnant women are an exception. The risk of pyelonephritis is too great to not treat a pregnant patient with asymptomatic bacteriuria.

50. Correct Answer: E (Chapter 64).
Oral medications such as metformin are now commonly used in the management of gestational diabetes. Although dietary management is part of all treatment, medications are often required, in the form of either oral hypoglycemics or insulin.

Macrosomia is a complication of gestational diabetes, not IUGR. IUGR is a potential complication of women with preexisting, often type 1 diabetes, who become pregnant. Macrosomic babies can have complications such as shoulder dystocia, cephalopelvic disproportion, and hypoglycemia in the neonatal period (secondary to fetal increase in insulin due to maternal hyperglycemia). Goals of therapy are to prevent the complications listed above as well as to maintain the mother's blood sugar levels in a normal range. Retinopathy and nephropathy are not generally concerns associated with gestational diabetes.

Concerns about diabetes do not vanish upon delivery and women should be followed-up and tested postpartum. A woman who has had gestational diabetes is at a higher risk for developing diabetes mellitus type 2 later on in life.

51. Correct Answer: C (Chapter 12).
With symptoms of fever and dyspnea and abnormal findings on lung examination, this patient most likely has pneumonia, and this may be documented by obtaining a chest x-ray. Sinusitis is not likely given the absence of nasal symptoms or headaches and a normal ear, nose, and throat examination. Symptomatic treatment with cough suppressants or incentive spirometry may be appropriate; however, evaluation and treatment of the underlying condition is the first priority in a patient with these signs and symptoms. Sputum cultures are generally not very helpful in the outpatient setting. However, if the patient does not respond to antibiotics, a sputum culture may be considered.

52. Correct Answer: B (Chapter 62).
Atrophic vaginitis is usually seen in postmenopausal women. Human papillomavirus infections are generally

asymptomatic and discovered by palpation or visualization of a wartlike lesion or by Pap smear testing. In menstruating women, *Trichomonas*, bacterial vaginosis, and *Candida* cause 90% of vaginitis symptoms. All three may cause itching, but the discharge seen in BV and trichomoniasis usually has a pH > 4.5. The diagnosis can be confirmed by examining a wet mount and then adding KOH to the slide, which will dissolve epithelial cells but not the spores and hyphae seen in candidal infections.

53. Correct Answer: B (Chapter 29).
The most common cause of chronic dyspnea in a smoker who presents like this patient, with no significant prior medical problems, is chronic obstructive pulmonary disease. In evaluating this patient, other causes for chronic dyspnea must also be considered. A chest x-ray and laboratory work can help to exclude causes such as pleural effusion, congestive heart failure, and anemia. When the diagnosis is in doubt, additional testing, including pulmonary function testing, may help in arriving at the diagnosis. Diabetes mellitus does not generally cause dyspnea except in association with ketoacidosis, which would present acutely in a younger patient than this. Patients with pneumonia, pulmonary embolus, and myocardial infarction present with acute dyspnea.

54. Correct Answer: D (Chapter 73).
Hypertrophic cardiomyopathy is an autosomal dominant trait with variable expression and is the most common cause of sudden death in those younger than 35 years. Most patients with this condition are asymptomatic, and sudden cardiac death may be the initial presentation. Definitive diagnosis is made via echocardiogram, which shows asymmetric septal hypertrophy and left ventricular outflow obstruction. In this condition, decreased venous return increases the obstruction and the intensity of the murmur. Squatting increases venous return, whereas standing increases venous pooling and limits venous return.

55. Correct Answer: E (Chapter 20).
Although a CBC, uric acid level, rheumatoid factor, and ESR are useful tests, a joint fluid analysis is critical to determine whether this patient has a septic joint and to detect uric acid crystals (gout) or calcium pyrophosphate crystals (pseudogout).

56. Correct Answer: D (Chapter 13).
The presence of WBCs and blood in the stool is consistent with an inflammatory process. Food poisoning, rotavirus, and irritable bowel are noninflammatory processes. Although Crohn disease can cause bloody stools with WBCs, there is no previous history of gastrointestinal complaints. The most likely cause is diarrhea from a bacterial infection, such as shigellosis.

57. Correct Answer: E (Chapter 16).
Migraine headaches are characterized by severe unilateral, throbbing pain, which is often accompanied by photophobia, nausea, and emesis. Migraines that are preceded by auras (transient neurologic abnormalities such as the sensation of flashing lights or strange odors) are called classic migraines, whereas those not associated with auras are called common migraines. A family history of migraines occurs in the majority of cases and is an important diagnostic clue.

58. Correct Answer: D (Chapter 19).
The subacute course, myalgias, fatigue, and elevated liver function tests are suggestive of hepatitis. Patients with appendicitis have nausea and vomiting along with right lower quadrant pain but do not have elevated liver enzymes. Although this patient does have risk factors for gallstones, patients with cholelithiasis typically present more acutely and have intermittent pain that is aggravated with food. Although hemolysis can cause jaundice, it is unlikely to be the cause of her problems, as the CBC is normal; in hemolytic disease, the unconjugated fraction of bilirubin is elevated. Painless jaundice is the classic presentation for pancreatic cancer involving the head of the pancreas. Supportive care is generally recommended for patients with hepatitis. Determining the specific viral cause may help in determining follow-up testing and the likelihood of developing chronic hepatitis as well as in counseling family members regarding testing.

59. Correct Answer: D (Chapter 53).
Herpes simplex virus causes painful genital ulcers, often with fever and dysuria. The ulcers of syphilis are painless. Urinary tract infections do not cause genital ulcers. Although women with cervicitis may note vaginal discharge, dysuria, or spotting, most are asymptomatic. Petechial or pustular skin lesions can be seen on the dorsal aspect on the distal extremity, ankles, or wrist joints with gonorrheal infections, but ulcers are not seen on the cervix.

60. Correct Answer: A (Chapter 19).
This patient most likely has cholelithiasis. She has risk factors for gallstone disease and her total and conjugated bilirubin levels are elevated, indicating that the stone may be obstructing the common bile duct. She may ultimately need endoscopy and endoscopic retrograde cholangiopancreatography (ERCP), but an ultrasound or CT scan is generally done prior to the ERCP to confirm the diagnosis. MRI and liver biopsy are not indicated in this situation. Peptic ulcers can sometimes present with right upper quadrant pain; however, they do not cause liver enzyme abnormalities.

61. Correct Answer: E (Chapter 36).
This patient has iron deficiency anemia, as indicated by low ferritin levels and increased total iron-binding capacity. The most probable cause of his anemia is a chronic gastrointestinal bleed, possibly from a colon cancer. Patients with thalassemia can have microcytic anemia; however, the iron-binding capacity and ferritin levels

would be normal. Similarly, the serum ferritin levels are normal or increased in anemia of chronic disease. Vitamin B_{12} or folate deficiency causes megaloblastic anemias.

62. Correct Answer: C (Chapter 34).
Most cases of acne are pleomorphic and include comedones, papules, pustules, and nodules. Topical agents such as tretinoin are often the first line of therapy. Other, milder comedolytics include salicylic acid, sulfur preparations, and azelaic acid. To reduce the follicular bacterial population, topical antibiotics such as erythromycin and clindamycin may be tried. Benzoyl peroxide also has bacteriostatic properties, which makes it effective for mild acne. The use of isoretinoin (Accutane) is reserved for severe acne and should not be used as the first line of treatment for this patient. It is teratogenic and should be used only in female patients with a secure means of birth control; its use should be restricted to dermatologists or those who are experienced with it.

63. Correct Answer: A (Chapter 23).
Nail pitting is commonly seen in psoriatic arthritis. Other skin lesions and associated diseases include tophi and gout, malar rash and mouth ulcers with lupus erythematosus, and erythema migrans with Lyme disease. Fingertip atrophy or ulcers along with calcinosis and telangiectasias are signs of scleroderma. Keratoderma blennorrhagicum, a hyperkerotic lesion on the palms and soles, and balanitis circinate, a shallow painless ulcer on the penis, are signs of Reiter syndrome.

64. Correct Answer: C (Chapter 36).
The patient has macrocytic anemia, as indicated by the high MCV. Thalassemia, iron deficiency, and anemia of chronic disease typically cause microcytic anemia. Both vitamin B_{12} and folate deficiencies may cause megaloblastic anemia; however, only B_{12} deficiency causes neurologic symptoms. The most common cause of B_{12} deficiency is pernicious anemia.

65. Correct Answer: C (Chapter 63).
Although this patient is sure of her last menstrual period (LMP), the physical findings do not correlate with the gestational age by LMP. At 10 weeks, the uterus is not palpable above the pubis, and it is unlikely that fetal heart tones would be detected by Doppler. Therefore an ultrasound is needed to confirm the gestational age as well as to document a single fetus and normal uterus. The incidence of chromosomal abnormalities does not exceed the risk of amniocentesis until after a maternal age of 35 years. Preeclampsia does not occur before 20 weeks of gestation. Abdominal x-rays should be avoided in pregnancy, as the radiation may affect the fetus.

66. Correct Answer: A (Chapter 47).
Graves disease is a common cause of hyperthyroidism and is the result of serum thyroid-stimulating antibodies. These antibodies act on the TSH receptors of the thyroid, which causes excessive release of thyroid hormone. As a result, TSH is low and free T4 levels are high. Thyroid scan shows diffuse uptake and thus helps differentiate between Graves disease and a nodular disorder. Fine-needle aspiration is performed to assess for cancer in patients with nodular lesions, but it would not be helpful in those with Graves disease.

67. Correct Answer: B (Chapter 8).
This patient has the typical symptoms and signs of allergic rhinitis. The nasal crease is a sign of chronic nasal itching, a common symptom associated with allergic rhinitis. Vasomotor rhinitis is characterized by chronic nasal congestion with pink nasal mucosa that is brought on by sudden changes in temperature, humidity, or odor. Although rhinitis occurs with sinusitis, it is unlikely that the patient has sinusitis. The nasal discharge in sinusitis is purulent rather than watery. Rhinitis medicamentosa is a condition caused by chronic use of cocaine or nasal decongestants. There is nothing in the history to suggest that the rhinorrhea may be secondary to rhinitis medicamentosa. Foreign body is associated with purulent, malodorous discharge and is unlikely in a patient this age.

68. Correct Answer: C (Chapter 10).
This patient has the classic signs and symptoms of costochondritis. The history and the fact that his pain is reproducible indicate that it is not cardiac but rather musculoskeletal. In pneumonia, patients can have chest pain worsened with inspiration, but they also have other symptoms, such as cough and fever, along with physical examination findings, such as inspiratory rales. Esophageal spasm is often associated with eating or drinking but is not affected by breathing.

69. Correct Answer: B (Chapter 44).
Patients with diverticular disease, colon cancer, or colon polyps can present with painless gastrointestinal bleeding, as in this patient. Diverticular bleeding is generally an acute episode; although the hemoglobin may decrease significantly, RBC indices are generally normal with acute blood loss. Colitis associated with rectal bleeding is generally not painless but associated with cramps and diarrhea. Although hemorrhoids can cause bleeding from the rectum, the bleeding is generally not enough to cause a significant anemia or the symptoms mentioned above. Before assuming that the bleeding is due to hemorrhoids, the patient should undergo diagnostic testing to eliminate other causes for his anemia. Colon cancer commonly presents with hypochromic microcytic anemia, and an acute bleeding episode may lead to laboratory testing that detects the chronic blood loss. Irritable bowel syndrome is a benign condition—where people feel cramping abdominal pain, relieved with a bowel movement—and is not associated with gastrointestinal bleeding.

70. Correct Answer: D (Chapter 63).
Triple marker screen should be offered to the patient in the second trimester. It includes the maternal serum AFP, estriol, and hCG. This is a screening test for neural tube defects and Down syndrome. High levels of MSAFP are associated with neural tube defects. Low levels of MSAFP are associated with trisomy 21. However, dating errors and multiple fetuses should be ruled out before ordering further testing for neural tube defects or trisomy 21. Not all women choose to have the triple screen performed. Counseling about the tests, possible test results, additional testing for abnormal results, and options available to the woman faced with an abnormal fetus should be provided to assist in her making the decision to be tested. All other listed tests are done in the first trimester except glucose screening, which is generally performed around 28 weeks' gestation.

71. Correct Answer: D (Chapter 50).
The first line of prevention for osteoporosis is lifestyle changes, although pharmaceutical agents are important for treatment. Smoking cessation, modest alcohol consumption, weight-bearing exercises, and the improvement of dietary habits should be stressed. Calcium intake should be 1000 mg/day for premenopausal women and 1200 mg/day for postmenopausal women. As patient's age, the risk for falls increases and measures to decrease falls—such as correcting visual problems, decreasing sedative medications, and initiating balance exercises—are beneficial. Medical management is indicated for women with a T score below −2.0 without risk factors and for those with a T score below −1.5 and risk factors, such as women above age 70 or those on long-term corticosteroids. The bisphosphonates must be taken on an empty stomach with at least an 8-oz glass of water while the patient remains upright, without eating, for at least 30 minutes. Though useful in treating menopausal symptoms, estrogen replacement therapy is no longer considered first line therapy for osteoporosis.

72. Correct Answer: B (Chapter 44).
This patient has diverticulitis. Although a barium enema or colonoscopy can help diagnose diverticular disease, these tests should not be done in acute diverticulitis because of the risk of perforation. In the acute setting, the test of choice is the CT scan. Ultrasound is useful in diagnosing appendicitis and other abdominal disorders but has not been shown to be a useful test for diagnosing diverticulitis.

73. Correct Answer: B (Chapter 12).
This patient had a viral illness prior to the onset of the cough. Postviral syndrome can cause cough for up to 8 weeks. It is unlikely that the patient has sinusitis without nasal congestion, headaches, or any other symptoms of sinusitis. Pneumonia is unlikely in the absence of fever, dyspnea, or sputum production. Psychogenic cough is a possibility, but the viral prodrome and the short duration of symptoms make it unlikely. Asthma is a chronic condition characterized by repetitive episodes of cough associated with wheezing on physical examination.

74. Correct Answer: C (Chapter 72).
This child has recurrent otitis media. Acute otitis media is often associated with a URI. Treatment should be initiated with antibiotics that cover *Streptococcus pneumoniae, Haemophilus influenzae,* and *Moraxella catarrhalis.* Children with recurrent otitis media should be started on prophylactic antibiotics for 6 months to suppress recurrent infections and allow fluid resolution. Otitis media tends to occur less frequently as children advance in age, and the prophylactic antibiotics may allow the child to grow and develop further while also suppressing recurrent infections. Myringotomy and tympanostomy tube placement is an option for those who fail suppressive therapy and for children with persistent otitis media with effusion, particularly when associated with hearing loss. Decongestant therapy has not been shown to be effective prophylactic treatment for otitis media.

75. Correct Answer: E (Chapter 29).
In patients with pneumonia, it is important to determine the best locus of care. Indications for hospitalization are (a) systolic BP less than 90; (b) pulse rate greater than 140; (c) O_2 sat less than 90% or PO_2 less than 60 mm Hg; (d) presence of abscess or pleural effusion; (e) marked metabolic abnormality; (f) age greater than 65; and (g) unreliable social situation. Underlying disease states such as CHF, renal failure, malignancy, diabetes, or severe COPD are also important factors in considering whether to hospitalize an individual with pneumonia.

76. Correct Answer: C (Chapter 40).
Patients with COPD are commonly treated with bronchodilators, anticholinergics, and inhaled steroids. During acute exacerbations, antibiotics, and oral steroids are commonly used for therapy. Nonmedication recommendations include smoking cessation and pulmonary rehabilitation, which includes exercise. Spiral CT scanning and bronchoscopy are not recommended routinely in patients with COPD except to assist in the diagnosis of suspected pulmonary embolus, lung cancer, or other structural lung lesions that may complicate or contribute to a patient's symptoms. Routine vaccinations recommended for patients with COPD include pneumococcal vaccine and an annual influenza vaccine. Hib vaccine is not recommended for patients with COPD.

77. Correct Answer: D (Chapter 24).
All of these conditions are diagnoses with palpitations as significant symptoms. Diagnostic testing is often warranted to evaluate patients presenting with a complaint of palpitations. Cardiac evaluation may include an

echocardiogram, 24-hour Holter monitor, or event monitor. The echocardiogram evaluates cardiac structure. A 24-hour Holter monitor may detect arrhythmias occurring on a daily basis, whereas an event monitor may detect those that occur more sporadically. A CBC, TSH, and FSH may help in diagnosing the other listed causes of palpitations. Panic disorder is diagnosed clinically; thus diagnostic testing, though useful in excluding other potential causes, does not diagnose panic disorder.

78. Correct Answer: C (Chapter 17).
Following therapy for gastric ulcers, ulcer healing must be documented to help ensure that the ulcer did not represent a gastric carcinoma. Once ulcer healing has been documented, observation for recurrence of symptoms is appropriate. Repeated therapy with antibiotics or extended use of proton pump inhibitors is not necessary in an asymptomatic patient provided that the EGD results are normal. If the ulcer persists and remains *Helicobacter pylori*–positive, a repeat course of antibiotics and proton pump inhibitors may be warranted. *H. pylori* antibody testing is not useful as a test of cure, since antibody levels remain abnormal for an indefinite time.

79. Correct Answer: A (Chapter 14).
A central cause is likely in this patient with vertigo in light of the physical finding of vertical nystagmus. Vertical nystagmus does not occur with peripheral etiologies. The lack of association of the patient's symptoms with positional changes and the normal findings on hearing evaluation also help to localize the process to a central etiology. Evaluation for possible multiple sclerosis should be performed with MRI scanning of the brain and possibly the use of brainstem auditory evoked responses. A psychiatric cause is unlikely and would not cause the finding of vertical nystagmus.

80. Correct Answer: B (Chapter 6).
The patient presented is undergoing vascular surgery, which is a high-risk surgery for concomitant coronary artery disease. Thus, a cardiac stress test should be ordered. A prothrombin time has been shown in several studies not to be warranted as a routine test, but it is indicated for those requiring warfarin therapy and for those with suspected liver disease. Pulmonary function testing may help to define the severity of lung disease but is not recommended as a screening test and does not define a prohibitive level of lung function for surgeries other than lung resection. An echocardiogram may help in assessing patients with known or suspected congestive heart failure or valvular heart disease. Venous duplex imaging is helpful in those suspected of having DVT but is not recommended as a screening test.

81. Correct Answer: A (Chapter 4).
Hepatitis A is generally a mild, self-limited infection in children. Vaccination for hepatitis A is currently recommended for all children. Hepatitis B is associated with chronic infection and can cause lifelong liver disease. Whereas most teens and adults develop immunity after infection with Hepatitis B, up to 90% of infants who are infected will develop chronic Hepatitis B infection. Oral poliovirus has been associated with vaccine-related infection and has led to recommendations for universal use of IPV, which has not had this association. Pneumococcal vaccine is recommended for all children as well as high-risk adults, although the vaccine for children is different than the one for adults. Individuals who require chronic aspirin therapy should receive influenza and varicella vaccines to limit the risk for developing Reye syndrome.

82. Correct Answer: C (Chapter 3).
Some controversy surrounds the issue of cholesterol screening in children, because childhood values are not predictive of future adult values. Cholesterol values tend to be variable and are affected by diet and level of physical activity; if they are elevated, therefore, they must be confirmed on one or more occasions. Elevated levels are those greater than 200 mg/dL, with values of 170 to 199 mg/dL considered borderline and those below 170 mg/dL normal. Screening is currently recommended for children above 2 years of age with a family history of premature cardiovascular disease (before age 55) in the parents or grandparents or with a parental history of hypercholesterolemia.

83. Correct Answer: C (Chapter 5).
Routine health care of a healthy 35 year old with no medical disease, no significant family or social history, and a normal physical examination including BP will involve minimal laboratory work. The primary focus of the examination is a review of risk factors, including those for accidents, injury, and exposures to sexually transmitted diseases, cigarettes, and drugs. Routine ECG, chest x-ray, and stress testing is not supported by the literature in any age group. Occult blood testing of the stool generally commences at age 50 but at age 40 in those with a family history of colon cancer. Lipid profile evaluation is recommended beginning at age 35 in men and at age 45 in women.

84. Correct Answer: B (Chapter 39).
Atopic dermatitis is a common disease affecting infants, with over 60% of cases diagnosed by 1 year of age and an additional 30% diagnosed by age 5. The lifetime incidence for atopic dermatitis is over 20%; however, many of these cases will spontaneously resolve by age 2, with most of the remaining cases resolving during the teen years. In infancy, the face and cheeks are commonly affected, along with other aspects of the trunk and extremities. In children and teens, atopic dermatitis spares the face and most commonly localizes to the flexural creases of the extremities. Atopic dermatitis is associated with other allergic

diseases, and children who develop atopic dermatitis may go on to develop allergic rhinitis or asthma.

85. Correct Answer: B (Chapter 38).
The patient described has mild intermittent asthma, for which short-acting beta agonists are recommended as needed for the acute exacerbations. Oral steroids may be used for acute exacerbations but are generally reserved for those with severe symptoms. Daily medication use is reserved for those with mild, moderate, or severe persistent asthma. Patients with persistent asthma have symptoms more than twice per week and/or nocturnal symptoms more than twice per month. Chronic oral steroids are reserved for those with chronic persistent asthma that is refractory to other therapies. Antibiotic therapy is not recommended for the treatment of uncomplicated asthma.

86. Correct Answer: B (Chapter 42).
Different classes of antidepressants are equally effective. The choice of medication depends on the patient's symptoms, current medications, and side effect profile. In a patient with insomnia, a tricyclic antidepressant, trazodone, or mirtazapine is a good choice. Buproprion is a good choice in patients with somnolence. If anxiety or agitation is a complaint, SSRIs should be avoided, since they can be energizing. The key to successful treatment is duration. For the first episode, depression should be treated for 6 to 12 months.

87. Correct Answer: A (Chapter 25).
The classic symptoms of infectious mononucleosis caused by heterophile-positive Epstein–Barr virus are fever, sore throat, malaise, lymphadenopathy, and splenomegaly. In adolescence, these symptoms are seen in 75% of the patients, whereas EBV infections in infants and young children maybe asymptomatic or present as a mild pharyngitis. The heterophile test is used for diagnosis in children and adults; however the mononucleosis spot test (Monospot) is more sensitive and more commonly used than the heterophile. All the above infections can produce a mononucleosis-like syndrome, but CMV is the most common. Patients with CMV mononucleosis are usually older and have fever and malaise as the major manifestations. Pharyngitis and lymphadenopathy are less common than with EBV mononucleosis.

88. Correct Answer: D (Chapter 38).
The patient described has moderate persistent asthma, for which daily therapy with inhaled steroids and long-acting beta agonists are recommended. The presence of daily symptoms requires daily medications to suppress the inflammation and reactivity of the airways of asthmatic patients. Oral steroids are reserved for severe persistent asthma and those with severe acute exacerbations. Nedocromil is useful for mild persistent asthma and may be used in combination with other therapies for more severe disease.

89. Correct Answer: C (Chapter 46).
Ninety-five percent of patients with a diagnosis of hypertension have primary or essential hypertension. Evaluation for secondary causes is generally reserved for those refractory to medical therapy or those presenting with hypertensive crisis. Although this patient may be at increased risk for cardiac disease in the future, screening cardiac stress testing is not routinely recommended for any patient. Testing is recommended to detect the secondary effects of hypertension, evaluate other cardiovascular risk factors, and help in choosing medical therapy. Recommended testing includes an ECG, chest x-ray, CBC, glucose, cholesterol, electrolytes, creatinine, calcium, uric acid, and urinalysis.

90. Correct Answer: B (Chapter 73).
An important part of the preparticipation evaluation (PPE) is to identify those at risk for sudden cardiac death. Although EKG, echocardiogram, or stress testing may be appropriate in those at risk for sudden cardiac death, these tests have not been shown to be effective in mass screening of those with a normal history and physical. Because the incidence of coronary artery disease increases with age, it is the most common cause of sudden cardiac death in athletes over the age of 40. Hypertrophic cardiomyopathy is the most common cause for death in athletes under age 40.

91. Correct Answer: A (Chapter 47).
Constipation, weight gain, depression, and fatigue are common in those with hypothyroidism and uncommon in those with hyperthyroidism. Geriatric patients may present with "apathetic hyperthyroidism" and appear clinically depressed due to the underlying hyperthyroidism, but younger patients do not generally present in this manner. Patients who complain of palpitations, unintended weight loss, loose stools, heat intolerance, nervousness, or have goiter, exophthalmos, or atrial fibrillation on physical examination should be evaluated for hyperthyroidism.

92. Correct Answer: E (Chapter 48).
The most appropriate next step is to determine the levels of free T4. TSH levels are useful to screen for thyroid dysfunction, whereas free T4 levels provide information about the amount of thyroid hormone being produced by the thyroid gland. If the free T4 levels are normal, this patient most likely has subclinical hypothyroidism, although if the levels of free T4 are low, she has overt hypothyroidism and requires medication.

93. Correct Answer: B (Chapter 16).
Sudden onset of a severe headache, especially the "worst headache of my life," should elicit concern about subarachnoid hemorrhage (SAH). Diagnostic steps include an emergent CT scan of the head. Because the CT scan will identify only 90% of all SAH, a negative scan should be followed up by a lumbar puncture to avoid

missing 1 out of every 10 subarachnoid hemorrhages. Empiric therapy without these tests would be inappropriate. Temporal arteritis is a consideration in evaluation of headaches, particularly in patients over age 50. ESRs are significantly elevated. If temporal arteritis is seriously suspected, steroid therapy should be started prior to results and arrangements made for temporal artery biopsy.

94. Correct Answer: C (Chapter 43).
The American Diabetes Association recommends screening high-risk individuals for diabetes with a fasting blood sugar and all patients over age 45 should be screened with a fasting blood sugar every 3 years. Hemoglobin A_{1C} is not one of the diagnostic criteria; it is rather a measure of blood sugar control. Fasting blood sugars greater than 126 on two or more separate occasions signify diabetes. Diabetic patients over age 30 need to be checked yearly for microalbuminemia.

95. Correct Answer: E (Chapter 27).
Inclusion conjunctivitis is seen in neonates and young adults with STDs. It is associated with a persistent watery discharge of the eye. With blepharitis, one sees chronic lid margin erythema, scaling, and loss of eyelashes. Bacterial conjunctivitis presents with a purulent discharge, whereas iritis is associated with pain, photophobia, pupillary constriction, and a cloudy cornea.

96. Correct Answer: D (Chapter 63).
In the second trimester, between 15 and 20 weeks, a MSAFP level should be offered as a screening test. Causes of an elevated MSAFP include an incorrect pregnancy date, twin pregnancy, and neural tube defects. Decreased levels are associated with pregnancy date errors or trisomy 21. Many physicians order an ultrasound to confirm the EDD established by the LMP in order to help in interpreting the MSAFP results.

97. Correct Answer: C (Chapter 72).
Middle ear effusions may persist for several weeks following an episode of acute otitis media. At 2 weeks, 60% of children will still have effusions. Further therapy may be indicated if the effusions persist and are associated with hearing loss. Although antibiotics and systemic corticosteroids have been studied and may be helpful as medical therapy, most effusions resolve spontaneously within 2 to 3 months. Thus, follow-up examination should be performed in 2 months to reassess for persistence of effusion. If the effusion is persistent, hearing evaluation should be considered. Bilateral effusions that persist for more than 4 to 6 months and are associated with bilateral hearing deficits of 20 decibels or more are indications for tympanostomy tube placement.

98. Correct Answer: D (Chapter 74).
Of those tests and vaccines listed, only pneumococcal vaccine is a part of the routine recommendations for health care in a 68-year-old man. The heptavalent pneumococcal vaccine is currently recommended for children. The 23-valent pneumococcal vaccine is recommended for all patients over age 65 and for high-risk individuals of other ages (e.g., those with asplenia, diabetes, asthma, or COPD). Chest x-rays are not routinely recommended in any age group. Hepatitis vaccine is recommended for children and for adults who are at risk. DEXA scanning is not routinely suggested for men. ECGs, although often routinely performed during physical examinations, are not recommended for routine screening.

99. Correct Answer: C (Chapter 29).
PE is high on the list of possible diagnoses in the patient presented. She has two significant risk factors for developing PE: history of recent travel and use of oral contraceptives. Fibromyalgia is a chronic non–life-threatening disease that may present with chest pains but will be associated with pain elsewhere as well as trigger points on physical examination. In addition, peripheral edema is not a characteristic of fibromyalgia. Costochondritis may cause chest pain and on occasion may be associated with dyspnea. The chest pain is typically reproduced by palpation of the costochondral margin. Both costochondritis and fibromyalgia are clinical diagnoses and there are no diagnostic tests for either. Varicose veins may be associated with the development of edema and are a risk factor for developing deep venous thrombosis and PE; however, varicose veins themselves are not life-threatening and do not cause dyspnea or chest pain. Lymphedema can cause swelling in the lower extremity but would not typically cause dyspnea.

100. Correct Answer: B (Chapter 10).
This patient has the classic presentation of stable angina. Typical cardiac pain is a substernal pressure with radiation to left arm, shoulder, or jaw. A distinguishing feature in this case is the duration of the pain. In MI, the pain usually lasts longer than 20 minutes. The pain in stable angina lasts less than 10 minutes. Unstable angina by definition occurs at rest or with increasing frequency or less strenuous activity. The pain of pericarditis and pleurisy is sharp and worsened with breathing. Both of these conditions are acute in nature and generally do not present with chronic symptoms, as described in this patient.

Appendix: Evidence-Based Resources

Chapter 1

Haggerty JL, Reid RJ, Freeman GK, et al. Continuity of care: a multidisciplinary review. *BMJ*. 2003;327(7425): 1219–1221.

Chapter 2

Bourgeut C, Gilchrist V, McCord G. The consultation and referral process: a report from NEON. Northeastern Ohio Network Research Group. *J Fam Pract*. 1998;46:47–53.

Bull SA, Hu XH, Hunkeler EM, et al. Discontinuation of use and switching of antidepressants: influence of patient-physician communication. *JAMA*. 2002;288: 1403–1409.

Emanuel EJ, Emanuel LL. Four models of the physician-patient relationship. *JAMA*. 1992;267(16):2221–2226.

Chapter 3

Agency for Healthcare Research and Quality. Put prevention into practice. A step-by-step guide to delivering clinical preventive services: a systems approach. Available at: http://www.ahrq.gov/ppip/manual/. Accessed September 8, 2004.

Canto JG, Iskandrian AE. Major risk factors for cardiovascular disease—debunking the "only 50%" myth. *JAMA*. 2003;290:947–994.

Clinician's Handbook of Preventive Services. Available at: http://www.ahrq.gov/clinic/ppiphand.htm#Adults. Accessed December 28, 2004.

Expert Panel on Detection, Evaluation, and Treatment of High Blood Cholesterol in Adults. Summary of the Third Report of the National Cholesterol Education Program (NCEP) Expert Panel on Detection, Evaluation, and Treatment of High Blood Cholesterol in Adults (Adult Treatment Panel III). NIH publication 01-3670. Bethesda, MD: National Institutes of Health; 2001.

Mosca L, Appel LJ, Benjamin EJ, et al. Evidence-based guidelines for cardiovascular disease prevention in women. *Circulation*. 2004;109:672–693.

Chapter 4

Campos-Outcalt D. Vaccine update: new CDC recommendations for 2007. *J Fam Pract*. 2008;57:181–184.

Centers for disease control and prevention: recommendations for childhood and adolescent vaccination schedule—United States; 2009. Available at: http://www.cdc.gov/mmwr//preview/mmwrhtml/mm5351-Immunizationa1.htm. Accessed September 16, 2009.

Hamlin J, Senthilnanthan S, Bernstein HH. Update on universal childhood immunizations. *Curr Opin Pediatr*. 2008;20:483–489.

Chapter 5

Iglar K, Katyai S, Matthew R, et al. Complete health checkup for adults. *Can Fam Physician*. 2008;54:84–88.

Chapter 6

ACC/AHA 2007 guidelines on perioperative cardiovascular evaluation and care for noncardiac surgery. Available at: www.guideline.gov. Accessed September 18, 2009.

Chapter 7

Nelson HD, Nygren P, McInerney Y, et al. U.S. Preventive Services Task Force. Screening women and elderly adults for family and intimate partner violence: a review of the evidence for the U.S. Preventive Services Task Force. *Ann Intern Med*. 2004;140(5):387–396.

Chapter 8

Bousquet et al. Algorithm for allergic rhinitis diagnosis and management. *Allergy*. 2008;63(suppl 86):8–160.

Rosenthal M. How a non-allergist survives an allergy clinic. *Arch Dis Child*. 2004;89(3):238–243.

Chapter 9

Chou R, Qaseem A, Snow V, et al. Diagnosis and treatment of low back pain: a joint clinical practice guideline from the American College of Physicians and the American Pain Society. *Ann Int Med*. 2007;147:478–491.

Speed C. Low back pain. *BMJ*. 2004;328(7448):1119–1121.

van Tulder MW, Touray T, Furlan AD, et al. Cochrane Back Review Group. Muscle relaxants for nonspecific low back pain: a systematic review within the framework of the Cochrane collaboration. *Spine*. 2003;28(17): 1978–1992.

Chapter 10

Jain A, Wadehra V, Timmis AD. Management of stable angina. *Postgrad Med J*. 2003;79(932):332–336.

Lauer MS. What is the best test for a patient with classic angina? *Cleve Clin J Med*. 2007;74(2):123–126.

Pollack CV Jr, Roe MT, Peterson ED. 2002 update to the ACC/AHA guidelines for the management of patients with unstable angina and non-ST-segment elevation myocardial infarction: implications for emergency department practice. *Ann Emerg Med.* 2003;41(3):355–369.

Wells PS, Anderson DR, Rodger M, et al. Evaluation of D-dimer in the diagnosis of suspected deep-vein thrombosis. *N Engl J Med.* 2003;349:1227–1235.

Chapter 11
Foxx-Orenstein AE, McNally MA, Odunsi ST. Update on constipation: one treatment does not fit all. *Cleve Clin J Med.* 2008;75(11):813–824.

Horwitz BJ, Fisher RS. The irritable bowel syndrome. *N Engl J Med.* 2001;344:1846–1850.

Locke GR III, Pemberton JH, Phillips SF. AGA technical review on constipation. *Gastroenterology.* 2000;119:1766–1778.

Chapter 12
Currie GP, Gray RD, McKay J. Chronic cough. *BMJ.* 2003;326(7383):261.

Morice AH, Kastelik JA. Chronic cough in adults. *Thorax.* 2003;58(10):901–907.

Pratter MR, Brightling CE, Boulet LP, et al. An empiric integrative approach to the management of cough: ACCP evidence-based clinical practice guidelines. *Chest.* 2006;129(1 suppl):222S–231S.

Chapter 13
Bartlett JG. Clinical practice. Antibiotic-associated diarrhea. *N Engl J Med.* 2002;346(5):334–339.

Gunn MC, Cavin AA, Mansfield JC. Management of irritable bowel syndrome. *Postgrad Med J.* 2003;79(929):154–158.

Otegbayo JA, Otegbeye FM, Rotimi O. Microscopic colitis syndrome—a review article. *J Natl Med Assoc.* 2005;97(5):678–682.

Poutanen SM, Simor AE. *Clostridium difficile*–associated diarrhea in adults. *CMAJ.* 2004;171(1):51–58.

Chapter 14
Baloh RW. Vestibular neuritis. *N Engl J Med.* 2003;348:1027–1032.

Chawla N, Olshaker JS. Diagnosis and management of dizziness/vertigo. *Med Clin North Am.* 2006;90(2):291–304.

Labuguen RH. Initial evaluation of vertigo. *Am Fam Physician.* 2006;73(2):244–251.

Chapter 15
Rosenthal TC, Majeroni BA, Pretorius R, et al. Fatigue: an overview. *Am Fam Physician.* 2008;78(10):1173–1179.

Whiting P, Bagnall AM, Sowden AJ, et al. Interventions for the treatment and management of chronic fatigue syndrome: a systematic review. *JAMA.* 2001;286(11):1360–1368.

Chapter 16
Cady R, Dodick DW. Diagnosis and treatment of migraine. *Mayo Clin Proc.* 2002;77:255–256.

Evans RW. Diagnostic testing for migraine and other primary headaches. *Neur Clin.* 2009;27(2):393–415.

Lake AE III, Saper JR. Chronic headache: new advances in treatment strategies. *Neurology.* 2002;59(5 suppl 2):S8–S13.

Trainor A, Miner J. Pain treatment and relief with primary headaches. *Am J Emerg Med.* 2008;26(9):1029–1034.

Chapter 17
Conroy RT, Siddiqi B. Dyspepsia. *Prim Care.* 2007;34(1):99–108.

Richter JE. The many manifestations of GERD: presentation, evaluation and treatment. *Gastroenterol Clin of North Am.* 2007;36(3):577–599.

Chapter 18
Choyke PL. Radiologic evaluation of hematuria: guidelines from the American College of Radiology appropriateness criteria. *Am Fam Physician.* 2008;78(3):347–352.

McDonald MM, Swaggerty D, Wetzel L. Assessment of microscopic hematuria in adults. *Am Fam Physician.* 2006;73(10):1748–1754.

Chapter 19
Beckingham IJ, Ryder SD. ABC of diseases of liver, pancreas, and biliary system. Investigation of liver and biliary disease. *BMJ.* 2001;322(7277):33–36.

Bansal V, Schuchert VD. Jaundice in the intensive care unit. *Surg Clin of North Am.* 2006;86(6):1495–1502.

Chapter 20
Earl JE, Vetter CS. Patellofemoral pain. *Phys Med Rehabil Clin N Am.* 2007;18(3):439–458.

Hunter DJ, McDougall JJ, Koefer FJ. The symptoms of osteoarthritis and the genesis of pain. *Rheum Clin North Am.* 2008;34(3):623–643.

Solomon DH, Simel DL, Bates DW, et al. Does this patient have a torn meniscus or ligament of the knee? Value of the physical examination. *JAMA.* 2001;286:1610–1620.

Chapter 21
Bozemore AW, Smucker DR. Lymphadenopathy and malignancy. *Am Fam Physician.* 2002;66:2103–2110.

Nield LS, Kamat D. Lymphadenopathy in children: when and how to evaluate. *Clin Pediatr.* 2004;43(1):25–33.

Twist CJ, Link MP. Assessment of lymphadenopathy in children. *Pediatr Clin North Am.* 2002;49(5):1009–1025.

Chapter 22
Magee LA, Mazzotta P, Koren G. Evidence-based view of safety and effectiveness of pharmacologic therapy for nausea and vomiting of pregnancy. *Am J Obstet Gynecol.* 2002;186(5 suppl):S256–S261.

Scarza K, Williams A, Phillips JD, et al. Evaluation of nausea and vomiting. *Am Fam Physician.* 2007;76(1):76–84.

Spiller RC. ABC of the upper gastrointestinal tract: anorexia, nausea, vomiting, and pain. *BMJ.* 2001; 323(7325):1354–1357.

Chapter 23
Kim PS. Role of injection therapy: review of indications for trigger point injections, regional blocks, facet joint injections, and intra-articular injections. *Curr Opin Rheumatol.* 2002;14:52–57.

Manek NJ. Medical management of osteoarthritis. *Mayo Clin Proc.* 2001;76:533–539.

Chapter 24
Hood RE, Shorofsky JR. Management of arrhythmias in the emergency department. *Cardiol Clin.* 2006;24(1): 125–133.

Snow V, Weiss KB, LeFevre M, et al. Management of newly detected atrial fibrillation: a clinical practice guideline from the American Academy of Family Physicians and the American College of Physicians. *Ann Intern Med.* 2003;139:1009–1017.

Chapter 25
Alcaide ML, Bisno AL. Pharyngitis and epiglottis. *Infect Dis Clin North Am.* 2007;21(2):449–469.

Choby BA. Diagnosis and treatment of streptococcal pharyngitis. *Am Fam Physician.* 2009;79(5):383–390.

Chapter 26
K/DOQI clinical practice guidelines for chronic kidney disease: evaluation, classification, and stratification. Kidney disease outcome quality initiative. *Am J Kidney Dis.* 2002;39(2 suppl 1):S1–S246.

Levey AS, Coresh J, Balk E, et al. National Kidney Foundation. National Kidney Foundation practice guidelines for chronic kidney disease: evaluation, classification, and stratification. *Ann Intern Med.* 2003;139(2): 137–147.

Stevens LA, Levey AS. Current status and future perspectives for CKD. *Am J Kidney Dis.* 2009;53(3 suppl 3): 517–526.

Chapter 27
Teoh DL, Reynolds S. Diagnosis and management of pediatric conjunctivitis. *Pediatr Emerg Care.* 2003;19(1):48–55.

Wirbelauer C. Management of the red eye for the primary care physician. *Am J Med.* 2006;119(4):302–306.

Chapter 28
File TM Jr, Garau J, Blasi F, et al. Guidelines for empiric antimicrobial prescribing in community-acquired pneumonia. *Chest.* 2004;125(5):1888–1901.

Moran GJ, Talan DA, Abrahamian FM. Diagnosis and management of pneumonia in the emergency department. *Infect Dis Clin North Am.* 2008;22(1):53–72.

Mucha SM, Baroody FM. Sinusitis update. *Curr Opin Allergy Clin Immunol.* 2003;3(1):33–38.

Chapter 29
Chunilal SD, Eikelboom JW, Attia J, et al. Does this patient have pulmonary embolism? *JAMA.* 2003;290(21): 2849–2858.

Gehlbach BK, Geppert E. The pulmonary manifestations of left heart failure. *Chest.* 2004;125(2):669–682.

Shiber JR, Santana J. Dyspnea. *Med Clin North Am.* 2006;90(3):453–479.

Torres M, Maayedi S. Evaluation of acutely dyspneic elderly patients. *Clin Geriatr Med.* 2007;23(2):307–325.

Chapter 30
Burbank KM, Stevenson JH, Czarnecki GR, et al. Chronic shoulder pain: part 1 evaluation and diagnosis. *Am Fam Physician.* 2008;77(4):453–460.

Burbank KM, Stevenson JH, Czarnecki GR, et al. Chronic shoulder pain: part 2 treatment. *Am Fam Physician.* 2008;77(4):493–497.

Stevenson JH, Trojian T. Evaluation of shoulder pain. *J Fam Pract.* 2002;51(7):605–611.

Chapter 31
Ballas CA, Staab JP. Medically unexplained physical symptoms: toward an alternative paradigm for diagnosis and treatment. *CNS Spectr.* 2003;8(12 suppl 3):20–26.

Kroenke K, Rosmalen JG. Symptoms, syndromes, and the value of psychiatric diagnostics in patients who have functional somatic disorders. *Med Clin North Am.* 2006;90(4):603–626.

Oyama O, Paltoo C, Greengold J. Somatoform disorders. *Am Fam Physician.* 2007;76(9):1333–1338.

Chapter 32
Cho S, Atwood JE. Peripheral edema. *Am J Med.* 2002; 113(7):580–586.

O'Brien JG, Chennubhotla SA, Chennubhotla RV. Treatment of edema. *Am Fam Physician.* 2005;71(11): 2111–2117.

Chapter 33
DeLegge MH, Drake LM. Nutritional assessment. *Gastroenterol Clin North Am.* 2007;36(1):1–22.

Robertson RG, Montagnini M. Geriatric failure to thrive. *Am Fam Physician.* 2004;70(2):343–350.

Rolland Y, Kim MJ, Gammack JK, et al. Office management of weight loss in older persons. *Am J Med*. 2006;119(12):1019–1026.

Chapter 34
Haider A, Shaw JC. Treatment of acne vulgaris. *JAMA*. 2004;292(6):726–735.

Rosen MP, Breitkopf DM, Nagamani M. A randomized controlled trial of second- versus third-generation oral contraceptives in the treatment of acne vulgaris. *Am J Obstet Gynecol*. 2003;188:1158–1160.

Tan HH. Topical antibacterial treatments for acne vulgaris comparative review and guide to selection. *Am J Clin Dermatol*. 2004;5(2):79–84.

Chapter 35
Asplund CA, Aronson JA, Hadassah EA. Three regimens for alcohol withdrawal and detoxification. *J Fam Pract*. 2004;53 (7):545–554.

Chapter 36
DeRossi SS, Raghavendra S. Anemia. *Oral Surg Oral Med Oral Pathol Oral Radiol Endod*. 2003;95(2):131–141.

Killip S, Bennett JM, Chambers MD. Iron deficiency anemia. *Am Fam Physician*. 2007;75(5):671–678.

Tefferi A. Anemia in adults: a contemporary approach to diagnosis. *Mayo Clin Proc*. 2003;78(10):1274–1280.

Chapter 37
Kroenke K, Spitzer RL, Williams JB, et al. Anxiety disorders in primary care: prevalence, impairment, comorbidity, and detection. *Ann Intern Med*. 2007;146(5):317–325.

Pigott TA. Anxiety disorders in women. *Psychiatr Clin North Am*. 2003;26(3):621–672.

Solvason HB, Ernst H, Roth W. Predictors of response in anxiety disorders. *Psychiatr Clin North Am*. 2003;26(2):411–433.

Chapter 38
National Heart, Lung, and Blood Institute, National Asthma Education and Prevention Program. Expert Panel Report 3: guidelines for the diagnosis and management of asthma. Summary report 2007:343. Available at: http://www.nhlbi.nih.gov/guidelines/asthma/asthgdln.htm.

Pollart SM, Elward KS. Overview of changes to Asthma guidelines: diagnosis and screening. *Am Fam Physician*. 2009;79(9):761–767

Chapter 39
http://www.fda.gov/bbs/topics/news/2006/NEW01299.html. Accessed December 14, 2009.

Boguniewicz M, Eichenfield LF, Hultsch T. Current management of atopic dermatitis and interruption of the atopic march. *J Allergy Clin Immunol*. 2003;112:S140–S150.

Chapter 40
Celli BR. Update on the management of COPD. *Chest*. 2008;133(6):1451–1462.

Highland KB, Strange C, Heffner JE. Long-term effects of inhaled corticosteroids on FEV_1 in patients with chronic obstructive pulmonary disease: a meta-analysis. *Ann Intern Med*. 2003;138:969.

Chapter 41
ACC/AHA 2005 Guidelines for the Diagnosis and Management of Heart Failure in Adults. Available at: www.guideline.gov. Accessed December 14, 2009.

Dosh SA. Diagnosis of heart failure in adults. *Am Fam Physician*. 2004;70:2145–2152.

Jessup M, Brozena S. Heart failure. *N Engl J Med*. 2003;348(20):2007–2018.

Morrison LK, Harrison A, Krishnaswamy P, et al. Utility of a rapid B-natriuretic peptide assay in differentiating congestive heart failure from lung disease in patients presenting with dyspnea. *J Am Coll Cardiol*. 2002;39:202–209.

Chapter 42
Kessler RC, Berglund P, Demler O, et al. The epidemiology of major depressive disorder: results from the National Comorbidity Survey Replication. *JAMA*. 2003;289:3095–3105.

Sharp LK, Lipsky, MS. Screening for depression across the lifespan: a review of measures for use in primary care settings. *Am Fam Physician*. 2002;66:1001–1008, 1045–1046,1048,1051–1052.

Using second-generation antidepressants to treat depressive disorders: a clinical practice guideline from the American College of Physicians. Available at: http://www.annals.org/cgi/content. Accessed December 14, 2009.

Chapter 43
Field S, Task Force Chair. The American Association of Clinical Endocrinologists. Medical guidelines for the management of diabetes mellitus: the AACE system of intensive diabetes self-management: 2002 update. *Endocr Pract*. 2002;8(suppl 1):40–86.

Institute for Clinical Systems Improvement (ICSI). Diagnosis and management of type 2 diabetes mellitus in adults. National Guideline Clearinghouse; 2008 Aug 13:12693.

Type 2 diabetes practice guidelines. Available at: www.guideline.gov; www.diabetes.org. American Diabetes Association.

Wild S, Roglic G, Green A, et al. Global prevalence of diabetes. Estimates for the year 2000 and projections for 2030. *Diabetes Care*. 2004;27:1047–1053.

Chapter 44

Martel J, Raskin JB. History, incidence and epidemiology of diverticulosis. *J Clin Gastroenterol.* 2008;42(10): 1125–1127.

Trivedi CD, Das KM. Emerging therapies for diverticular disease. *J Clin Gastroenterol.* 2008;42(10):1145–1151.

Chapter 45

Centers for Disease Control and Prevention. Advancing HIV prevention: new strategies for a changing epidemic—United States, 2003. *MMWR.* 2003;52:329–332.

Gallant JE. HIV counseling, testing, and referral. *Am Fam Physician.* 2004;70:295–302.

Hogg R, Lima V, Sterne JA, et al. Life expectancy of individuals on combination antiretroviral therapy in high-income countries: a collaborative analysis of 14 cohort studies. *Lancet.* 2008;372(9635):293.

Lohse N, Hansen AB, Pedersen G, et al. Survival of persons with and without HIV infection in Denmark, 1995–2005. *Ann Intern Med.* 2007;146(2):87.

Panel on Antiretroviral Guidelines for Adults and Adolescents. *Guidelines for the use of antiretroviral agents in HIV-1-infected adults and adolescents.* Bethesda (MD): Department of Health and Human Services (DHHS);2008 Nov 3:139. [558 references]

Chapter 46

Chobanian AV, Bakris GL, Black HR, et al. The seventh report of the Joint National Committee on Prevention, Detection, Evaluation, and Treatment of High Blood Pressure: the JNC 7 report. *JAMA.* 2003;289:2560–2572. Available at: http://www.nhlbi.nih.gov/guidelines/hypertension/express.pdf. Accessed August 2, 2003.

The ALLHAT Officers and Coordinators for the ALLHAT Collaborative Research Group. Major outcomes in high-risk hypertensive patients randomized to angiotensin-converting enzyme inhibitor or calcium channel blocker vs. diuretic: the Antihypertensive and Lipid-Lowering Treatment to Prevent Heart Attack Trial (ALLHAT). *JAMA.* 2002;288:2981–2997.

Chapter 47

Cooper DS. Antithyroid drugs in the management of patient with Graves disease: an evidence-based approach to therapeutic controversies. *J Clin Endocrinol Metab.* 2003;88(8):3474–3481.

Chapter 48

Fatourechi V. Subclinical hypothyroidism: an update for primary care. *Mayo Clin Proc.* 2009;84:65–71.

Stathatos N, Wartofsky L. Perioperative management of patients with hypothyroidism. *Endocrinol Metab Clin.* 2003;32(2):503–518.

Chapter 49

Bray GA. Medical consequences of obesity. *J Clin Endocrinol Metab.* 2004;89(6):2583–2589.

Greenwood JL, Stanford JB. Preventing or improving obesity by addressing specific eating patterns. *J Am Board Fam Med.* 2008;21(2):135–140.

Slentz CA, Duscha BD, Johnson JL, et al. Effects of the amount of exercise on body weight, body composition, and measures of central obesity: STRIDE—a randomized controlled study. *Arch Intern Med.* 2004;164:31–39.

Chapter 50

Bonura F. Prevention, screening, and management of osteoporosis: an overview of the current strategies. *Postgrad Med.* 2009;121.

NIH Consensus Development Panel on Osteoporosis Prevention, Diagnosis, and Therapy. Osteoporosis prevention, diagnosis, and therapy. *JAMA.* 2001;285:785–795.

Writing Group for the Women's Health Initiative Investigators. Risks and benefits of estrogen plus progestin in healthy postmenopausal women: principal results from the Women's Health Initiative randomized controlled trial. *JAMA.* 2002;288:321–333.

Chapter 51

Dimitrakov JD, Kaplan SA, Kroenke K, et al. Management of chronic prostatitis/chronic pelvic pain syndrome: an evidence-based approach. *Urology.* 2006;67:881–888.

Lin K, Lipsitz R, Miller T, et al. Benefit and harms of prostate-specific antigen screening for prostate cancer: an evidence of update for the US preventive services task force. *Ann Int Med.* 2008;149:192–199.

Chapter 52

Centers for Disease Control and Prevention. Sexually transmitted diseases treatment guidelines 2002. *MMWR.* 2002;51(RR-6):1–77.

Corey L, Wald A, Patel R, et al. Once-daily valacyclovir to reduce the risk of transmission of genital herpes. *N Engl J Med.* 2004;350:11–20.

Kropp R, Latham-Carmanico C, Steben M, et al. What's new in management of sexually transmitted infections? *Can Fam Physician.* 2007;53:1739–1741. Update to CDC's sexually transmitted disease treatment guidelines, 2006: fluoroquinolones no longer recommended for treatment of gonococcal infections. *MMWR Weekly.* April 13, 2007;56(14):332–336.

Chapter 53

Bernard P. Management of common bacterial infections of the skin. *Curr Opin Infect Dis.* 2008;21:122–128.

Silverberg NB, Lim JK, Palter AS, et al. Squaric acid immunotherapy for warts in children. *J Am Acad Dermatol.* 2000;42:803–808.

Chapter 54
Aveyard P, West R. Managing smoking cessation. *BMJ.* 2007;335:37–41.

Rigotti NA. Treatment of tobacco use and dependence. *N Engl J Med.* 2002;346(7):506–512.

Chapter 55
Foxman B. Epidemiology of urinary tract infections: incidence, morbidity, and economic costs. *Am J Med.* 2002;113(suppl 1A):5S–13S.

Mori R, Lakhanpaul M, Verrier-Jones K. Diagnosis and management of urinary tract infection in children: summary of NICE guidance. *BMJ.* 2007;335: 395–397.

Wagenlehner FM, Weidner W, Naber KG. An update on uncomplicated urinary tract infections in women. *Curr Opin Urol.* 2009;19:368–374.

Chapter 56
Fromer L. Treatment options for the relief of chronic idiopathic urticaria symptoms. *South Med J.* 2008;101(2): 186–192.

Kaplan AP. Chronic urticaria: pathogenesis and treatment. *J Allergy Clin Immunol.* 2004;114(3):465–474.

Morgan M, Khan DA. Therapeutic alternatives for chronic urticaria: an evidence-based review, part 1. *Ann Allergy Asthma Immunol.* 2008;100:403–412.

Chapter 57
Solomon D, Schiffman M, Tarone R, The ALTS Study Group. Comparison of three management strategies for patients with atypical squamous cells of undetermined significance: baseline results from a randomized trial. *J Natl Cancer Inst.* 2001;93:293–299.

Valdini A, Vaccaro C, Pechinsky G, et al. Incidence and evaluation of an AGUS Papanicolaou smear in primary care. *J Am Board Fam Pract.* 2001;14:172–177.

Wright TC, Cox JT, Massad LS, et al. 2001 consensus guidelines for the management of women with cervical cytological abnormalities. *JAMA.* 2002;287: 2120–2129.

Chapter 58
Albers JR, Hull SK, Wesley RM. Abnormal uterine bleeding. *Am Fam Physician.* 2004;69(8):1915–1926.

Apgar BS, Kaufman AH, George-Nwogu U, et al. Treatment of menorrhagia. *Am Fam Physician.* 2007;75: 1813–1819.

Chapter 59
Master-Hunter T, Heiman DL. Amenorrhea: evaluation and treatment. *Am Fam Physician.* 2006;73:1374–1382.

Schlechte JA. Clinical practice. Prolactinoma. *N Engl J Med.* 2003;349(21):2035–2041.

Chapter 60
Morantz C. American Cancer Society. ACS guidelines for early detection of cancer. *Am Fam Physician.* 2004;69(8): 2013.

Smith RA, Cokkinides V, Eyre HJ. American Cancer Society. American Cancer Society guidelines for the early detection of cancer, 2004. *CA Cancer J Clin.* 2004;54(1):41–52.

Stein L, Chellman-Jeffers M. The radiologic workup of a palpable breast mass. *Cleve Clin J Med.* 2009;76(3): 175–180.

Chapter 61
Amy JJ, Tripathi V. Contraception for women: an evidence based overview. *BMJ.* 2009;339:b2895.

Herndon EJ, Zieman M. New contraceptive options. *Am Fam Physician.* 2004;69(4):853–860.

Chapter 62
Centers for Disease Control and Prevention. Diseases characterized by vaginal discharge. Sexually transmitted diseases treatment guidelines. *MMWR.* 2002;51(RR-6):42–48.

Egan ME, Lipsky MS. Diagnosis of vaginitis. *Am Fam Physician.* 2000;62(5):1095–1104.

Farage MA, Miller KW, Ledger WJ. Determining the cause of vulvovaginal symptoms. *Obstet Gynecol Surv.* 2008; 63(7):445–464.

Spence D, Melville C. Vaginal discharge. *BMJ.* 2007; 335:1147–1151.

Chapter 63
Atrash H, Jack BW, Johnson K. Preconception care: a 2008 update. *Curr Opin Obstet Gynecol.* 2008;20: 581–589.

Gregory KD, Davidson E. Prenatal care: who needs it and why? *Clin Obstet Gynecol.* 1999;42(4):725–736.

Chapter 64
Gabbe SG, Graves CR. Management of diabetes mellitus complicating pregnancy. *Obstet Gynecol.* 2003;102(4): 857–868.

Henry CS, Biedermann SA, Campbell MF, et al. Spectrum of hypertensive emergencies in pregnancy. *Crit Care Clin.* 2004;20(4):697–712.

James AH. Venous thromboembolism in pregnancy. *Arterioscler Thromb Vasc Biol.* 2009;29:326–331.

Koch KL, Frissora CL. Nausea and vomiting during pregnancy. *Gastroenterol Clin.* 2003;32(1):201–234.

McLaughlin SP, Carson CC. Urinary tract infections in women. *Med Clin North Am.* 2004;88(2):417–429.

Nicholson W, Bolen S, Witkop CT, et al. Benefits and risks of oral diabetes agents compared with insulin in women with gestational diabetes. *Obstet Gynecol.* 2009;113: 193–205.

Chapter 65

Dildy GA. Postpartum hemorrhage: new management options. *Clin Obstet Gynecol.* 2002;45(2):330–344.

Shaw E, Kaczorowski J. Postpartum care-what's new? *Curr Opin Obstet Gynecol.* 2007;19:561–567.

Chapter 66

Dennery PA, Seidman DS, Stevenson DK. Neonatal hyperbilirubinemia. *N Engl J Med.* 2001;344(8):581–590.

Fulhan J, Collier S, Duggan C. Update on pediatric nutrition: breastfeeding, infant nutrition, and growth. *Curr Opin Pediatr.* 2003;15(3):323–332.

Immunization schedules. Available at: www.cdc.gov/vaccines/recs/acip. Accessed September 14, 2009.

US Preventive Services Task Force Pocket Guide to Clinical Preventive Services. Available at: www.ahrq.gov/clinic/pocketgd.htm. Accessed September 14, 2009.

Chapter 67

Immunization schedules. Available at: www.cdc.gov/vaccines/recs/acip. Accessed September 14, 2009.

US Preventive Services Task Force Pocket Guide to Clinical Preventive Services. Available at: www.ahrq.gov/clinic/pocketgd.htm. Accessed September 14, 2009.

Chapter 68

Goldstein MA. Preparing adolescent patients for college. *Curr Opin Pediatr.* 2002;14(4):384–388.

Hornberger LL. Adolescent psychosocial growth and development. *J Pediatr Adolesc Gynecol.* 2006;19:243–246.

Chapter 69

Block RW, Krebs NF, Comm on Child Abuse, Comm on Nutrition. Failure to thrive as a manifestation of child neglect. *Pediatrics.* 2005;116:1234–1237.

Buchhalter JR, Jarrar RG. Therapeutics in pediatric epilepsy: part 2: epilepsy surgery and vagus nerve stimulation. *Mayo Clin Proc.* 2003;78(3):371–378.

Jarrar RG, Buchhalter JR. Therapeutics in pediatric epilepsy: part 1: the new antiepileptic drugs and the ketogenic diet. *Mayo Clin Proc.* 2003;78(3):359–370.

Russell K, Wiebe N, Saenz A, et al. Glucocorticoids for croup. *Cochrane Database Syst Rev.* 2004(1):CD001955.

Sobol SE, Zapata S. Epiglottis and courp. *Otolaryngol Clin North Am.* 2008;41:551–566.

Chapter 70

Banks JB. Childhood discipline: challenges for clinicians and parents. *Am Fam Physician.* 2002;66:1447–1452.

Daughton JM, Kratochvil CJ. Review of ADHD pharmacotherapies: advantages, disadvantages, and clinical pearls. *J Am Acad Child Adolesc Psychiatry.* 2009;48:240–248.

Hamilton SS, Glascoe FP. Evaluation of children with reading difficulties. *Am Fam Physician.* 2006;74:2079–2084.

Chapter 71

McCarthy PL. Fever without apparent source on clinical examination. *Curr Opin Pediatr.* 2004;16(1):94–106.

Sur DK, Bukont EL. Evaluating fever of unidentifiable source in young children. *Am Fam Physician.* 2007;75:1805–1811.

Chapter 72

Dagan R, Garau J. Appropriate use of antibiotics: focus on acute otitis media. *Clin Pediatr.* 2004;43(4):313–321.

Spiro DM, Arnold DH. The concept and practice of wait-and-see approach to acute otitis media. *Curr Opin Pediatr.* 2008;20:72–78.

Chapter 73

Giese EA, O'Connor FG, Depenbrock PJ, et al. The athletic preparticipation evaluation: cardiovascular assessment. *Am Fam Physician.* 2007;75:1008–1014.

Joy EA, Paisley TS, Price R Jr, et al. Optimizing the collegiate preparticipation evaluation. *Clin J Sport Med.* 2004;14:183–187.

Wingfield K, Matheson GO, Meeuwisse WH. Preparticipation evaluation: an evidence-based review. *Clin J Sport Med.* 2004;14:109–122.

Chapter 74

CDC Adult Immunization Schedule. Available at: http://www.cdc.gov/mmwr/PDF/wk/mm5753-Immunization.pdf. Accessed December 14, 2009.

Leipzig RM. Update in geriatric medicine. *Ann Intern Med.* 2003;139(12):1003–1008.

Spalding MC, Sebesta SC. Geriatric screening and preventive care. *Am Fam Physician.* 2008;78(2):206–215.

Chapter 75

Amin SH, Kuhle CL, Fitzpatrick LA. Comprehensive evaluation of the older woman. *Mayo Clin Proc.* 2003;78(9):1157–1185.

Caprio TV, Williams TF. Comprehensive geriatric assessment. In: Duthie EH, Katz PR, Malone ML, eds. *Practice of Geriatrics.* 4th ed. Philadelphia: Saunders Elsevier ; 2007.

Devons CA. Comprehensive geriatric assessment: making the most of the aging years. *Curr Opin Clin Nutr Metab Care.* 2002;5(1):19–24.

Chapter 76

Bogardus ST Jr, Yueh B, Shekelle PG. Screening and management of adult hearing loss in primary care: clinical applications. *JAMA.* 2003;289(15):1986–1990.

Gohel PS, Mandava N, Olson JL, et al. Age-related macular degeneration: an update on treatment. *Am J Med.* 2008;121:279–281.

Hauser RA. Levodopa: past, present and future. *Eur Neurol.* 2009;62:1–8.

Chapter 77
Blennow K, deLeon MJ, Zetterberg H. Alzheimer's disease. *Lancet.* 2006;368:387–403.

Knopman DS. An overview of common non-Alzheimer dementias. *Clin Geriatr Med.* 2001;17:281–301.

Chapter 78
Huggins ME, Bhatia NN, Ostergard DR. Urinary incontinence: newer pharmacotherapeutic trends. *Curr Opin Obstet Gynecol.* 2003;15(5):419–427.

Martin JL, Williams KS, Abrams KR, et al. Systematic review and evaluation of methods of assessing urinary incontinence. *Health Technol Assess.* 2006;10(6):1.

Chapter 79
Charette SL. Hospitalization of the nursing home patient. *J Am Med Dir Assoc.* 2003;4(2):90–94.

Ferrell BA. The management of pain in long-term care. *Clin J Pain.* 2004;20(4):240–243.

King MS, Lipsky MS. Evaluation of nursing home patients. A systematic approach can improve care. *Postgrad Med.* 2000;107(2):201–204, 207–210, 215.

Index

Index note: page references with *a b, f,* or *t* indicate a box, figure or table on the designated page; page references in bold indicate discussion of the subject in the Question and Answers sections.